Rehabilitation/Restorative Care in the Community

Rehabilitation/Restorative Care in the Community

Shirley P. Hoeman, PhD, MPH, RN, CNAA, CRRN

Consultant, Private Practice,
Health Systems Consultations,
Long Valley, New Jersey

Contributing Authors
Nancy H. Glenn, RN, MSN, CRRN

Charlotte Mecklenburg Hospital Authority,
Charlotte Rehabilitation Hospital,
Charlotte, North Carolina

Alice Stymacks, RN, CRRN

Rehabilitation Consultant,
West Orange, New Jersey

The C. V. Mosby Company

St. Louis • Baltimore • Philadelphia • Toronto 1990

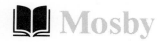 **Mosby**

Executive Editor: Richard A. Weimer
Assistant Editor: Adrianne H. Cochran

The intent of this text is to provide training materials applicable to health care workers practicing in a rehabilitation capacity in the home setting. Since there is no common terminology that reflects precisely what the scope of home health or rehabilitation is, it is intended that the materials enclosed be directed for proper utilization by user agencies in conjunction with local regulation, laws, and guidelines.

In no way is either the Publisher or Author liable for actions by anyone who has studied this text.

Printed in the United States of America

The C.V. Mosby Company
11830 Westline Industrial Drive, St. Louis, Missouri 63146

Library of Congress Cataloging-in-Publication Data

Hoeman, Shirley P.
  Rehabilitation/restorative care in the community / Shirley P.
Hoeman; contributing authors, Nancy H. Glenn, Alice Stymacks.
    p.   cm.
  Includes bibliographical references.
  ISBN 0-8016-2415-0
  1. Home care services. 2. Home nursing. 3. Handicapped—Medical
care.   I. Glenn, Nancy H.   II. Stymacks, Alice.   III. Title.
  [DNLM: 1. Home Care Services. 2. Rehabilitation. WY 115 H694r]
RA645.3.H62   1990
362.1'4—dc20
DNLM/DLC
for Library of Congress   89-13514
                                                                CIP

CG/GW/VH   9 8 7 6 5 4 3 2 1

TO DENNY

They that wait upon the Lord shall renew their strength;

they shall mount up with wings as eagles;

they shall run, and not be weary;

and they shall walk, and not faint.

Isaiah 40:31

Preface

This book was prepared as a contribution toward improving the daily care and quality of life for persons with chronic or disabling conditions. It was written to promote dignity and self-care for those who live with their families or other caregivers and reintegrate into their communities. The same concepts and principles apply to long-term care settings, home health programs, respite or day care programs, rehabilitation units, and other residences or services. The knowledge, skills, and attitudes achieved by caregivers are major factors in each client's potential outcomes for restoration, rehabilitation, or habilitation.

Increasingly clients receive care, often lifelong care, in their homes and communities rather than in institutions. Advanced preparation and training of all levels of health workers as well as advances in technology and equipment enable clients to survive conditions and traumas that would have been fatal in the past. As a result, community reintegration occurs more frequently and earlier in the course of recovery, and clients return home with acute care needs and technology. Families and community caregivers provide a great deal of sophisticated long-term care to clients. It is important that the care be aligned with the goals of rehabilitation and the individual client goals. Each client has individual needs and abilities as well as different deficits that must be brought together in the plan for care.

Thus the tone of the book centers on the client as a whole person, not on his condition or disability. The goals are to prevent further disability or complications; to assist with maintaining independent functioning; to promote wellness, abilities, strengths, resources, and enabling activities over losses; to encourage self-directed care; and to remember the combined worth of body, mind, and spirit.

Although some procedures are given, they are guides. This is not intended to be used as a basic text for aides. This book builds on basic text materials so that caregivers can assist with tasks and procedures under direction and supervision of a nurse supervisor and according to each client's individual abilities and deficits. Each state and agency has its own procedures and scope of duties for each level of caregiver that take precedence over information suggested in the book. No one should perform any task for which he or she is not legally licensed or certified, that has not been supervised and directed by the nurse supervisor, that is against the client's will, or that is unsafe or unethical at any moment.

Shirley P. Hoeman

Acknowledgments

This book was created and written because of encouragement and support from many friends, our families, and colleagues too numerous to list. Special acknowledgments are extended to Mary Ann Solimine, Carl and Sharon Nilsen, Debbie Winters, Joyce and Marvin Friedman, and Craig and Heather Norris for their on-going assistance and encouragement. We thank Janet LaMantia, Phyllis Passarella, Evelyn Savage, and Ann Liebers for their reviews and comments; Mosby editors Richard Weimer, Adrianne Cochran, and Lin Dempsey; and the representatives for the companies who contributed photographic materials. We appreciate our families—Denny, Chris, Tim, and Jon Hoeman, Bernie Pollock, and Joe Stymacks—for their unconditional support and belief in our commitment to the book.

Contents

1 Principles Of Rehabilitation, 1
2 Responding To Basic Needs And Emergency Situations, 26
3 Sensory and Communication Deficits, 61
4 Turning, Moving, and Positioning, 84
5 Equipment for Clients with Disabilities, 145
6 Activities of Daily Living and Assistive Devices, 178
7 Care for the Client who has had a Stroke, 206
8 Care for Client with a Traumatic Brain Injury, 217
9 Care for the Client with a Spinal Cord Injury, 224
10 Care for the Client with an Amputation, 240
11 Care of Clients who have Chronic Conditions, 261

Appendix A Traveling with a Disability, 319
Appendix B Therapeutic Diets and Nutrition, 323
Appendix C Exercise, 328
Appendix D Glossary, 338

CHAPTER 1

Principles of Rehabilitation

*O*BJECTIVES:

When you have studied this chapter and practiced the procedures it describes you will be able to:

1. Define disability.
2. List the roles of the key members of the rehabilitation team.
3. Learn about the importance of maintaining the confidentiality of clients and their families.
4. Identify several important considerations when the client is a child.
5. Discuss the stages of the grieving process commonly observed following disability.
6. Respond correctly to negative situations involving abuse and anger, as instructed.
7. Perform proper infection control techniques, as instructed.
8. Maintain personal and client safety in the home, including preventive measures.

*O*VERVIEW

What is a disability? Disabilities are physical or mental conditions that prevent clients from performing functions or activities for daily living and self-care. Functional abilities may be absent, impaired, or diminished. Psychosocial difficulties and emotional changes may accompany physical disabilities. In most cases, the client's disability affects the entire family. For example, whenever a family member cannot do things for himself, perform his role in the family structure, or even communicate with the family, many responsibilities change within the family.

Although some disabilities are related to illness, a disability is not the same as a disease. Certain disabilities and chronic conditions commonly occur as part of the normal aging process. Older people become more far-sighted, tend to move more slowly, and lose some of their sense of taste. These changes do not mean that the person cannot function and contribute. Similarly, diseases like diabetes and hypertension require care and health maintenance to keep the person functioning at the highest level possible and prevent complications. Understanding how to help your clients continue to be as independent as possible is a key part of your job. In many cases, your client will be able to direct you in the specifics of his care. Listen to your client.

Only perform the tasks and activities specified by your nurse supervisor in the care plan. Only perform tasks, activities, and duties that you are trained, qualified, and if applicable, licensed to perform in the state where you work.

Disability can be caused by traumatic accidents, diseases, strokes, and congenital (birth) or developmental defects. A great many elderly people become disabled after falling, often in their own homes. Each person's disability is unique according to his particular situation, resources, the kind and severity of the disability, and how well he can cope and adapt. It is important to understand that a person may have a disability but still be essentially healthy.

A loss of ability in one area does not mean that the person himself is disabled. The disability is only a part of the whole person. Think about persons as having disabled parts or decreased functional abilities rather than labeling them by the name of the disability. Words like cripple and stroke victim should not be used because they are offensive, negative labels that demean and devalue the client as a whole person. Be careful with the word handicapped; some think of it as a negative label while others are not offended. A person may be handicapped whether or not he has a disability. It is essential that you learn to view your client first as a person, and then as a person with a disability, but never as a "diagnosis."

For example, your client is not an old amputee; rather he is an elderly person who has circulatory problems that led to the removal of his left leg—the man is not the amputation and the amputation is not the man. Your client may have a physical disability but this does not by itself mean that he has mental problems, or that he is retarded or hard of hearing. Many persons speak loudly and slowly to a person with a disability as if the impairment of a leg caused hearing loss.

Persons with disabilities have the same basic health care needs as other clients, such as good nutrition, a safe and clean environment, and proper personal hygiene. They also need rehabilitation activities designed to keep them as independent as possible and to encourage self-care. *The goal of rehabilitation is to enable the person to live to the fullest capacity possible, focusing on the achievements rather than the disability.*

Many of the conditions that require long-term care are not curable. Chronically ill persons have many of the same health care needs as those with other physical disabilities. Chronic long-term health needs affect individuals and their families in many of the same ways that physical disabilities do. In fact, they often occur together in the same person. Today's most advanced medical treatments cannot cure chronic problems of persons who are disabled. Their greatest needs are for care.

The causes of chronic conditions are not always clear. Factors that influence the cause of any chronic condition include:

—age;
—sex;
—health behaviors, including risk factors;
—cultural background, including race and ethnic factors;
—diet;
—exposure, such as in the workplace or environment;
—general health and tolerance level;
—access to preventive measures or treatment;
—inherited traits;
—habits, including smoking, substance abuse, or others; and
—geographic location.

Thus many factors combine to produce chronic conditions. This process has been described as a web or multiple cause system for developing a particular condition. No one factor causes the problem. One person may develop a disease while another does not, even in the same basic circumstances.

Chronic conditions may lie hidden for many years before their signs or symptoms become evident, which makes their cause or causes even more difficult to trace. We rarely know when the disease or condition first started, even after it becomes a problem. Often the cause remains unknown.

Chronic conditions and diseases do require long-term care. Sometime a large portion of a client's health and functioning can be restored or rehabilitated. Often he must work to maintain his level of health.

Rehabilitation does not claim to cure disabilities, but it can "restore the individual to the fullest physical, mental, social, economic, and vocational capacity of which he is capable." As a home caregiver you can use rehabilitation and restorative care techniques and procedures to benefit your client in important ways. You will:

—help prevent further disabilities or complications,

—follow care plan directions precisely to restore as much functional ability as possible,

—maintain activities of daily living and self-care,

—assist clients to meet their basic needs,

—provide a safe environment,

—assist in new techniques as directed by your nurse supervisor, and

—encourage the family and client to work toward rehabilitation goals.

You have a special responsibility to know which activities your client can perform for himself and which areas require your assistance. Remember that a disabled body does not mean a disabled person. Sometimes it may be faster and easier for you to do the care for the person than to wait for him to complete it on his own. Family members may question why you do not perform certain services for the client. Strive to involve your client to some degree in as many activities as possible. Make him an *active partner* in the activity instead of a *passive receiver.* For example, if he cannot complete an activity alone, place your hand over his to guide him through the task. Give him choices and allow him to make decisions whenever possible, even for small things. He will benefit from having a sense of control over a part of his life. Be sure you refer to the care plan and clearly understand the type and amount of assistance you are to provide for your client and how much he is to do for himself. You must also know the safe and proper ways to assist your client. The plan for his care will be developed, directed, coordinated, and supervised by a registered nurse.

*T*HE REHABILITATION TEAM

A team of rehabilitation professionals may work with your client. (Figure 1-1) The purpose of the team is to provide comprehensive rehabilitation services precisely designed for each client. Most clients do not have a full rehabilitation team visit their homes. Team members make visits to provide services as needed for set lengths of time. One team member may begin services after another team member has completed his services. For example, your client may have a nurse and physical therapist in addition to your services in the home, while other clients may visit a physical therapist at an outpatient clinic.

Members of the rehabilitation team may include you, the client and his family, and a registered professional nurse, plus one or a combination of health care professionals.

KEY MEMBERS OF THE REHABILITATION TEAM
The Client and His Family

The client and his family are key members of the rehabilitation team. Each family will differ in the amount of involvement members have in the client's care. There will be differences in families as well. Some clients may have large, extended families that include grandparents, aunts, uncles, and their children. Others may have one or two family members, or have families who live in other parts of the country. For some clients, members of their social groups, fellow church members, or close friends may serve in some family roles. (Figure 1-2)

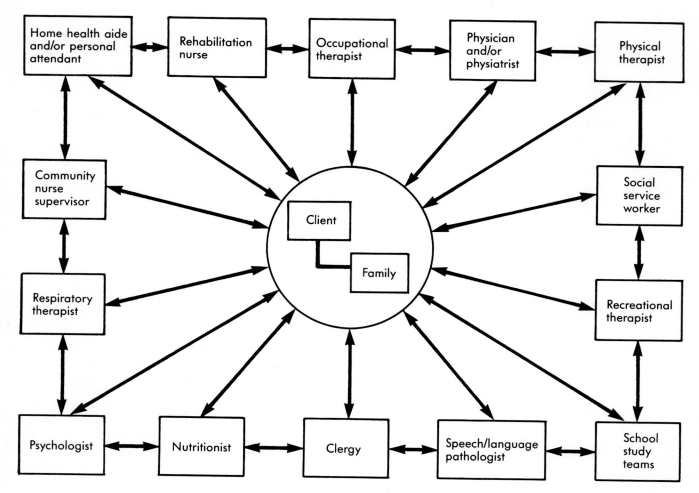

Figure 1-1.   *Members of the interdisciplinary rehabilitation team include the client as an active participant.*

Health Care Professionals Involved in the Rehabilitation Team

physical therapist	occupational therapist
speech pathologist	dietitian/nutritionist
social service worker	home health aide/attendant
physiatrist/physician	vocational counselor
clergy	psychologist
child study team	prosthetist/orthotist
equipment/supply vendors	recreation therapist
respiratory therapist	rehabilitation/insurance nurse

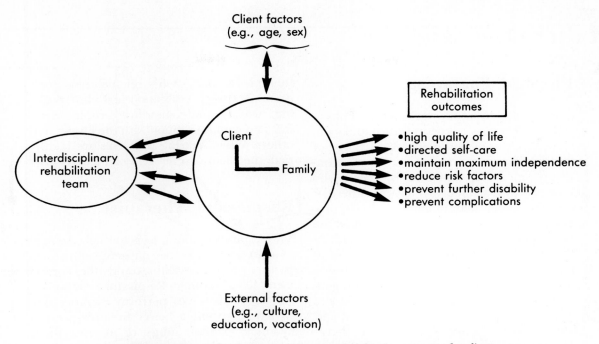

Figure 1-2. *Multiple factors influence rehabilitation outcomes for clients.*

Clients' families are taught about the client's condition. They learn how to perform his care and to manage his equipment. Ideally, a client will direct as much of his care as possible.

The Registered Professional Nurse

The registered professional nurse is the coordinator of care and rehabilitation team activities in clients' homes and communities. The nurse provides direct physical care to clients and psychosocial interventions for clients and families. The nurse works in conjunction with the team, clients, and their families to assess and evaluate unmet needs, to plan for clients' overall care, to set standards and goals for care outcomes, and to identify existing or needed resources. You will always have regular supervision from a registered nurse because a nurse oversees and monitors a client's care. The amount of direct supervision you receive from the nurse will depend on each client's needs, and on your ability and training.

Ideally, a certified rehabilitation nurse (C.R.R.N.) will be available for supervision and consultation. The *rehabilitation insurance nurse* is the case manager for clients with private insurance or insurance such as no-fault accident coverage. Her job is to advocate for the client's highest level of needed care, services, and equipment while providing a cost-effective settlement for the company. This is an increasingly important role for nurses in the community and for quality aftercare or lifelong care for clients.

The Home Health Aide

The home health aide or personal care attendant is a trained paraprofessional health worker who provides direct services to clients in their homes. Increasing numbers of aides are becoming certified and seeking further training and education. The home health aide spends more time with clients than other team members do, and is often alone with the client or family. Aides provide care for clients under the direction and supervision of a registered professional nurse and within the established policies and procedures of their employing agencies. A home health aide may accompany a client to therapy sessions or to workshops for testing and vocational work experiences. There is an increasingly important role for aides in the home setting, especially for clients who require rehabilitation or long-term care.

HEALTH PROFESSIONALS

Physical Therapist

The physical therapist works under a physician's orders to assist clients with ambulation, transfers, use of equipment, and range of motion. Physical therapists may provide ongoing supervision and care for clients who have braces or a lower extremity prosthesis, if ordered. They may establish exercise programs, apply hot or cold treatments, and use equipment such as TENS or ultrasound. In the home setting, therapists participate in the plan of care in many ways, such as teaching gait and crutch walking or ambulating up and down stairs, transferring clients on and off the toilet, or ways to move clients in and out of doors. Occasionally, a physical therapist will supervise certain aspects of care by a home health aide if the nurse is no longer directly supervising the client; however, there must be a designated nurse supervisor to contact if needed.

Occupational Therapist

The occupational therapist works with clients under the direction of a physician and usually in close collaboration with the nurse and physical therapist. The occupational therapist may work with your client to evaluate functional abilities of his upper extremities and trunk, to assist with any lower extremity weakness, for endurance and homemaking activities, to evaluate and develop a driver training program, and to work with certain vocational skills. The therapist checks for weakness, level of endurance, and degree of performance. If a client has an upper extremity prosthesis or a splint for weakness, the occupational therapist will supervise its use and care, and may make the splint.

Speech-Language, Hearing Therapist (Speech Pathologist)

The speech therapist evaluates clients' communication needs. A client who has difficulty eating or swallowing may work with a speech therapist as part of his rehabilitation program. A speech evaluation includes speaking, hearing, understanding, writing, reading, and communication with the family and others. When hearing problems are identified, the client is referred to an audiologist.

Respiratory Therapist

The respiratory therapist is specially trained to assist clients who use oxygen, ventilators, positive pressure machines, and other equipment for breathing. Respiratory therapists also assist clients to perform exercises designed to promote better breathing, clear mucus from their lungs, or increase their lung power. Many times the respiratory therapist will work closely with or directly for the vendor that supplies the equipment or oxygen.

Physiatrist (Physician)

The physician who specializes in rehabilitation services is called a physiatrist. The physiatrist is a medical doctor who instructs and supervises other members of the team in the rehabilitation program for each client. Not all clients will use a physiatrist as the primary physician. For example, many clients will visit their family physicians, others will have orthopedic surgeons or neurosurgeons supervise their care. Clients may also have specialists if they have chronic conditions, such as a cardiologist for a heart condition. Physical and occupational therapists may receive orders for care directly from these physicians. In a rehabilitation center, each rehabilitation professional contributes an assessment and evaluation of a client's abilities and needs which enables the physician to give medical approval to one comprehensive plan for care. In the home setting, the physician is less visible, may not be a physiatrist, and there may be more than one physician. A primary physician should be designated by the family; the nurse supervisor will direct you accordingly.

Dietitian (Nutritionist)

The dietitian may not personally visit the home, but will provide dietetic services in collaboration with the nurse. Whenever a client has a special diet or food need, the dietitian will establish a dietary plan. The dietitian may also recommend dietary measures to assist a client who experiences bowel problems, skin breakdown, swallowing difficulties, or similar problems. You may be a part of the dietary plan when you keep diet diaries, measure food intake, or prepare foods in certain ways for your client.

Social Service Worker

A community social service worker may visit your client for several reasons. Social workers assist clients and families to secure resources to pay for and supply health care needs. They also provide counseling about adjustments to disability, alternatives for care and housing, and information about community resources and services.

Prosthetist/Orthotist

The prosthetist designs, makes, and fits a wide variety of prosthetic devices and appliances. The orthotist designs, makes, and fits braces. Many prosthetists are also orthotists who work with a physiatrist and other members of the team to produce the prosthetic product that best suits each client's needs. You may work with these professionals if your client has prosthetic equipment or braces that need adjustment or repair, requires a body jacket or must have a solid seat formed for his support.

Vocational Counselor

The vocational counselor evaluates and counsels clients about obtaining jobs or education. If a client is physically and emotionally able to become employed, the vocational counselor will assist both the client and the potential employer to define the job and the client's work abilities. If a client wishes to return to school or college, the counselor assists in finding a suitable and satisfactory educational opportunity accessible for the client.

Clergy

Each client and family will have a different approach to clergy in their lives according to their particular religious beliefs and patterns. When a client and family chooses clergy as part of their rehabilitation team, you may have regular visits in the home from the clergy or other representatives of the religious group. Many clients and families rely on prayer, support, and assistance from their religious organizations and friends. The spiritual side of health care is often ignored or avoided by health professionals. As you work with clients you are likely to discover that spiritual health is a vital factor in quality of life, whatever the disability.

Psychologist

Most psychologist's activities in the home setting involve in-depth counseling and treatment for the client and his family. The psychologist does not make visits to the home except to conduct sessions there when it is more accessible for the client. The psychologist is often involved in designing or conducting support groups and peer groups for clients and families.

Equipment and Supply Vendors

Vendors are not members of the professional rehabilitation team in many agencies. However, many vendors do have professional health staff, especially respiratory therapists, dietitians, and nurses. If your client requires equipment, replaceable supplies such as oxygen or nutritional supplements, or assistive devices, among other items, you will have contact with a vendor delivering to or servicing the home. Many times the vendors will have current information about products and services that the client and family will need to know. They are also important for making emergency repairs and deliveries.

SPECIAL CONSIDERATIONS FOR CARE OF CLIENTS IN THE HOME

CONFIDENTIALITY

You must remember to keep the events that occur in your client's home confidential except for those things that you must report to the supervising nurse. You are a guest in the home even though you provide important and necessary functions for the client and family.

Confidentiality means not discussing your client's condition, not telling others, even your co-workers, about incidents that occur in the home even when they are seemingly innocent, or gossiping about the client's or family's conversations and activities. It may require a conscious effort on your part to keep confidentiality; it is easy to let information "slip out," especially when something exciting or humorous has happened. Respect and protect your client's confidentiality just as you would his physical well-being.

Do not give out information about the client or his condition to callers on the telephone, callers at the door, insurance representatives or other official agencies, or even to the client's relatives and friends.

Keep confidential information about your client confidential. Make it a rule that whatever happens in your client's home is confidential. You may have to remind yourself about this whenever you think of telling an interesting story about what happened during your day. This means that you do not talk about your client after work hours, even among people who do not know him.

A second rule is to tell things only to persons who have a *need to know* about them. Very few people need to know what happens at your client's home, or what his medical condition is. The client himself, the family, and the nurse supervisor are people who may need to know; most other people do not.

CHILDREN AS CLIENTS

When the client is a child you have additional duties and responsibilities (Figure 1-3). Although you may have different ideas about childrearing, you must take care to support the family pattern of childraising as long as

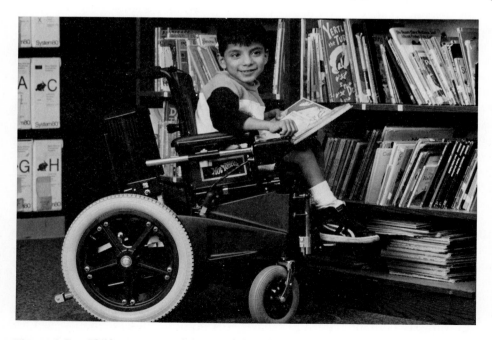

Figure 1-3.   *Children are not miniature adults. They require care and equipment designed especially for their growth, development and disabling disorders.*
Courtesy Everest & Jennings, Inc.

no one is being harmed. You are legally required to report any abusive or neglectful incident, whether the client is a child or an adult. However, family discipline and ideals can be very different, especially if the family comes from a background that is not like your own. Consider the whole family and how they do things as you carry out procedures and give assistance. What you do and say should fit in with the family and encourage the child as he grows and develops.

In many families, the home caregiver spends the greatest amount of time with the client and becomes a guide for how things should be done. You have opportunities to help the family prepare a disabled child for the future. However, you must be sure that the guidance you are offering is consistent with the plan of care directed by the nurse supervisor and is the appropriate level of care for you to perform.

THE GRIEVING PROCESS

Clients who have disabilities or loss of functions mourn the loss of those abilities. They must resolve these losses as they cope and adapt to the changes in their lives and in themselves. Some of the reactions that your client may experience are:

---

*The Stages in Grieving
and Loss Reactions*

—denial or disbelief,
—anger and "why me?",
—bargaining or pleading for changes
—depression and realization of loss,
—acceptance or decision to cope, and
—finding ways to go on.

It is important not to make judgments about the grieving of the client or his family. Each person will progress through these stages in his own way and at his own speed. Sometimes clients do not follow this exact order or seem to go back through stages, returning to depression and anger as they mourn losses of previous lifestyles and abilities. Families may go through their own grieving stages for the client. However, one member of the family may be angry while others are denying the crisis. Not everyone will mourn the same way or at the same time.

Feelings of Fear, Lack of Power or Control, or Frustration

- These feelings may be very real to the client because of his disability, living arrangements, dependence on other people, finances or the like.
- Give the client as much control as possible over his self-care activities, how and when his care is performed, the menu for meals, and general household rules.
- Let him decide where things are placed in his room, what goes on in his environment, what music or program is played.
- Get the client up in his wheelchair, and out-of-doors if possible. Encourage rides to the shopping mall, to sports events or concerts, or other recreational activities as he is able.
- Provide positive encouragement for any studies or work projects that may be available to him.
- Create a sense of his private personal space even when performing personal care for him. Respect his dignity and need for self-esteem.

Concerns about a meaningful future:

- Your client must adjust to a changed image of his body and how it functions. Adjustment to his new body may reduce his self-esteem and sense of worth.
- Be aware of how you refer to his body and his abilities; he may not show you how sensitive he is about his disability.
- Assist him to have good hygiene and a positive appearance, especially in social settings. He should wear clothing and hair styles that are comfortable for his group.
- Respect his sexuality and needs for relationships with others.

COMMUNICATE WITH THE NURSE SUPERVISOR

Tell your nurse supervisor if your client or his family have questions or misinformation about his care or disability. Inform the nurse supervisor if your client or family ask you questions about the client's care, abilities, or functions. Also report questions that you are not qualified to answer.

Report changes in your client's attitude, especially unusual depression or hopelessness.

Report important information to the nurse. Good reporting to the nurse supervisor about what is happening with your client is essential.

- Practice writing down information for your nurse supervisor by using simple words to describe what happened.
- Write down information before you forget to do it or forget exactly what happened.
- Use special forms as directed for recording specific measurements and time of day.
- Know what needs to be reported immediately.
- Be accurate and complete in your reports.

KNOW YOUR CLIENT

You should take time to review specific information in the care plan with your nurse supervisor. This information about your client, his family, and his home can help you avoid problems and is important to have on hand for quick reference in case of emergency. The hospital or rehabilitation center may have sent instructions, teaching materials, and assistive devices or equipment home with the client. The nurse supervisor will instruct you and the client about using these materials in the home. The care plan will include the following information, at a minimum, that you need to know about your client.

- What is the rescue squad number? Are there other emergency numbers?
- What things cause problems for your client—does a full bladder cause a reaction?

- What things does the client do for himself and what do others do, such as intermittent catheterization?
- What kinds of devices does the person have—a catheter, phrenic pacemaker?
- What are repeated problems for your client, such as constipation or high blood pressure?
- What is the special equipment and how does it work?
- Think of other questions and ask your client and the nurse.
- Be prepared and write the information where you can find it.

ABUSE, ANGER, AND FRUSTRATION

Abuse and Neglect

Unfortunately, some clients become so frustrating to work with that family members or caregivers physically or verbally abuse them. This may begin when a family member becomes upset and frustrated with a client because they cannot communicate. Often incidents of abuse happen when someone is using alcohol or when there are a lot of other problems going on in the home. Abuse of the elderly, disabled persons, or children, a sad situation in any home, is occurring at high rates in the community. Any single instance of abuse may lead to future instances.

Physical abuse is more readily apparent than verbal or psychological abuse. Shouting, screaming, threatening, name-calling, and negative "put-down" comments are all forms of verbal and psychological abuse. Whenever you see or suspect that a client is being abused, report it immediately to the nurse supervisor.

Neglect is similar to abuse and often accompanies abusive actions. Clients may be well treated and cared for in most areas of their lives while one or two areas of care are neglected. You will be in a position to notice such outright physical neglect as soiled bedding or bruises on his body. Ignoring the client, leaving him isolated or alone in another room, omitting parts of care such as mouth care, failing to provide adequate food, or putting off repair of glasses are examples of neglect.

Dealing with Your own Anger or Frustrations

If you ever become so upset or angry with a client that you feel you want to strike him, remove yourself to another room and take several deep breaths. Remember the reasons for your client's behavior and what you are to do to help him. You can change the way you feel and react in stressful situations. Talk to the nurse supervisor about attending an educational program or inservice on this topic. Most home health agencies arrange for staff to attend regular educational inservice programs to keep them informed or to brush up on former skills.

Here are some ways to handle your anger:

- Try to keep from letting a situation or comment get to the point of anger—prevent anger from surfacing. One way to do this is to know what things make you angry and recognize them early.
- When you feel yourself becoming angry, remove yourself from the situation if possible. Think about doing things that keep you from becoming angry instead of dwelling on the situation. Tell yourself that you are becoming angry and have to think through the next steps.
- Think about positive things, things that make you feel better about yourself. Think about times you have successfully avoided becoming angry and how much this helped your self-esteem; congratulate yourself.
- Try to take as much time as possible before you speak or act. The more time you can put between the situation and your action, the less apt you are to be violently angry. Anger should ease as other thoughts enter your mind.
- Work with your nurse supervisor on ways to develop positive coping patterns to control your anger, and ways to relax and ease the tension you feel. If a client continues to upset and frustrate you, ask for a reassignment. You are not the first caregiver to become frustrated with a client, but it should not continue to happen.

INFECTION CONTROL

You are the first line of defense in preventing the spread of disease to yourself and to your clients. This means you must understand how diseases are caused and spread from one person to another. *Frequent handwashing, using the proper technique, is the easiest and best way to prevent the spread of diseases.* This is so easy that it seems too good to be true. And health care workers do not always pay attention to this simple fact.

Our environment is filled with invisible microorganisms. They are in water, soil, air, food, and on our bodies. Some microorganisms are useful, helping to break down our environment so we can use it. For example, microorganisms in our digestive systems help us to digest food. Other microorganisms are used to convert milk products into yogurts or cheeses. They also break down garbage into compost and are even used to make some pharmaceutical products.

Other microorganisms, which we call germs or viruses are disease-causing "pathogens." Even a useful microorganism can become a pathogen if it becomes active in the wrong place. For example, the microorganism that lives in our digestive system to break down food does not cause illness. This microorganism leaves the body in the stool or feces. But when it enters the body elsewhere—outside the digestive system—it becomes a pathogen. It causes infection if it enters through an open sore or if it gets into the bladder. Simple handwashing kills this microorganism and stops it from entering the body improperly.

Viruses cause most colds. We pick up many viruses from the environment by getting them on our hands. Viruses do not enter the body through the hands, but our hands deliver the viruses to other parts of our bodies. For example, if you have a virus on your hands and rub your eyes or your nose, eat your sandwich, or scratch a mosquito bite, you can introduce the virus into your body.

Unless, of course, you wash your hands before doing any of these things. Handwashing is also important because it can *control or stop* one of the steps in the infection process.

Steps in the Infection Process:

An infectious disease must go through six steps to travel from one person or place to the person it will try to infect (Figure 1-4). If any one of these steps is eliminated, there is a good chance to prevent the infection from spreading. Think about how many steps can be eliminated by good handwashing. There must be:

Step 1—a pathogenic microorganism present.

Step 2—a source in the environment for the microorganism to come from, such as another person, food, water, equipment, body fluids, insects, plants, or animals.

Step 3—a way for the microorganism to leave the source. For example, if the source is a person, the microorganism can leave his body in the spray of droplets when he sneezes or coughs. Or it can leave in urine, feces, blood, vomit, or fluids from wounds.

Step 4—a way for the microorganism to travel from the source to its target. This is called transmission. Transmission through direct contact occurs when one person touches another person or object and transfers the microorganism directly. Other transmission is through the air, through food that is spoiled or improperly washed or cooked, contaminated drinking water, or by insects or animals.

Step 5—a way for the microorganisms to get into the body. The body has many protective barriers to stop organisms from entering and causing disease. The skin is a strong barrier to pathogens. However, any break or opening in the skin creates an easy doorway for pathogens to enter the body. Other easy entry points are: inhaling pathogens that are in the air, including airborne droplets from other persons' coughs and sneezes; eating or drinking foods or liquids containing pathogens; putting unwashed objects or fingers into the mouth; or having contaminated objects enter the blood stream.

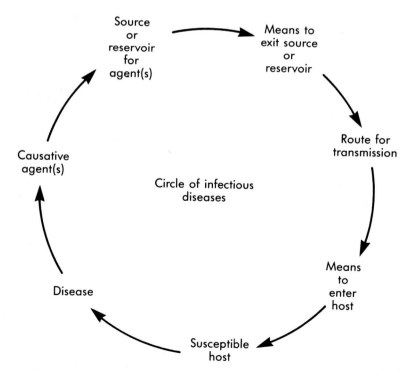

Figure 1-4. *These steps must be present in order to further the spread of infection.*

Step 6—a person who cannot fight off the microorganism. The microorganism must be able to multiply itself and grow strong enough inside the person to cause an infection or illness. If the person's immune system is stronger than the microorganism, it will fight off the infection or disease. This is why we are immunized against certain infectious diseases. The immunization causes our bodies to build up antibodies or defenses in readiness against an invasion by a specific organism. Unfortunately, there are no immunizations available for many diseases.

Some factors make a person weaker and more apt to get an infection or disease. These include:

- Stress: Stressful events occurring over a long period of time lower the body's resistance.
- Nutrition: Persons with poor nutritional status cannot build the healthy body tissues they need to ward off illness.
- Fatigue: The person who is tired and worn out does not have the strength to fight against disease.
- Gender: Some diseases occur more often in men and others more often in women.
- Inheritance: Our family, ethnic, and racial background all affect our genetic makeup and make us susceptible to certain illnesses or conditions.
- Age: Some diseases affect only the very young or the elderly. Multiple sclerosis is a disease of young-middle-aged adults. As a rule, the very young and very old are more apt to have serious responses to illnesses or infections because of their less efficient immune systems.

Steps in Universal Infection Control

Although there are several ways to reduce the chances of getting an infection or of giving one to others, *the single most important prevention is proper handwashing.* This means knowing *when* and *how* to wash your hands. (Figure 1-5)

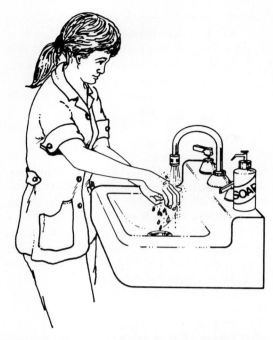

Figure 1-5. *Hand washing is the most important step in preventing the spread of infection.*

When:

Wash your hands *after:*

- —going to the bathroom;
- —direct contact with your client;
- —removing gloves following a procedure or task;
- —sneezing or blowing your nose;
- —handling soiled linen, laundry, or garbage; and after
- —they become soiled with any body fluids.

Wash your hands *before:*

- —all direct contact with your client,
- —preparing food,
- —performing a personal task or procedure for your client, and
- —assembling equipment or items for your client's use.

Keep your hands away from your face, eyes, and mouth. Think about the cleanliness of your hands before you touch yourself anywhere on your body.

How:

1. Use plenty of soap and warm running water. The nurse supervisor may ask

you to use a special soap if necessary for your client's protection.

2. Rub your hands together briskly. Friction will assist in removing pathogens from your skin.
3. Clean underneath your fingernails. Use a nailbrush.
4. Wash between your fingers and around the cuticles.
5. Wash for at least 1 minute.
6. Rinse your hands and leave the water on until you dry your hands.
7. Use a clean towel to dry your hands. Holding the towel, turn off the faucets so that your hands do not touch the faucets. You touched the faucets with dirty hands before washing. Do not put your clean hands on the dirty faucets.

OTHER INFECTION CONTROL MEASURES

These procedures are important for you to follow personally and for you to perform for or with your client.

- Regular daily bathing—daily grooming including hairwashing as needed.
- Dental and oral hygiene several times daily.
- Personal care for clients:
  —daily, more often if the situation merits;
  —cleansing "front to back" following bowel or bladder movements for female clients; and
  —cleansing under foreskin for male clients.
- Changing clothes and bedlinens daily or when soiled.
- Changing and cleaning cushion covers, liners, binders or other materials whenever soiled or as directed.
- Keeping the environment clean, especially kitchen and bathroom areas.

Knowing What is Clean

An object is clean when all pathogens that potentially cause disease are removed or eliminated. Pathogens are eliminated in different ways from objects. The following instructions list how to clean pathogens from most household objects and supplies. Your nurse supervisor may give you other directions for special cases. Those listed here are considered universal methods today. From time to time new discoveries can change the ways in which pathogens are eliminated. The nurse supervisor can review these with you and make any necessary adjustments.

To clean an object such as clothing, the toilet, sink, or floor:

1. Put on gloves and secure your clothing or sleeves out of the way.
2. Rinse the object in COLD water to remove any organic material. Do not rinse in the food preparation sink. Organic materials include blood, feces, drainage from a sore or wound, or urine. Organic materials contain protein. Hot water will cause the protein to clump and stick to the object.
3. Wash the object using HOT soapy water. Most household detergents will provide sufficient cleaning action. If there are isolation precautions, use bleach or other disinfectants as directed by the nurse supervisor.
4. Use a stiff bristled brush to scrub out any grooved areas, corners, or hard-to-clean open areas.
5. Wash and rinse your hands, wearing the gloves.
6. Rinse the object in HOT water. Rinse until all soap residue is removed.
7. Remove and dispose of your gloves. Wash your hands.
8. Dry with a clean cloth. Clothing or linens can be machine dried or hung on the line, especially if it is a sunny day.

Sterilizing

Sterilizing is a means of destroying all microorganisms from an object. There are many ways to sterilize. The methods discussed here are commonly used in the home setting. Follow your nurse supervisor's directions.

The most familiar kind of sterilization is chemical sterilization. Contact with certain household chemical mixtures destroys microorganisms by poisoning their body systems.

Universal Cleaning Techniques

- The following universal cleaning techniques apply to disease control and prevention in any home health setting.
- Clean all pots, pans, and dishes that have not been used for a long period of time.
- Clean counter tops and sinks with scouring powder.
- Supply your client with clean glasses or cups during the day.
- Rinse the lids of cans before opening them.
- Wash fruits and vegetables before preparing them.
- Cook all meat thoroughly. All poultry and pork products especially should be cooked until well done.
- Wash all areas, utensils, cutting boards, or cooking pans where uncooked poultry or meats have been prepared before using them for any other purpose. Use hot soapy water or scouring powder and rinse. Wash your hands before touching other things.
- Refrigerate all foods after cooking and eating. Do not allow foods to sit out after cooking.
- Clean the refrigerator with soap and water to remove molds or food spills. Rotate food and remove outdated products.
- Eggs with cracked shells, raw eggs, and unpasteurized milk products are not considered safe for your client because they may cause food-related infections such as salmonella.
- Wash and dry all dishes before leaving for the day. Do not let dirty dishes sit overnight.
- Do not use sponges or cloths to wash dishes or clean food preparation areas for any other use. **Never** clean the floor or any body fluids with a dish sponge or dishcloth.
- Wear an apron or gown when working with soiled linen or bathing your client. Remove the apron before beginning food preparation activities.
- Never wash out mops or pour mop or nfloor cleaning water down the kitchen sink where food is prepared or dishes washed. Mop kitchen floor or if carpeted, vacuum daily.
- Wash mops at least weekly by soaking them in the 1:9 bleach solution for 10-20 minutes. Use a separate bucket to soak the mops. Then launder apart from other linens or kitchen linens.
- When dusting, use a slightly dampened cloth and dust away from your body.
- When touching dirty linens or clothing, wear gloves. Handle the cleanest part or the part that is farthest from the dirty part. Keep dirty items away from your body. Change your apron if necessary.
- Dispose of all garbage and recyclable materials. Remove them from the home at the end of your day there.
- Each person should have his own personal care items which are not shared with any other person. These include razor, toothbrush, bar soap, douching devices, enema equipment, sexual devices, cosmetics, hairbrushes or combs, waterpiks, and similar personal items.
- Each person must have his own thermometer and other health related supplies.
- Each person should have his own towels, washcloths, and bed linens.
- Bathrooms should be cleaned after each use by the client. Any feces, urine, or other body fluids must be cleaned immediately, using disposable towels or wipes. Disinfect the area with the 1:9 bleach solution.
- Bathroom sponges or cloths are never used to clean in the kitchen or elsewhere.
- Bathroom fixtures, showers, tubs, floors, toilet seats, and basins must be cleaned regularly. Mop floors. Wash other fixtures with soap and water, then disinfect with 1:9 bleach solution after each use by the client.

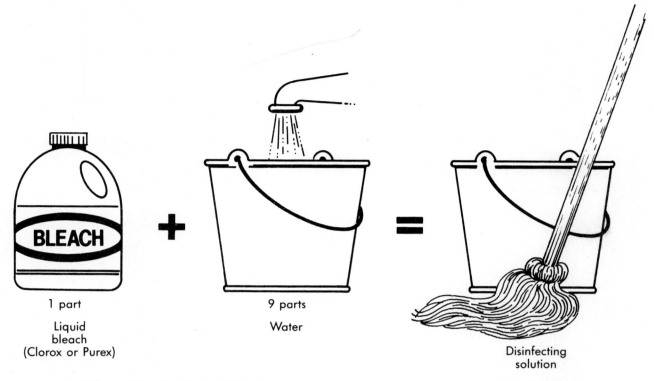

1 part

Liquid
bleach
(Clorox or Purex)

9 parts

Water

Disinfecting
solution

Figure 1-6. *Regular liquid bleach can be mixed with tap water to make an effective disinfectant.*

1. Liquid bleach and water (Figure 1-6):
   a) 1 part liquid chlorine bleach (Use Clorox or Purex liquid bleach to be sure of the proper strength)
   b) 9 parts of water
   c) Put the water in the container first, then add the bleach. This will keep the bleach from splashing out (any splashes will be water). Do not splash bleach into your eyes or onto your skin. If you do so, wash with large amounts of clear running water. If bleach gets in your eyes, also call the nurse supervisor for assistance. If she cannot be reached, go to your physician or the nearest emergency room immediately.
   d) Ask the nurse supervisor to approve the measuring, mixing, and storing of this solution.
   e) Make this solution *fresh each day. DO NOT STORE.*
   f) DO NOT mix with any other solutions or cleansers.
2. Boiling water:
   a) Ask the nurse supervisor to approve

the vessel or pot to be used for boiling.
   b) DO NOT leave a heating element, open flame, or pot of boiling water on the stove unattended.
   c) Be sure the object can be safely boiled.
   d) Be sure the object is immersed or submerged under the water.
   e) Boil for 20 minutes.
   f) Use a timer. Start to time when the water has begun a full and rolling boil.
   g) Be careful not to burn yourself when removing the object. You may be instructed to boil tongs with the object. You would then use the sterilized tongs to remove the object so it will not become contaminated when you remove it from the water.

Isolation Precautions

Another way to control microorganisms, beyond preventing them from spreading from place to place or from person to person, is to confine them. Special techniques are used to confine or isolate microorganisms in one area and keep them from spreading outside of that area. This section describes the various kinds of isolation procedures. Use them as a guide, but follow the directions of your nurse supervisor if they differ in some ways.

Respiratory Isolation Precautions

Respiratory isolation precautions are taken when the pathogen is spread from the respiratory tract of one person to that of another. The pathogen is carried by the water droplets that are sent into the air when the infected person coughs, sneezes, or breathes. Precautions to prevent the spread of infection are directed at the means of transmission; that is, keeping the respiratory droplets from reaching others. (Figure 1-7)

Respiratory isolation precautions are used when a client has active pulmonary tuberculosis or a staphylococcal pneumonia.

Certain clients may have weakened immune systems. These clients are prone to getting even minor infections and becoming very ill. In these cases, the isolation precautions would be reversed. *You would protect your*

Respiratory Isolation Precautions

- Place a supply of disposable or washable facial masks outside the client's room. The masks should be large enough to cover the nose and mouth.
- Keep a supply of facial tissues on hand.
- Line a trash container with a plastic bag.
- Make sure that each person wears a facial mask when entering the client's room.
- Make sure that the client wears a facial mask whenever he must leave his room.
- See that the client uses several layers of facial tissues to cover his mouth and nose whenever he coughs or sneezes. He should collect all secretions and droplets into the tissues.
- Directly and immediately dispose of all tissues into a prepared trash container. The container can be lined with a plastic bag liner for easy disposal.
- Wear gloves to empty the trash or handle the tissues.
- Wash your hands and have the client wash his hands.

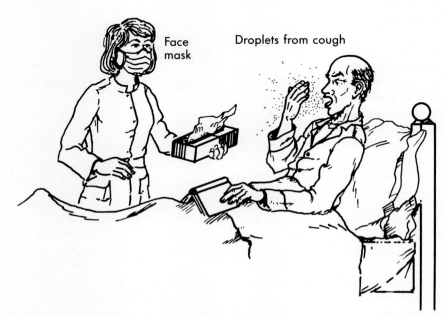

Figure 1-7. *The spread of many infectious diseases can be prevented by using gloves and facial masks.*

client from your microorganisms by wearing a mask if you had a runny nose or a cough. You would also use the layers of tissues to collect droplets and wear gloves to care for your client. Good handwashing is essential to successful respiratory isolation precautions.

Enteric or Fecal Isolation Precautions

Enteric isolation procedures are used when the pathogen is spread through contact with the client's feces. This contact can be direct or indirect. The pathogen from the feces must somehow be taken in through the mouth. Feces, and in some cases throat secretions and emesis (vomitus) may be contaminated with the pathogen. Handwashing is essential.

Enteric or Fecal Isolation Precautions

- Make sure that the client uses his own bathroom. No one else should use the bathroom.
- If the bathroom must be shared with others:
  —Clean after each use by the client.
  —Wear gloves and a gown while cleaning.
  —Clean all surfaces of the commode, basin, and floor. Clean even if commode seat covers or other preventive materials are used.
  —Collect all items or linens that may have come into contact with the client's feces, urine, or emesis.
  —Use 1 part Clorox or Purex liquid bleach to 9 parts of water to clean (or solution as directed by the nurse supervisor).
- Wash linens and gown according to directions listed in this section or as the nurse supervisor directs.
- Dispose of gloves in special lined trash container.
- Wash your hands. Have client wash his hands.

Wound or Skin Isolation Precautions

The client's skin, a break in his skin, or a wound can be infected by a pathogen. The infection can be spread directly to you and to others if you come into contact with it. Dressings or coverings from the infected area carry the pathogen. The client's gowns, clothing, or linens may also be contaminated by drainage from the infected wound. You can become infected from contact with these items.

Precautions are as for other isolations.

- Wear gloves and gowns when changing or handling wound dressings.
- Wear gloves and gowns when handling clothing or linens that may have wound drainage on them.

Blood Isolation Precautions

This isolation is to prevent the spread of pathogens that infect a client's blood. Follow your nurse supervisor's directions carefully.

- Wear gloves and a gown whenever there is a chance of coming into contact with:
  —a client's blood.
  —items that have, or may have had, blood on them.
  —sharp objects or needles, to prevent being stuck accidentally.

SAFETY

Safety in the Home Setting

Giving care to a client in the home differs from giving care in a hospital or other institution. Some of the day-to-day practical differences are related to safety measures. This section discusses safety in several areas:

—keeping yourself and your client safe during care activities,
—practicing safe use and disposal of products and supplies,
—practicing safe use and care of home equipment,
—maintaining a safe home environment, and
—reducing hazards.

Personal and Client Safety During Care

Falls are one of the greatest safety concerns in the home. Injuries incurred by caregivers are another concern. A common cause of back injuries among caregivers is the improper use of body mechanics when lifting and moving clients or equipment. Both client falls and caregiver injuries are preventable. Throughout this book, safety precautions and procedures are stressed and discussed. Read the section on body mechanics and pay close attention to the safety messages that accompany procedures, care activities, and use of products and equipment.

Never attempt to perform a level of care or procedure for a client if you are not trained, licensed, or qualified to do so. **Always** ask the nurse supervisor when in doubt. The next sections of this chapter continue with specific safety concerns for the care of the clients in their homes. Client safety must be one of your primary concerns.

Supplies and Products

The types and amounts of supplies that are available in the home often differ from the supplies and products available in institutions. Clients and families may not choose to use disposable supplies at home or be able to obtain them as readily as they did in the institution. Purchased assistive devices and equipment and facsimile homemade adaptations for equipment can be very useful for your client's self-care and well-being. Some products may be made at home, using readily available materials, for a very small investment. Many home adaptations are suggested in this book; carefully read the safety precautions for each one. An item that can be made inexpensively and easily at home must be safe as well as solve the problem.

Do not:

—attempt to reuse or resterilize items that are intended for disposable, one-time-only use;

—use equipment or supplies that are not in good working order, or have parts loose or missing;

—use equipment or supplies without training and practice in their use;

—use equipment or supplies without clear instructions for use;

—attempt home repairs on equipment unless you have been specifically instructed by the nurse supervisor, or

—use any equipment that you or the client believes to be unsafe, even if you cannot identify the problem.

Homemade products or supplies are not necessarily less expensive than purchased commercial items. Many high quality, functional products that are available commercially are illustrated in this book. Some items may be purchased in local variety stores or from mail order catalogues at lower cost than from medical supply houses. Their quality and safety must be carefully checked before purchase and use. Purchasing a high quality safe product or piece of equipment may be less expensive in the long run than using a poorly constructed homemade item. The cost of basic raw materials and the availability of workers and tools must be considered as part of cost comparisons. Moreover, commercial products have been tested and evaluated and equipment vendors provide service for repairs and adjustments, often on short notice or 24 hours a day.

Be sure the item is needed and useful. Sometimes families buy too many devices, supplies, and equipment without considering their real value to the client. Each piece of equipment or assistive device, whether purchased, adapted for home use, or homemade, must be evaluated by the nurse supervisor or the therapists before it is used with the client. Although an item may not be dangerous in itself, if it does not work in harmony with the client's rehabilitation goals, it may not be right for him.

Each item must be examined in terms of its merit, cost, and usefulness. What might be appropriate for one client may not be for the next person, even if both have similar problems to solve. Have the nurse supervisor examine and approve all items before using them. The nurse supervisor will evaluate each item according to the client's and family's:

—budget,
—care needs,
—preferences,
—available space,

—time for assisting with care,
—energy level and coping abilities,
—functional and self-care abilities, and
—safe environment for use.

Some items will be safely reusable. Be sure you understand the instructions for maintaining the reusable items. For example, if an item is to be boiled, write down the instructions about how long, how to place the item into the water, and how to remove and store it. If an item is to be soaked in a solution, have the nurse supervisor help select the soaking vessel, decide on what will be used to measure the solutions, and to label and store the solutions. Know how and where to store the item until its next use, and write down specific instructions.

If you use household cleaning supplies, be sure you do not create accidental chemical hazards in the home. Never mix solutions unless directed by the nurse supervisor. For example, toxic fumes are released when household chlorine bleach is mixed with ammonia. All supplies or products, whether purchased or homemade, must be carefully handled for disposal. Whenever products or supplies are disposed of, ask the nurse supervisor about proper ways to prepare and package items for disposal to prevent infection, leakage, contamination, poisoning, and possible toxic fumes or explosions. Ask the client or his family about proper disposal sites to be sure that you adhere to local recycling laws.

Equipment in the Home

Much of the preceding information about supplies and products also applies to equip-
ment. Most clients who have home equipment also have an equipment vendor to supply their needs and arrange for repairs. The equipment in clients' homes will vary from complex state-of-the-art equipment scaled to home sizes, to modifications for solving client problems, to the most basic standard equipment. However, home equipment is frequently constructed and operated differently from institutional equipment. Read the precautions and instructions for safe use of equipment and safety for yourself and your client in Chapter 5. Read each section carefully and practice before using any new equipment and again the first time you use equipment with a new client.

A Safe Home Environment

This section is a checklist for home safety. Use it to check the home of a client under the supervision and direction of the nurse, the client, the family, and possibly the therapists. Be sure that any safety violations or hazards are reported, investigated, and fixed or corrected.

Housewide Check

Architectural barriers:

—Doorways should be wide enough to permit wheelchairs to go through without hitting the person's hands.
—Ramps should allow wheelchairs to safely reach the outdoors; never take a wheelchair down stairs with a person in the chair.

Things to Know When Handling Household Supplies and Products

the proper solution
how to handle it
what the hazards are
how to prepare it
how long to prepare and use it
what to prepare it in
how to measure
what to measure it in
whether to wear gloves
temperatures for use and storage

how to apply or use it
protection for the client
emergency actions
how to store it
where to store it
what to store it in
how and where to label it
how to clean up spills
when not to use it
how to dispose of it

In The Home Setting:

Do not use equipment or supplies that are not in full working order.

Do:
—have the nurse supervisor review your use of the equipment and direct you in its use with each client,
—make sure you and the client are both ready to use the equipment and feel safe and comfortable using it,
—have other persons available to assist you if there is a problem with the use of equipment,
—know how to contact someone for help,
—be sure that the equipment works,
—know how to work the equipment,
—know the rules for safe use,
—use proper body mechanics,
—know how to handle other assistive devices the client may have while using the equipment,
—check client safety at each step of a procedure,
—use equipment in the place and manner in which it is designed to be used,
—clear enough space to use the equipment properly,
—know basic things to check before requesting repairs, and
—know emergency measures.

—Kitchens should be fitted with safety devices along with any adaptive or assistive devices.

Smoke Detectors and Fire Extinguishers:

—Both devices should be on every level of the home.
—Check that the operating signal (usually a red light) is lit on the smoke detector, indicating that the battery is operating, or follow manufacturer's instructions for checking operating condition.
—Matches, lighters, and other flame-producing items should not be carried about the house. A client may keep a few cigarettes with him if he smokes and have you light them in safe areas where he is supervised.

Rugs, Carpets, and Runners:

—All floor coverings should be non-slip or have rubber matting.
—Rugs should not be frayed or have loose loops.
—Take up throw rugs if possible.
—Ends and edges should not roll or turn up; use double-edged tape or tack down edges if the rug must stay where it is.
—Rugs should not obstruct wheelchairs, canes, or walkers.
—Rugs should not be placed in front of an open fire or near a heat source.
—Check stair carpet runners or stair pads for loose ends or pieces that might catch a shoeheel or cause someone to trip.

Electrical Cords, Telephone Cords, Appliance Cords:

—Do not use multiple extension cords on the same outlet.
—Cords should not extend through walking areas.
—Frayed or damaged cords should be replaced.
—Use only three-pronged outlets for three-pronged plugs.
—Cords should not run under carpets, or near heat sources.
—Do not stretch cords across the room, even temporarily.
—Do not leave toaster ovens, irons, curling irons, hair dryers, and similar small appliances plugged in when not in use.
—If children are in the home, use plug protectors to seal off wall sockets.
—Do not let cords trail over the edges of tables or desks.
—Exposed wiring or switches without cover plates must be repaired.

Lighting:

—Light bulbs should illuminate dark areas, stairs, hallways, and passageways.

Use nightlights to provide guides for bathroom use and security lighting.
—Lightbulbs should be the correct wattage for the lamp.
—Glaring overhead lights are not recommended; they add heat to a room and are unpleasant.
—Nighlights in good repair are recommended even if the client does not regularly get up at night.

Heat Sources:

—Woodburning stoves should be installed by professionals and inspected by the fire department or building code inspector.
—Woodburning stoves must be carefully tended and the doors tightly shut to keep logs from accidentally rolling out.
—Woodburning stoves and their pipes and chimneys must be cleaned at least annually. Only dry non-resinous wood is safe to burn. The family must check the stove, pipes, and chimney for creosote buildup (the tarlike residue from burned wood) every two to three weeks.
—Never store gasoline, kerosene, paint thinners, or other flammable products in the house. Store them in properly labeled containers made for that purpose, never in glass containers. Keep these products away from heated areas. The fumes or vapors can carry 6–10 feet and even a warm heat source may ignite a flammable product. Fumes or vapors may be toxic or cause people to feel sick.
—Rags or papers that have been used with flammable products can also ignite spontaneously. They should not be stored in the house or garage or rolled together in an unventilated area.
—Heating plates should never be used as heaters or placed near a bed or window curtains.
—Ovens and stove top burners should not be turned on as heat sources.
—Never use gasoline as a cleaning fluid for anything.
—Kerosene heaters must be located where they cannot be turned over and where there is excellent ventilation.
—Only fuel recommended by the manufacturer in the manual (usually white, top-grade kerosene) should be used to fuel kerosene heaters. Cool down heaters before refueling and refuel heaters out of doors and avoid inhaling the vapors or spilling fuel.
—Kerosene heaters must be vented according to directions to prevent carbon monoxide buildup in the house. Never use kerosene heaters in a tightly closed room. Never leave a kerosene heater burning when you go to sleep. Turn off the heater if you leave the house unattended.
—Gas pilot lights should be kept burning without odors.
—Charcoal should not be burned indoors because of the fumes that build up without outside ventilation.
—Furnaces should be checked each year and cleaned if soot has built up in the system.

Cooling System:

—Air conditioning units should be checked each year for proper operation and for cleaning.
—Air conditioners require their own electrical three-pronged outlets.
—Nothing should obstruct the outside of the air conditioner or the area around the main air conditioning system if central air conditioning is used.

Rooms:

The Kitchen:

—Keep vents and fans clean and free of grease and dust buildups.
—Clothing should not hang over the stove or have loose sleeves, sashes, or other parts that could catch fire from the burners. This happens with electric burners as easily as with gas flames.
—Potholders should be thick and flame resistant, without holes, and available for quick use but not stored near heat.
—Do not place papers, plastic utensils or containers, kitchen towels, or flammable sprays on or near the stove.

—Do not allow curtains or towels to hang over the stove or where a stovetop fire could easily spread to them.

—Do not store items over the stove so that you have to reach over the heating elements to get them. Keep foods or treats that may tempt children away from that area.

—Keep baking soda near the stove to use for grease fires.

—Do not line ovens, burners, or toaster ovens with aluminum foil.

—Do not turn burners up to high unless the cookware is designed for high heat.

—Do not leave a stove unattended when cooking. This means do not start cooking and then leave the room. If you need to attend to your client, turn the stove off.

If a fire starts while you are cooking:

—Turn off the stove.

—Smother the fire with a pan lid.

—Add baking soda to cover the flames.

—Never use a towel to cover the fire.

—Do not touch handles that may be hot.

—A fire extinguisher should be nearby. Know how to use it.

—Never, never, move a fire in a pan or other utensil out of doors or to the sink. It may spread or flare up suddenly.

—Never put water on a grease fire or hot greasy pan.

—Steam can cause burns if it rises onto the skin, as it can when pouring steaming hot liquids from a pot or into a strainer.

—Keep cooking areas well-lit.

—Do not empty ashtrays or throw cigarette ends directly into the wastebasket. Smoldering ashes can erupt into flames in trashcans, wheelchair cushion seats, bedclothing, and in folds of bathrobes.

—Do not place knives or other sharp objects into dishwater where they cannot be seen.

—Do not add water to hot cooking utensils, especially if they have oil or grease in them. Do not immerse hot cooking utensils in water.

—If you use a step stool, use one with a hand rail or a front guard rail; it should be no more than two or three steps high. Be sure it is stable, has non-slip footing, and no loose parts. Be sure the stool is fully open before climbing on it.

—Do not climb on chairs, table tops, or counters.

—Do not touch or operate electrical appliances with wet hands or where the cord or appliance might touch water.

—Do not allow trash or food scraps to accumulate in the kitchen. Follow local recycling laws and keep garbage out of the house.

—Clean spills or food off the floor to prevent slipping.

—Plumbing problems such as water leaks, poorly draining sinks, or bad odors from the drains should be checked by a plumber. Report such plumbing problems to the nurse supervisor and family.

Bathroom:

—Bathtubs, showers, and floors should have non-slip rugs, mats, or surfaces. Wet, soapy tiles, toilets, and tubs are dangerously slippery and hard.

—Grab bars should be placed by tubs, showers, and toilets. They must be stable and strong, attached to studs in the wall, and properly placed beside the fixtures.

—Chlorine bleach should not be mixed with cleaning products, particularly with those containing ammonia.

—Water temperatures should not exceed 120 degrees. Water temperature is usually controlled at the hot water heater. Some showers and tubs have temperature-controlled faucets.

—Always check the water temperature before using the tub or shower. Use a thermometer.

—Use ground fault circuit-interrupters, which are simple devices that prevent electrical shock from water and electricity by interrupting the electric current.

—Household cleansers, medications, over-the-counter items and other products stored in the bathroom should be safely out of the reach of children, even if the children only visit the home.

—Store medications in high places and use childproof caps. Assist your client if necessary with the caps.

Be sure that all medications are shown to the nurse supervisor, who will check the dates and types of medications. Some clients stock-pile medications and con-

tinue to take them after their expiration dates or after they are no longer necessary. Occasionally, clients will attempt to trade medications with other persons. Many medications and over-the-counter preparations deteriorate over time or when exposed to heat, light, moisture, or air. Notify the nurse and do not use products if they have:
—developed an unusual odor,
—changed color,
—become cloudy,
—formed a residue,
—crumbled (or crumble when handled; e.g., tablets),
—separated or discolored (ointments),
—developed specks or spots, or passed their expiration dates.

Bedroom:

—Never allow smoking in bed.
—Ash trays, hot plates, portable heaters, or other heat sources should not be near the bed or where the bedclothes or linens might touch or hang over them.
—Hot liquids or foods should not be near the bed where they could spill, causing burns.
—Electric blankets should not be used unless they are ordered by the nurse supervisor. Electric blankets must be in good condition, kept on low heat, and have safe plugs. Do not place other blankets on top of an electric blanket and do not tuck in edges; heat could build up and cause fire.
—Use siderails when ordered. Place the head of the bed and one side against the wall if a light and a telephone can be placed within reach. This will make the person get in and out of bed on the same side and lessen confusion if he tends to be disoriented upon arising.
—Lamps, telephones, or other signaling devices should be within operating distance or easy reach of the bed.
—A smoke detector should be near each bedroom.
—If oxygen is stored in the home or bedroom, follow the instructions given by the nurse supervisor and the oxygen supply vendor. Read about oxygen storage in the home in Chapter 11.

Stairs:

—Stairs should be well-lit from both top and bottom.
—Do not store or collect items on the stair steps.
—Stair runners should be secure and tacked down.
—Handrails should be at proper height for support, securely attached to the wall, and preferably on both sides of the steps.
—Stairsteps should not be loose or warped. Steps should be even in size.
—Block stairs with childproof gates to prevent falls by children or unwary adults.

General Information:

—Post telephone numbers for emergencies near the telephone. Include numbers for the Poison Control Center, Rescue Squad and emergency room, nurse supervisor, family members, any responders to communication alert systems such as Lifeline, and any numbers related to the client's special needs.
—Know where the fusebox or electrical circuit breaker box is located. Some homes have circuit breakers that can be reset by pushing a button. Older homes usually have fuseboxes. If a fuse blows, it must be replaced with a fuse of the same size and wattage. Check with the family or the nurse supervisor about fuses.
—Small objects such as buttons, safety pins, marbles, or loose screws should be kept out of reach of children and others who might put them in their mouths and swallow or choke on them.
—Alcoholic beverages should be stored out of reach.
—Practice a fire evacuation plan under the supervision and direction of the nurse. Other persons in the home should practice with you as much as possible. Everyone should be informed of and aware of the evacuation plan and several escape routes.
—Know how to move the client, especially if he is unable to move himself. For example, use a blanket to drag a person out of a room or building rather than try to carry him.

—Have a family member round off or move objects that have sharp corners or edges.

—Check latches, knobs, locks, and handles to make sure they are securely in place and in working order.

Communication Safety:

—Keep a whistle near the bed or in the wheelchair.

—Fire alarm systems as well as telephones are available with flashing lights or other visual alarms for persons who are hearing-impaired.

—Keep a flashlight with working batteries, candles, and matches near candle-holders, and similar supplies available in case of power failure.

You must be sure that the environment you are working in is safe and that you are using preventive behaviors and actions.

CHAPTER 2

Responding to Basic Needs and Emergency Situations

*O*BJECTIVES:

When you have studied this chapter and practiced the procedures it describes, you will be able to:

1. Define terms relating to the basic health needs of clients.
2. Assist your clients with self-care and basic needs, as directed.
3. Discuss your role and tasks in providing or assisting with clients' basic needs.
4. Care for clients' basic needs while maximizing their independence and self-care.
5. Work with clients, families, and other health caregivers in programs designed to manage basic needs, such as bowel programs.
6. Use basic needs programs and techniques when caring for clients who have various disabilities or conditions.
7. Perform selected activities and make certain supplies for home care basic needs.

*O*VERVIEW

This chapter discusses needs that are basic parts of a client's rehabilitation. Taking care of these basic needs will prevent many complications for your client and improve his quality of life. The basic needs discussed here are skin care, oral care, nutrition, bladder training programs, bowel training programs, range of motion exercises, safety in the home, and emergency techniques. Exercises and diets for special purposes are addressed in the Appendices.

SKIN CARE

Care of the skin is a very important responsibility that rarely receives the attention it deserves. You must be very concerned about the care you give your client's skin every day. Skin care begins with good hygiene and inspection of the total skin condition. Skin is a living part of the body, just like the heart and lungs (Figure 2-1). It is the body's largest organ and can breathe, stretch, and replace its layers. The skin is the body's first barrier against infections from the outside world. Skin holds nerves, blood vessels, and hair roots, and helps the body to:

—keep cool by sweating and stay warm by insulating with fatty tissues;
—stay healthy by carrying blood vessels, lymph, and nutrients, oil for lubrication, and carrying off wastes; and
—stay protected from the outside threats posed by sun and wind, insect bites, cuts and scrapes, and dirt and infection.

One of your most important jobs is to prevent skin problems. This means preventing pressure areas on the skin that can develop into pressure sores. Other names for pres-

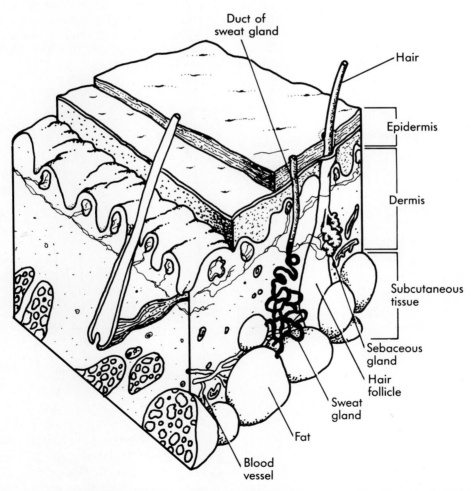

Figure 2-1. *The skin is the largest organ in the body. The epidermis or outer layer contains the pigment that give color to the skin. This layer is continually sloughing off old cells and replacing them with new cells. The dermis layer of the skin holds the blood vessels, hair roots, and oil and sweat glands. Subcutaneous fatty tissues lie under the dermis.*

sure sores are bedsores and decubitus ulcers. A pressure sore can cause your client to have to stay in bed. It can also lead to infection, other medical problems, and even a hospital stay. An important thing to remember is that *pressure sores are preventable.* If one starts, it must be detected and stopped at its earliest stage, while only a reddened area of skin. Although you may only see a reddened area on the skin surface, a larger area of skin tissue below the surface has already been damaged. If enough damage has occurred below the outer layer of the skin, the skin surface may open into a sore. This is why it is essential to remove pressure immediately from a seemingly small reddened area.

Certain areas of the body are vulnerable to development of pressure sores. These are the places where you will always look for potential problems. For example, pressure sores develop readily where the skin is stretched over a bony prominence or where weight is placed on the body for lengthy periods of time. Figure 2-2 shows sites on the body where pressure sores most frequently develop.

PREVENTION OF PRESSURE SORES

1. **Observation.** The first step in prevention is observation of the skin by you, your client, the family, and other caregivers. Observation of the entire body should be done at least twice daily; a good routine is to do it in the morning and at bedtime. Pressure areas may be observed more often if a regular schedule is planned. Clients are taught to use a mirror to inspect areas of their bodies they cannot visualize directly (Figure 2-3).

You and your client are looking for:

—any localized reddened areas, beginning with pink and progressing to redness;
—localized warmth and/or swelling;
—open areas, cracks, or breaks in the skin;
—blisters or rashes;

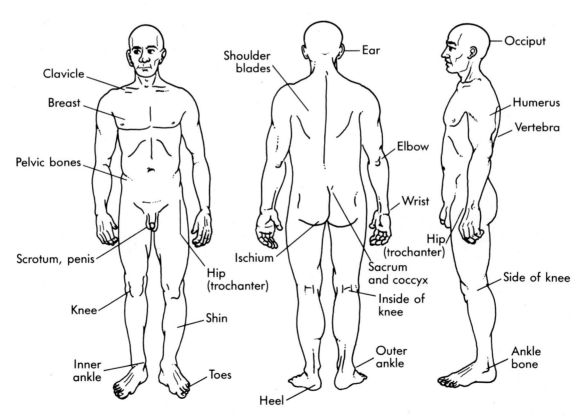

Figure 2-2. *Certain areas of the body are at risk for developing pressure areas that may lead to decubitus ulcers. Bony prominences and pressure points must be inspected regularly to detect reddened skin, signs of friction or tearing, or other skin damage. Early identification and prevention of skin problems are an important goal of care.*

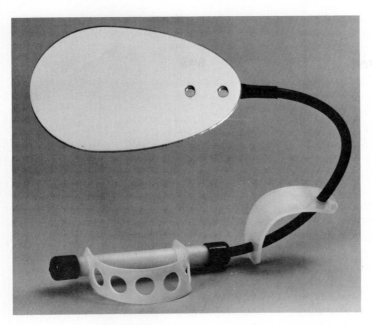

Figure 2-3. *Specially designed mirrors can help clients view areas of their bodies that they are not otherwise able to inspect. This is one way to assist a client to be active in his own care.*

—weeping, flaking, or scaling areas;
—cuts, bruises, scrapes, bites;
—dry skin; and
—soiled skin such as urine-soaked areas.

2. **Preventing Pressure on the Skin.** The most common way to place pressure on the skin is to remain in one position too long. Your clients are not always able to realize that they have been in one position too long. They may not feel their arm "going to sleep," or sense the pressure of one leg lying on the other, or have the need to stretch. They must learn to shift and move their bodies every 20–30 minutes. Circulation to disabled areas of their body may be decreased and these areas may be undernourished. They may not be able to sit very long without causing pressure areas on their skin.

Skin pressure is greatest on the body parts highlighted on the diagrams. Where the possibilities for pressure are strongest, it takes the least amount of time for a problem to start. Pressure can also come from sources like equipment, shoes, and braces. Inspect your client's skin carefully each time you turn him, whenever you remove a piece of equipment he has been using, or when you take off his shoes. If possible, remove any pressure-causing materials. Report any signs of pressure to the nurse. Each time you turn your client you must also check his positioning and body alignment.

The nurse will give you a written program for scheduled position changes and turns. The schedule should consider the client's other activities, such as bowel and bladder programs, meals, and therapy sessions. Initially, **weight shifts** for the person in a wheelchair should be scheduled every 20 minutes. There are several ways to do weight shifts, depending on the client's abilities and reliability. If he is dependent, you must assist him to lift his weight out of the chair for approximately 20 seconds at a time. If he is able, have him lean from side to side to shift the weight off his buttocks. Ideally, a client will perform wheelchair pushups. He does these by straightening his elbows and placing his hands on armrests of the wheelchair. He pushes down with his hands, lifting his buttocks off the seat of the chair.

When the person is in bed, he should be turned on a schedule of every 2 hours. He will be turned more often if he has reddened areas on his skin. Turning becomes less frequent as the person's tolerance, or ability to stay in one position, increases. Tolerance does not increase beyond a certain point for any individual. No client should sit in a wheelchair or keep one position in bed for longer than 4 hours. There may be exceptions to this interval if the person is placed prone in bed or has one of the specialized beds. The nurse supervisor will direct you if the turning time is changed. The person's body position and alignment must be corrected after each turn.

Once he has an established routine, your client should assume responsibility for shifting his weight and turning, if he is able. Observe how often he does this and remind him when he is overdue for a position change. If he cannot shift weight or turn, you are responsible for turning him on schedule. Check his skin every time he is turned, or at least twice each day. Watch for such silent problems as a dangling leg, arm, or hand that may swell while hanging in a dependent position. Dangling limbs cause swelling in the hands and lower arms that can quickly damage the skin tissues. Dangling hands may also be caught in the spokes of the wheelchair.

Friction and Shearing

These two terms describe skin damage that can occur with or without pressure on the skin. **Friction** is the heat caused by rubbing two surfaces together. For example, friction is produced when a person's spastic leg rubs against a piece of equipment. **Shearing** is like friction except that the skin tissues slide over each other. This is especially likely to be a problem over bony prominences. Shearing causes stretching and pressure on the skin and underlying tissues. It affects a larger area than that indicated by signs of pressure. Persons who are very heavy, unconscious, have paralyzed limbs, or are spastic are more difficult to move and transfer. They therefore need special attention to avoid friction and prevent shearing damage to the skin.

If a pressure area has already started to develop, the only way to stop further damage is to remove all pressure from the area. Inform the nurse supervisor of any red areas on the client's skin. You may be instructed to use one of the paddings designed to lift the areas receiving pressure. The most commonly used paddings include foam rubber (4"), pillows, water or gel pillows, water and air mattresses, eggcrate foam mattresses, and rubber rings or foam rolls. Sometimes equipment that is intended to solve one problem for the client can cause other problems.

Basic Rules for Skin Care

- Keep his skin clean. Pay special attention to folds and creases in the skin and where there is urine or fecal soiling.
- Prevent dry skin that may crack and peel. Massages with lotion will aid circulation to the skin and keep the skin supple. Do not use powder and lotions together as they form a paste.
- Avoid contact with harsh chemicals such as unrinsed laundered clothing and sheets, and solutions that may irritate some individuals.
- Prevent burns from:
  —overexposure to sun and wind,
  —contact with soap residues,
  —adhesive tapes that may actually "burn" the skin,
  —sitting near an open fire, and
  —burns from such sources as heating elements, car seat or seatbelt buckles that have been heated by the sun, hot water pipes beneath a sink, and car or home radiators.
- Protect the skin from too much moisture. Moisture can cause the growth of bacteria and contribute to softening and breakdown of tissues. Heavy perspiration, draining wounds or tubes, urine and fecal materials, spilled foods, and solutions should be cleaned and dried promptly.

For example, stomach tubes or restraints can cause pressure or friction spots.

Trochanter rolls, sandbags, footboards, and other equipment designed to maintain good alignment and positioning may cause pressure areas on the skin. Elastic hose, bandages, ace wraps, and bindings can all cause pressure points. Do not allow them to be wrinkled, too tight, poorly wrapped, fastened with lumpy tails or metal clips, or left in place too long. The skin under these devices should be checked at least four times a day. Observe the skin for color, temperature, condition, pulse, and swelling. You may be instructed to use adhesive tape to secure any wrappings. If so, the tape should not extend completely around the client's limb. This could constrict circulation or produce pressure on the skin.

Some clients select sheepskins for their beds and the seat of their wheelchairs. Sheepskins are washed in cold water with a wool soap and allowed to dry. Drying may take overnight. There are also many wheelchair cushions from which to choose. There are designs to suit each client's individual needs for comfort, position, function, and prevention of pressure areas.

There is no substitute for prevention of pressure sores.

To help prevent problems, the skin should be:

—kept clean,
—well-nourished,
—free from traumas, and
—inspected regularly.

You and your client have a great deal of control over the outcomes of his skin care. It is important to follow these procedures:

CARE OF HANDS, FEET, FINGERNAILS, AND TOENAILS

Care of the hands, feet, toenails, and fingernails is important for all clients. For example, ingrown toenails can cause infections, skin breakdown, and in some cases, autonomic dysreflexia. (See Chapter 9 on spinal cord injury.) Clients who cannot feel their feet or who have diabetes and circulatory problems are at risk for foot troubles. Likewise, clients who have foot problems may have difficulty wearing shoes.

Care of Your Client's Hands and Feet

- **Never** cut a client's nails. Inform your nurse supervisor of any ingrown nails or other nail problems.
- Soak his hands in mild, soapy water every day, gently cleaning between his fingers, the palm of his hand, and around the nails;
- Use a fine-grained emery board to gently smooth any snags or rough areas on fingernails;
- Ask your nurse supervisor to show you how to relax your client's hand when it is clenched or paralyzed;
- Inspect the skin of the feet twice daily as part of his skin care.
- Soak both his feet for about 20 minutes in warm, *not hot,* soapy water. Clients who have diabetes will require daily foot baths; other persons may soak their feet 1–3 times per week according to the care plan.

- Rinse his hands or feet well and dry them thoroughly.
- Gently rub any dry or calloused areas with a soft washcloth.
- Massage a moisturizing lotion into the skin of his hands and feet, including heels and elbows, to keep them soft and to aid circulation.
- Look for any reddened areas, cracks, inflammation, corns, swelling, or pustules.
- Tell the nurse or family about any of the client's foot problems. This includes ill-fitting shoes, thickened and deformed nails, or areas that rub against equipment.

MOUTH AND DENTAL CARE

Care for the mouth and teeth is often neglected by both clients and caregivers. Some clients have not taken good care of their mouths and teeth over the years. They may have poorly fitting dentures, tooth decay, or gum disease. Moreover, whenever the body is stressed or weakened, there are increased stresses on the mouth and teeth. Oral hygiene must be scheduled, just as skin care and positioning activities are scheduled. You must allow time for the client to use assistive devices and do as much of his own oral care as possible.

Three parts of the mouth require attention: the teeth, the gums, and the mouth tissues.

The *teeth* must be brushed at least daily,

ideally both after meals and at bedtime. The purpose of toothbrushing is to remove plaque and bacteria from the surfaces of the teeth. Otherwise they build up, causing tooth decay and gum deterioration. Built-up plaque contains bacteria that cause swelling, infection, decay of the teeth and gums, and offensive breath odors.

If your client cannot brush his own teeth, you will have to do this for him. Before you start, check on the correct brushing technique with the nurse supervisor.

Discuss any suspected mouth or dental problems with your nurse supervisor so arrangements can be made for dental work, if indicated.

Some clients wear **dentures.** Note how well

Helping Your Client with Mouth and Dental Care

- Wear gloves to give oral care. Refer to the information about Universal Infection Control in Chapter 1. Wearing gloves will reduce the chance of you or your client spreading bacteria or viruses. Explain to your client that you are wearing gloves to prevent the spread of infection.
- Brush your client's teeth with a soft toothbrush that is in good condition. Use your client's choice of toothpaste.
- Think about what you are trying to accomplish as you brush.
- Brush all three sides of the teeth in small circles. Be gentle, but firm. Do not scrub at the gums.
- Keep the brush angled down 45 degrees toward the gums. This stimulates the gums as you brush.
- Rinse thoroughly after brushing.
- Use a waterpik and unwaxed dental floss if your client wishes. Ask the nurse supervisor about these items.
- Let your client do everything he can for himself, using assistive devices if needed.

- Try having a family member or friend brush your teeth for you. This will give you a better idea about how to approach your client. It will also help you understand some of the needs he may have as you brush his teeth.
- Look at the condition of your client's mouth.
  —Does he have good oral hygiene?
  —Do his gums bleed easily?
  —Are there obvious deposits of plaque and tartar on the teeth?
  —Are there sores, ulcerations, or white patches on the gums or cheeks?
  —Are any teeth missing or loose?
  —Is the gum tissue firm up to the teeth?
- Check the lips and tongue for dryness, cracks or fissures, crusty coverings, or changes of the tongue.
- Note if he has peculiar or bad breath odor.

they fit and if they are worn regularly. Ask the client about any pain, chewing problems, or other difficulties with his dentures. For example, dentures often do not fit well when clients have had strokes. A dentist must refit the dentures for these clients. Also, poorly fitting dentures may cause eating difficulties. Dentures must be removed and cleaned daily. They are not replaced until the mouth has been cleaned. Brush dentures with a soft brush, using the client's choice of dental powder. Some clients soak their dentures to clean them.

If your client cannot remove his own dentures, you can do so for him. Use a gauze square or clean cloth so you will have a firm grasp on the dentures. Place the gauze to cover the front teeth portion of the upper dentures, grasping in front and behind the teeth with the gauze. Then gently lower the upper dentures from the front, then sides, of the client's mouth and remove them from his mouth. Repeat the procedure for lower dentures, except lift the front portion of the dentures, using the gauze.

Your client may lack feeling in parts of his mouth, have trouble with moving food around in his mouth, chewing, swallowing, or may be neglecting one side of his mouth. Pay close attention to instructions from the nurse supervisor about care. Find out if the client has any particular food habits, such as "pocketing" food in his cheeks.

NOURISHMENT AND EATING

Everyone needs to eat and drink fluids in order to live. But as we all know, just eating food does not mean that we are being nourished properly. Your client has a chronic or disabling condition that requires certain nutrients and fluids. He must take the amounts and kinds of nourishments necessary for meeting his energy needs, and rebuilding and repairing his body. Nutrition is important for a variety of reasons. Well-nourished skin helps fight infections and resist pressure sores. A client must balance his diet so that he has protein to rebuild tissues. The client who has both diabetes and heart problems will require a low sodium, low fat, and calorie-controlled diet. These special diets do not require unusual or expensive foods or difficult preparations. They do require thought and planning.

Include your client in the planning of his meals. The person with a disability is no different from the rest of us in that we all like to choose what we eat and decide how the food is prepared. The person with a disability may view food selection as an activity that he can control. After receiving instructions from the nurse, you may be responsible for preparing the food and feeding your client. Or the client may be learning self-feeding techniques.

Consider these things when planning a diet with your client:

The Dietary Instructions

Your nurse supervisor and the dietitian will give you diet instructions that are specific for your client. You may be asked to weigh or measure food and to record the amounts your client eats and drinks. If food is to be prepared a certain way, do not vary this unless you ask the nurse. For example, do not fry food if it is to be steamed. He may be on a low-fat diet that does not allow fried foods, even if he likes them best.

Clients who are rebuilding body tissues—those with pressure sores, for example—need extra protein. The protein must be balanced with bulk, fluids, and roughage to prevent constipation. The person needs enough calories to build himself up. But he must be very careful to keep his weight under control. Sweets, processed foods, and snacks offer high calories but little nutritional value. Obesity is especially undesirable for a person with a disability. The overweight individual has more difficulty moving his body from place to place.

The foods a person eats can increase or decrease the effects of many medications. Food and medication combinations can influence the therapeutic effects of the medications or cause unpleasant side effects for the person. Over-the-counter medications, as well as prescription drugs, can produce food-drug interactions. Some medications are ordered to be taken with food; others are to be taken "on an empty stomach."

Clients who do not eat a balanced diet while taking long-term drug therapies may develop nutritional deficiencies. In these cases, the medication interferes with the clients' nutritional status. This is because medications are designed to perform specific functions within the body, but may cause an imbalance or reaction for another body function.

Clients who take many medications may have different dietary restrictions for each medication; the side effects and reactions are multiplied. Be particularly alert to the client who uses alcohol and takes medications. Each medication a client takes should be reviewed by the nurse supervisor in conjunction with his diet, habits, and other medications. Any dietary instructions should be written out for you to use in preparing meals for the client. The client or family can also call the pharmacist or physician who prescribed the medication for this information.

Report any changes in your client's health, mental attitude or alertness, or side effects your client experiences while on a medication to the nurse supervisor. Also report changes in your client's diet, amount of food intake, or alcohol intake. You may be asked to keep a food diary or record of your client's intake.

The Amount and Kinds of Fluids

Fluids are very important to keep body functioning in balance and to eliminate body wastes. Some clients will need to "force" fluids while others must "limit or restrict" fluids. You will often be told to offer fluids that are high in acid and low in calcium (see charts in the appendix) in order to prevent kidney and bladder stones. Similarly, you may be instructed to avoid fluids that concentrate the urine. Examples include coffee, tea, and soft drinks.

Your client may choose to drink alcoholic beverages. If so, he should drink an equal amount of water. Alcohol is dehydrating and the fluid must be replaced. Talk to your nurse about alcohol restrictions for your client because of medications he may be taking.

Both you and your nurse supervisor need to be aware of clients who abuse alcohol or other substances. Appropriate actions must be taken. Inform your nurse supervisor. The nurse will discuss alcohol use with your client and give you specific instructions.

Most of the time you will be asked to force fluids with your client (13 eight-ounce glasses). The kinds of fluids will be specified if this is necessary. Some medications are taken with fluids or require extra fluids. Body fluids assist in carrying away wastes from infection and controlling body temperature.

Some clients are on bladder training programs, intermittent catheterizations, or take certain medications. You may have instructions about giving fluids in certain amounts at specific times during the day. If possible, fluids are often restricted after 10 p.m. or two hours before the client's bedtime. This restriction reduces nighttime toileting needs. You may be asked to offer fluids on a schedule. You must be sure to measure them correctly and record what has been taken each time. You may also be asked to measure and record the times and amounts of urinary output.

Clients with Difficulty Chewing or Swallowing Foods

Clients who have had strokes or head trauma may have difficulty chewing and swallowing their food. Their food must be prepared in a form that lets them feed themselves, chew, and swallow. They do best with semi-solid foods the consistency of mashed potatoes. It is difficult for them to drink liquids or eat hard solids. However, they require a balanced and appealing diet. The nurse, dietitian, and speech therapist will plan a diet for these clients. You are responsible for observing how well your client eats and for serving food that is properly hot or cold, good to look at, and manageable for your client.

If your client has difficulty swallowing **(dysphagia)**, follow the nurse's instructions carefully. The following list will assist you in working with this client:

- *Know what to do if your client chokes.* Refer to the Emergency measures in this chapter. Post the directions for performing the Heimlich Maneuver in the room where your client eats his meals.

- Create a calm, quiet eating area so the client can concentrate on eating.
- Take the client to the bathroom before the meal.
- Sit the client comfortably at a table or erect in his wheelchair.
- Place arms on armrests padded with pillows.
- Stand in front of your client so he can see you.
- Communicate with him about food choices and eating. However, do not distract or exhaust him.
- Encourage the client to feed himself if he can. If necessary, cut foods and pour liquids. Allow the client to choose which foods are to be eaten for each bite.
- Set up assistive devices if he uses them.
- Allow enough time for the meal and be understanding of his problem.
- Be sure your client is scanning if he has visual deficits and cannot see one half of the plate. Remind him to scan if necessary.
- Take precautions for poorly fitted dentures.
- Season with herbs and spices to his liking or to stimulate diminished smell and taste.

Do the following if your client has difficulty swallowing:

- Offer small spoonfuls of food at a time.
- Use foods that are semi-solid or of a soft consistency.
- Place food in the unaffected side of the client's mouth.
- Remind the client to chew and swallow.
- Repeat instructions if he has memory or recall problems.
- Check his cheeks after each bite for food that he may trap between his jaw and cheek.
- Give liquids in small sips. Clients have the most difficulty with liquids. Check with the nurse supervisor for tips on how best to do this. For example, start with crushed ice or spoonfuls of liquids at a time.
- Offer fluids during the day to prevent low fluid intake and dehydration. Milk may cause increased mucus production in some clients, but slightly thickened liquids may be more easily swallowed. These include tomato juice, pear nectar, or foods pureed with added liquid.
- Give good mouth care to the client after each meal. His appetite may be increased with oral hygiene before his meal as well as after eating.
- Give several small meals throughout the day if he tires. Clients who have difficulty swallowing may tire from the work of eating.

CULTURAL CONSIDERATIONS

These three factors are important to consider when planning a diet with a client and his family:

—*client and family food habits and budget,*
—*religious or ethnic diets, and*
—*the meaning of food to the client.*

A client may want particular ethnic foods or favorite foods. Write these down and have the nurse supervisor or dietitian determine whether they can be included in your client's diet. You may be responsible for food shopping for your client. Work with the dietitian to identify budget-wise foods and the use of food stamps or coupons for nutritionally sound, inexpensive meals.

Some clients begin to lose their appetites following a disabling event. They become depressed and frustrated with their situation and do not like the foods they are told to eat. Other persons eat excessive amounts of food and gain weight. Weight gains affect their health and make it more difficult for them to transfer and move. Discuss a client's weight changes with the nurse supervisor. She may work with you, the client, and his family to develop an agreement about the food. Do not "preach" about diets or foods.

THE CLIENT'S ABILITY TO FEED HIMSELF

One of the most important daily activities a disabled person can achieve is to feed himself. If a person can feed himself with or without assistive devices, he has taken a big step toward feeling more independent. You can help your client toward this goal by working with the occupational therapist and the nurse supervisor. They may order devices for your client that will assist him with self-feeding. Insurance coverage may pay for them. Many devices can be easily made at home.

Ideas for self-help devices and homemade assistive devices are included in Chapter 6 about Activities of Daily Living. Many organizations print information about assistive devices. There are also specialty catalogues that advertise merchandise for the disabled.

BLADDER FUNCTION AND DYSFUNCTION

BLADDER TRAINING

Bladder training is used to help a client control when and where he urinates. Clients who have neurological impairments following strokes, multiple sclerosis, spinal cord injuries, brain trauma, and the like frequently have difficulty controlling their urine. You can be more patient and helpful to your client when you understand why he is incontinent.

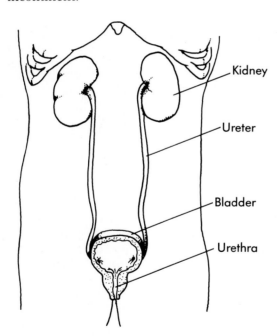

Kidney

Ureter

Bladder

Urethra

Figure 2-4. *The urinary system excretes waste products from the body in the form of urine. Urine flows from the kidneys through the ureters and into the bladder. Urine empties from the bladder through the urethra and out of the body at the meatus. Many clients have bladder programs designed to maintain fluid balance in their bodies and assure complete emptying of the urine from their bladders. When urine "backs up" in the ureters and into the kidneys or settles in the bladder, infections or other complications may develop.*

When urine flows from the kidneys into the bladder it stretches the bladder muscles. When the bladder is full, nerve impulses signal the brain that the bladder should be emptied. The person has the sensation that it is time to go to the bathroom. The person has to release the muscles that keep the urine in the bladder. Once the muscles relax, urine flows out of the bladder (Figure 2-4).

IMPAIRED BLADDER FUNCTION

When the signals are destroyed or interrupted, the bladder, brain, and muscles do not work together. Urine flow is not controlled. The person may not be able to go to the bathroom when he wants or may go when he is not prepared. A person may not be able to control his bladder once the signal to urinate is received. Or he may not receive the signal that the bladder is full.

When it is possible, the best way to control bladder incontinence is by bladder training. Training means that you must be very prompt when your client needs to go to the bathroom. If he does not ask within every two hours, you must offer to help him to the bathroom. You are helping him to teach his bladder to empty at certain times. The goal is for him to use the commode without soiling himself and his clothing. Training means paying close attention to something that you take for granted. That is, the nerves in your bladder signal your brain that it is time to go to the bathroom. Your client does not receive that signal and he is not reminded to go to the bathroom in time.

If your client does not have a catheter, is willing, and is able to cooperate, there is a good chance that the nurse can teach him

---

Teaching Your Client Bladder Training

- See that he has an opportunity to go to the bathroom (or use the commode) at the same times every day.
- Encourage him when he has successful training times.
- Remind him to go to the bathroom every two hours or on whatever schedule is set by the nurse. (This time will change as the bladder training program progresses.)
- Provide a quiet, private environment for bladder training.
- Offer the bedpan or assistance to the commode as soon as possible. This is especially important at night if the client is up to go to the bathroom or to use a bedside commode.
- Assist the client to promptly and safely transfer to the commode or toilet.
- Assist him to stand to urinate or her to sit, if this is possible for the client.
- Offer liquids one hour to one-half hour before the scheduled time to urinate.

- Offer 6–8 glasses of liquids each day.
- Dress your client so that it is easy for him to undo clothing.
- Keep the genital and buttocks areas clean, dry, and in good condition.
- Change his protective pad or pants frequently, if he wears them. Cleanse the genital area to prevent skin breakdown, odors, and infections.
- Remind your client to do bladder exercises, if he has been instructed in these by the nurse supervisor.
- Keep a record of when the client goes to the bathroom. Record the time of any accidents.
- Note the color and odor of the urine. Report changes to the nurse supervisor.
- Measure the amount of urine.
- Note whether the client was upset, tired, or otherwise excited when any accidents occurred.
- Do not blame or shame him if he has an accident.

---

bladder training. You have an important role in the success of bladder training. It usually takes about 7 to 10 days of bladder training before the person's own routine is set. The length of time can vary a great deal depending on the person.

Report to the nurse if your client has:

> —an increase in the number of times he urinates each day,
> —cloudy, strong, or foul-smelling urine,
> —sandy or gritty urine,
> —complaints of pain or burning when urinating,
> —tea-colored urine,
> —blood-tinged urine,
> —a decreased amount of urine each day,
> —signs of a fever or other discomfort,
> —reddened or broken skin in the genital areas,
> —any family problems with the bladder training, or
> —any concerns about the bladder training program.

SPECIALIZED URINARY DEVICES
Absorbing Devices

Many clients use devices designed to absorb urine into a pad or absorbent fibers. These devices are used by many persons who do not require a urine-collecting device, but who have some degree of urinary incontinence. Effective absorbent devices:

> —absorb the amount of urine the client eliminates.
> —separate the urine away from the client's skin.
> —enable the client or caregiver to change and fasten the device in a reasonably easy manner.
> —do not cause skin rash, allergic reactions to the materials, or lead to skin breakdown. If the materials do not allow air to circulate, they may cause skin breakdown and odors.
> —are affordable.

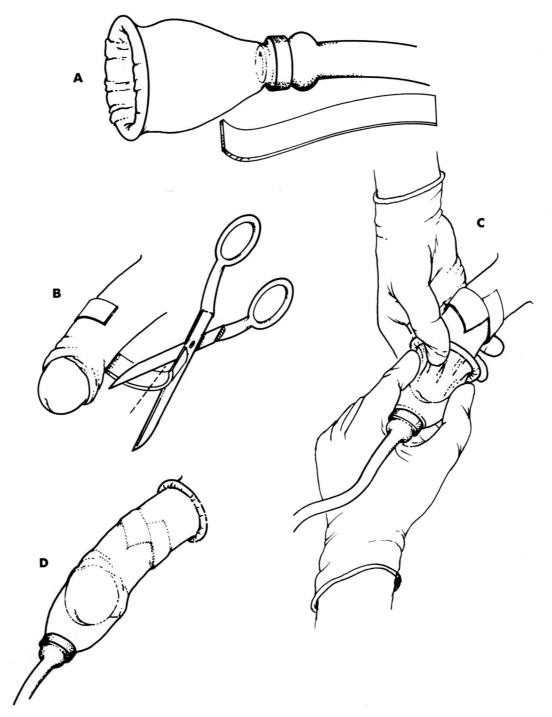

Figure 2-5.   *Read the instructions before applying a commercial urinary sheath to a male client.*

A, *Wear gloves and assemble the urinary sheath, double-sided skin tape, and skin shield solution.*

B, *Apply the skin shield solution and double-sided skin tape around the middle of the penis shaft.* **Do not** *overlap the tape edges. This may cause constriction of the penis. Remove any excess length of tape.*

C, *Roll the urinary sheath onto the penis as if applying a condom. Continue to roll the sheath, covering the double-sided tape, until it reaches the base of the penis.*

D, *There should be 1 to 1¹/₂ inches of space between the head of the penis and the tubing of the urinary sheath. After the sheath is completely rolled down over the penis, gently squeeze it into place, securing it to the double-sided tape. Check the tubing and drainage bag.*

—must be kept clean or readily disposable.

—do not interfere with a urine control or bladder training program.

—do not promote client dependency on the device instead of on independent bladder functions.

The client or family may have purchased absorbing devices from a catalogue or the local pharmacy on their own. The nurse supervisor will be able to inspect the absorbent device to be sure it is appropriate for the client's needs.

Absorbent products may be disposable or designed for reuse or refills. Disposable products include pads that line undergarments, disposable incontinence pants, and diaper-like pants that have disposable fillers. These are not usually disposed of in a flush toilet. Reusable products can be laundered and reused. These products may be combinations of paddings or liners and underpant garments. Some may also have vinyl liners.

Urinary Sheaths

A commonly used urinary device is a *urinary sheath*. There are several styles of urinary sheaths for men available on the market. Commonly used names are urinary sheaths, Texas catheters, or external catheters. Sheath-like appliances that work well for women are not available, although many products are tested from time to time. Sheaths

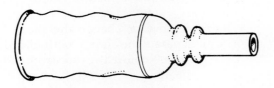

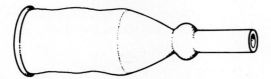

Figure 2-6. *A self-adhesive commercial urinary sheath is applied in the same manner as other sheaths, except the adhesive is already inside the sheath. Roll the sheath down the penis as if applying a condom. Be sure the self-adhesive portion is on the inside of the sheath and properly positioned on your client for comfort, safety, and function.*

provide protection from incontinent leaks for clients who use intermittent catheterization or for those who simply dribble urine. Your client may wear one of the commercial sheaths. Each brand has specific directions for application and use. Some brands use two-sided tape on the penis to secure the catheter. Others use cements or are self-adhesive (see Figures 2-5 and 2-6).

As an alternative, a sheath may be made at home, using inexpensive supplies. Figure 2-7 describes how to make a homemade sheath. Work with your nurse supervisor, the client and his family to construct sheaths until everyone is satisfied with the results.

To construct a urinary sheath at home you will need the following supplies:

—a rubber condom,

—3–4 inches of ½" rubber tubing, and

—scissors.

Practice constructing a urinary sheath until you are able to construct a sheath approved by your nurse supervisor and your client. Have spare sheaths available. Figure 2-8 demonstrates how to place the homemade version of a urinary sheath on your client.

1. Wash your hands and put on gloves before you assemble the supplies. You will need:

   —soap, water, and a scissors,

   —the prepared condom sheath with 3–4 inches of ½" rubber tubing,

   —skin cement and tincture of benzoin,

   —a disposable napkin or paper towel,

   —a urine drainage bag or leg bag with connectors, and

   —non-allergenic silk tape.

2. Wash your client's genital area, retracting the foreskin to cleanse if present, then rinse and dry. Check the condition of the skin. Ask your nurse supervisor to remove any body hair that would pull or collect cement and tape residue.

3. Place your client's penis through a hole in the disposable napkin or paper towel. Use a cotton-tipped applicator to apply tincture of benzoin solution to the shaft of his penis.

4. Allow the benzoin to dry until it becomes sticky. At this point, place the condom portion of the sheath over the

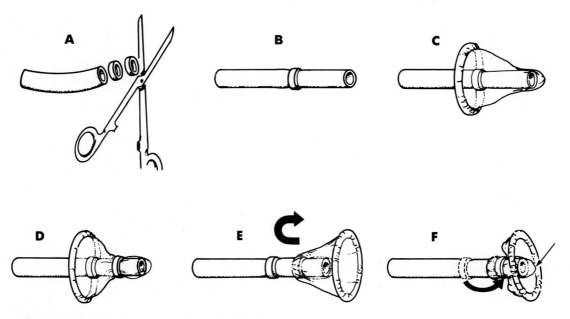

Figure 2-7.   *How to make a urinary sheath at home.*
   A, *Cut two rings (¹/₄ inch each) from the end of a piece of rubber tubing.*
   B, *Insert the tubing through one of the rings.*
   C, *Insert the tubing partially into the condom. Do **not** unroll the condom any further than necessary.*
   D, *Place the remaining tubing over the end of the tubing that is covered by the condom.*
   E, *Reverse the condom back over the second tubing ring.*
   F, *Slide the first tubing ring over both the condom and the second ring. This will secure and tighten the fit. The condom will have to be punctured where it fits over the tubing opening.*

tip of his penis. Do not unroll the condom. Use the condom to hold the penis away from his body.

5. Use a second cotton tipped applicator to apply a ³/₄ to 1-inch wide coating of skin bond cement to the shaft of the penis. Circle the shaft of the penis with the cement at about the midpoint. This will hold the condom in place after it is applied. **DO NOT** allow cement onto the tip of the penis or into the area where the penis joins the scrotum.

6. The cement will set in about one minute. Then unroll the condom portion of the sheath to cover the cemented area of the penis shaft.

7. Check that there is 1–1¹/₂ inches of space between the tip of his penis and the opening for the rubber tubing to prevent abrasion.

8. Secure the sheath around the penis using non-allergenic tape folded as shown. This will make changing the sheath easy to do.

9. Connect the urinary sheath to the clear plastic extension tubing of a urinary drainage bag.

10. Change the sheath at least every other day. Remove it before baths or showers.
    —To remove or change the sheath:
    a) Separate the ends of both folded tapes. Remove the tube from the sheath.
    b) If necessary, use adhesive tape remover pads at the top opening of the condom.
    c) Cleanse the genital area with soap and water. Dry thoroughly.

Catheters

One way of controlling bladder incontinence is for the nurse to insert a **catheter** to drain urine from the bladder into a collection bag. Some catheters are left in place for a while and others are inserted to drain the urine and then removed. The nurse performs this

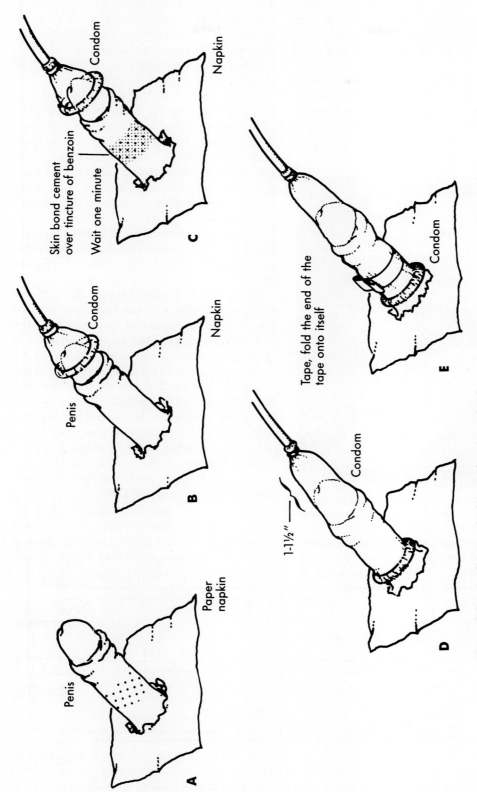

Figure 2-8. *Application of a homemade urinary sheath.*
A, *Apply tincture of benzoin solution and allow it to dry until sticky.*
B, *Place condom portion of sheath over penis. Do not unroll condom.*
C, *Apply skin bond cement to shaft of penis over tincture of benzoin.*
D, *Unroll the condom. The tip of the penis should be 1 to 1½ inches from the opening of the rubber tubing.*
E, *Secure the sheath by taping as pictured.*

procedure, although with the use of a special mirror, some clients or their families have been taught to insert their own catheters (Figure 2-9). Your client may talk about a catheter he had in the hospital before he came home.

An **indwelling urinary catheter** (indwelling Foley catheter) may be inserted into your client's bladder to drain urine *continually*. Catheters are hollow plastic or rubber tubings that come in various styles and sizes (Fig-

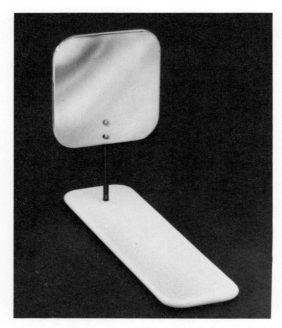

Figure 2-9.   *This type of standing mirror is useful for many female clients who perform their own catheterization.*

Reprinted by permission of © Bissell Healthcare Corporation/Fred Sammons, Inc.

ure 2-10). The indwelling catheter is styled with two hollow tubes inside the outer covering. One tube is open on both ends to drain urine; the other tube has an inflatable balloon above the drainage holes. The balloon is inflated after the catheter is in place for use (Figure 2-11).

Using the end with the deflated balloon, the nurse inserts the catheter through the client's urethra and into the bladder (Figure 2-12). Then the nurse inflates the balloon with sterile water. The inflated balloon keeps the catheter from slipping out of the bladder. The free end of the catheter is connected to the clear plastic extension tubing of a urinary drainage bag.

The indwelling catheter should be taped to one leg to help prevent tension on the catheter and irritation to the bladder (Figure 2-13).

Urine drains freely through the catheter tubing and collects in the bag. Bags may be attached to the frame of the bed or wheelchair (Figure 2-14). The bags are marked in increments of approximately 100 cc. These provide a quick and easy measurement of the amount of urine that has drained into the bag. When an exact measurement is needed the urine must be drained from the bag and measured in a calibrated container. This would be done for clients who need to have an exact report of their intake and output.

The nurse supervisor will have a scheduled time for changing a client's indwelling catheter. The catheter should also be changed if it becomes plugged, if urine leaks around the catheter, or the client has pain or discomfort. When your client is out of bed,

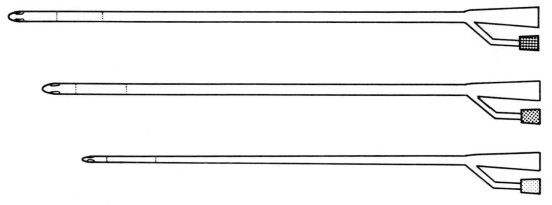

Figure 2-10.   *Urinary catheters are produced in various sizes and shapes to suit the specific needs of individual clients. Clients may arrange for their local pharmacies to keep their specific urinary catheters in stock if the necessary size or type is not readily available.*

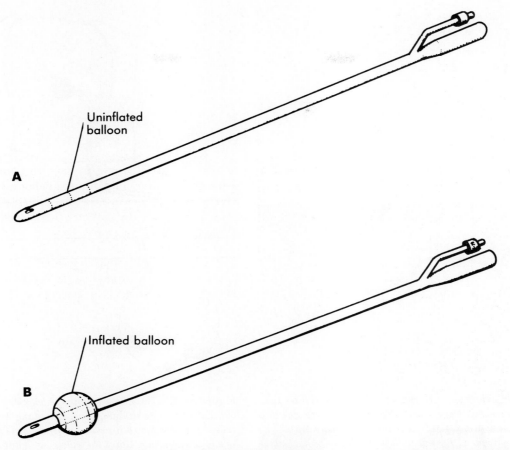

Figure 2-11. *Indwelling urinary catheters have an inflatable balloon tip that retains the catheter inside the bladder.* **A** *shows an indwelling urinary catheter with the balloon tip uninflated. The catheter is inserted before the balloon is inflated.* **B** *shows the same catheter with the balloon tip inflated. The nurse inflates the balloon after the tip is properly positioned inside the bladder.*

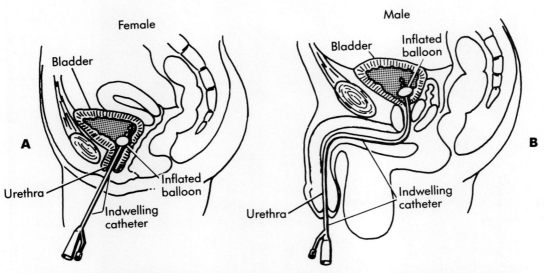

Figure 2-12. *The inflated indwelling urinary catheter positioned inside the bladder of a female* **(A)** *and a male* **(B).** *Notice how the inflated tip holds the catheter inside the bladder; at the same time notice how pulling or pressure on the tubing could cause discomfort or injury to a client.*

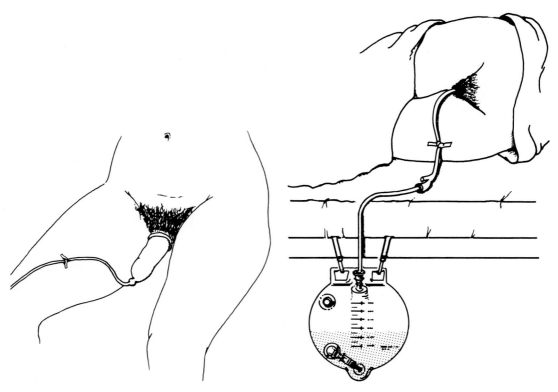

Figure 2-13. *An indwelling urinary catheter tubing is taped to a client's leg using the technique illustrated in this figure. Use the crossed-over tape technique to prevent pulling or tension on the catheter tubing that would cause discomfort or injury to the client.*

Figure 2-14. *The urinary drainage bags that collect and hold urine draining from indwelling urinary catheters can be attached to the bed frame or to the side of a wheelchair. Check the tubing so that it is not looped or kinked; in a wheelchair attachment, keep the tubing free from moving parts and the revolutions of the wheels.*

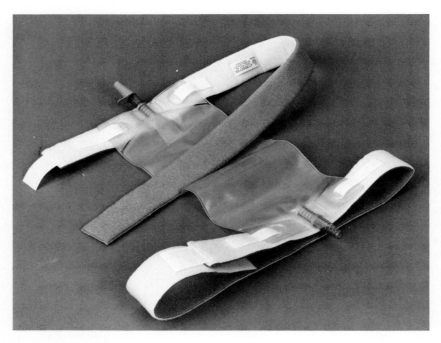

Figure 2-15. *A urinary leg bag.*
Permission to reproduce this copyrighted material has been granted by the owner, Hollister Incorporated.

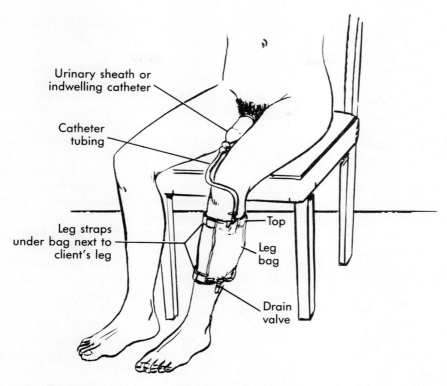

Figure 2-16. *A client can become more mobile when he can take his urinary drainage system with him. Attaching the tubing from a urinary sheath so that it will drain into a leg bag can improve a client's mobility.*

the indwelling catheter may be disconnected from the bed drainage bag and reconnected to a leg bag (Figures 2-15 and 2-16).

Care of Urinary Drainage Bags

—*Wear gloves and wash your hands before and after care.* Use a new pair of gloves for each procedure. Discard used gloves into the trash as you are directed by the nurse supervisor.

—Empty bags before they are 2/3 full so the urine can continue to flow into the bag and not back up.

1. To empty a drainage bag:
   —Before removing the cover from the drain at the bottom of the bag, drain urine from the tubing into the leg bag or drainage bag.
   —Completely empty the bag of air and urine.
   —Use an alcohol swab or cotton ball dipped in alcohol to wipe the drain at the bottom of the bag. Then replace the cover over the drain tube.

2. To clean a leg bag:
   —Leg bags are cleaned each day.
   —Disconnect the bag from the catheter (connect the catheter to another bag).
   —Rinse bag with water.
   —Soak bag, connectors, tubing, and caps in solution of:
     * 1 oz. liquid bleach (Clorox or Purex) to 20 oz. water (2 1/2 cups). Have your nurse supervisor help you measure these amounts and mark them for future measures.
     * Use a funnel to fill the inside of the leg bag.
     * Place all parts under the solution, completely covered and filled with solution.
     * Soak for 20 minutes.
     * Rinse with water and dry with a towel.
     * Soak any crusted parts in white vinegar overnight (up to 24 hours) to soften and remove crust.

3. To disinfect leg bag or drainage bag caps and connectors:
—Rinse parts with water.
—Place in a cup or small ceramic dish with either:
   a) 1 oz. Clorox or Purex bleach with 1 pint (16 oz.) water, OR
   b) ½ cup white vinegar and ½ cup boiled water.
      —Soak 20 minutes.
      —Change soaking solutions every 10–14 days. Date the solutions when you make them so they are changed on time.
4. To change a catheter from a bed drainage bag to a leg bag:
—Drain urine from the tubing into the drainage bag.
—Hold the end of the catheter. Wipe the end of the catheter and the leg bag connector with an alcohol swab.
—Connect the catheter to the leg bag.
—Wipe the end of the drainage bag tube with alcohol and cover it with a disinfected cap. Do not let the uncovered drainage tube end drop onto the floor or touch anything.
—Empty and clean the leg bag.

Occasionally, a client will have a catheter that inserts into the **supra pubic** area (Figure 2-17). This means that he has had a surgical bypass of part of his urinary system so that the urine leaves his body at the supra pubic area instead of through the urethra. The nurse supervisor will instruct you in specific actions about this catheter.

Some of your clients will use a catheter to **intermittently drain urine** from their bladders. This catheter does not have an inflatable balloon because it is inserted into the bladder to drain the urine and is removed again. It is important to note the amount of urine that is drained and the time when each catheterization is done. You may have to assist a client to gather his supplies and remove the urine. Only the client, his family or the nurse supervisor will perform the catheterizations. You *do not* perform catheterizations.

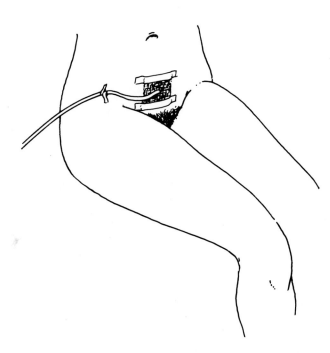

Figure 2-17. *A suprapubic catheter is inserted through the abdominal wall and enters directly into the bladder to drain urine. The tubing from the suprapubic catheter can be attached to tubing, leg bags, or drainage bags.*

Care for the Client with an Indwelling Catheter

- Wear gloves and use infection control procedures.
- The drainage bag must be kept in a position **lower** than the client's bladder. This is necessary for the urine to drain from the bladder into the bag. If urine is allowed to flow back up the tubing, it may reenter the client's bladder, leading to infection and other problems.
- The catheter and any tubing must be kept straight, without kinks or twists in the tubing. Tubing that becomes blocked will halt drainage. Urine may back up through the tubing and into the bladder.
- Tape the tubing to the inside of your client's leg, allowing enough slack for movement. Your nurse supervisor will show you how to do this. If the catheter is not taped, the catheter will pull on the bladder and urethra, causing pain and tissue damage. Use skin-sensitive tape; some clients are allergic to adhesive tapes.
- Do not allow catheter tubing or drainage bag to touch or drag on the floor.
- Do not disconnect the catheter from the drainage bag or close off the drainage, except when you empty and clean the drainage bag. Ask your nurse supervisor about specific instructions for emptying and cleaning the many different types of drainage bags.

- Record the amount of fluid intake and the amount of urine output for your client as directed.
- Keep your client's skin clean and dry, especially around the urinary meatus (wear gloves).

Report to your Nurse Supervisor if:
- There is a decreased amount or no urine draining into the bag over several hours time.
- The urine contains blood, particles, or sediment, or develops a strong odor. The urine in the bag may appear darker when collected in a bedpan. If the urine appears darker, your client may not be drinking enough fluids and the urine is more concentrated.
- Your client complains of pain or discomfort, feels as if his bladder is too full or that he needs to urinate, or leaks urine around the catheter.
- Your male client has erections. The catheter may stimulate male clients to have erections. You should not become concerned and can assure him that this is not a problem. Discuss the situation with your nurse supervisor to prevent you or your client unnecessary embarrassment.

*B*OWEL FUNCTION AND DYSFUNCTION

BOWEL FUNCTION

Bowel training is much like bladder training except that it involves fecal material. Fecal material (stool) is the waste that is left over from the food a person eats. Once food is chewed, it passes to the stomach, where digestive juices reduce the food so it can pass into the bowel (colon). The bowel uses wavelike motions to push the partly digested food along. As the food moves along, the bowel pulls out the liquids and nutrients the body

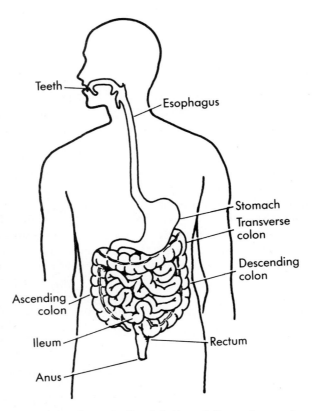

Figure 2-18.   *The digestive system takes in food and fluids and digests them so they can be used as nourishment for the cells. The cells use the foods to make energy and heat to operate the body function (metabolism). Finally, the body eliminates the solid waste products from metabolism as feces. The anatomy of the digestive tract shows the pathway of foods through the body.*

needs. The rest of the food is waste and becomes the stool (Figure 2-18).

Once the stool reaches the end of the bowel it causes pressure on the muscles around the rectum. If it is not a time when the person wishes to go to the bathroom, the muscles tighten and he waits to pass the stool. When it is time to go, the brain signals the muscles to pass the stool out of the rectum and he has a bowel movement. Some clients have an interruption in this communication system. They may have problems controlling when and where they have bowel movements. This may result in constipation and diarrhea. Most persons have a bowel movement at least every other day.

IMPAIRED BOWEL FUNCTION

Constipation is a bowel problem that happens when the fecal material or stool takes too long to pass through the colon (bowel). The stool becomes hard and dry when the colon takes out too much water. The stool then becomes hard to pass through the colon. It may pile up and become stuck (impacted). Constipation is a problem that can worsen over time. Persons who are not active enough, do not drink enough liquids, or eat sufficient fiber are likely to have constipation more often than others. Your client may not have the proper nerve signals for moving his bowels. Some persons who have long-term or chronic constipation are given medicines called stool softeners. They soften stools so they will pass more easily. A successful bowel program does not routinely use medicines.

Diarrhea occurs when the bowel hurries the stool along without taking enough water from the stool mass. Often diarrhea begins when there is something irritating the bowel. This irritation could be an infection, a reaction to a medicine, or something the person has eaten. Diarrhea may occur while the cli-

---

Establishing Your Client's Bowel Training Program

- Assist your client at a regular time each day so he can have a bowel movement. Common times for bowel movements are after breakfast or after dinner at night.
- Assist your client to a comfortable place for the bowel program. The best choice is the bathroom toilet or a bedside commode. If the bowel program must be done in bed, position him to lie on his left side or on a bedpan.
- Provide at least 6–8 glasses of liquids each day. These should be spaced throughout the day until 7 p.m.
- Prepare the prescribed diet for your client, one that is high in fiber and low in fat.
- Note which foods cause him to have gas, constipation, diarrhea, or stomach ache.
- Learn what helps your client to start the bowel movements, such as a cup of warm liquid before the program.
- Record the time, amount, description, odor, and color of stool as directed by the nurse.

- Discourage clients and family from use of laxatives and enemas unless the physician orders them.
- Allow the client enough time to chew food and relax at meals.
- Take the client to the commode or toilet 15–30 minutes after a meal (use a set meal each time once the program is established) to attempt a bowel movement.
- Encourage regular activity or help the client to move about to prevent a sluggish bowel.
- Provide a safe, comfortable, private place for the bowel program. Be sure to stay within hearing distance.
- Remove the client from the commode as soon as he has completed the bowel movement.
- Clean his skin and buttocks after a bowel movement to reduce irritation and odors.
- Encourage your client; do not shame him for accidents.
- Follow the client's directions and desires as much as possible. Discuss any differences with the nurse supervisor.

---

ent is still constipated. When this happens, the person has a fecal impaction. Loose stool seeps around the solid impacted mass of stool resulting in a small amount of diarrhea. Tell the nurse if your client has diarrhea or soiling with loose stool.

If your client cannot control his bowel movements he will not be comfortable around other people or want to go out in public. He will be concerned about having an accident or about bad odors. Helping your client establish a bowel program that works will give him extra freedom and self-confidence. The nurse supervisor can instruct you about your client's bowel training program.

Notify the nurse if:

—constipation or diarrhea is severe or lasts more than two days;
—any signs of blood or excessive mucus show in stool;
—client does not take food and liquids properly;
—has difficulty eating or swallowing food;
—client complains of pain, distension, or fullness in his stomach;
—has redness or other signs of skin breakdown; or
—the client or family has questions or concerns about the bowel program.

The Ostomy and Ostomy Devices

An **ostomy** is a surgically created opening. It may open into the colon, ureter, or ileum so that body wastes can be eliminated without the usual body functions. An ostomy that excretes feces from the body by bypassing the colon and rectum is an **ileostomy** or a **colostomy.** A **ureterostomy** excretes urine,

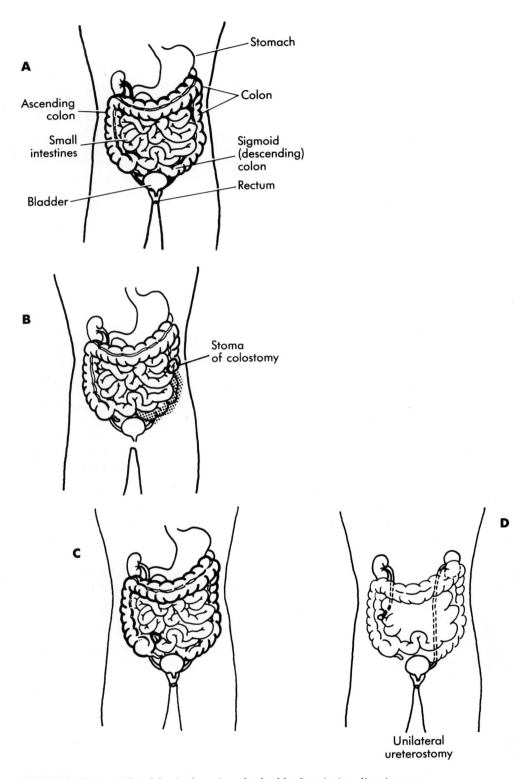

Figure 2-19.   A, *The abdominal portion of a healthy functioning digestive tract.*

B, *Following surgical colostomy, one end of the intestine or bowel is separated from the distal portion of the bowel and brought to the surface of the skin. The shaded portion of the bowel may have been surgically removed or will not handle waste material.*

C, *An ileostomy is similar to a colostomy, but the locations of the surgery and stoma are in the upper bowel.*

D, *When the bladder and urethra are bypassed, urine is excreted through a stoma in the abdominal wall. A ureterostomy can be unilateral or bilateral. (This view shows a conduit through the ileum).*

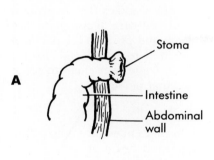

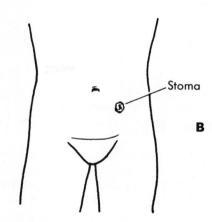

Figure 2-20.   **A,** *A side view of the abdominal wall shows the bowel with a stoma opening to the skin.*
    B, *A stoma opening onto the abdomen appears on the skin as a small, raised, gathered, or puckered edge around an opening.*

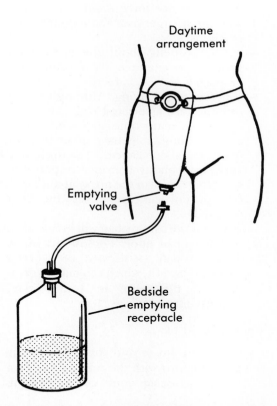

Figure 2-21. *A wide range of ostomy supplies and appliances are available for each client's special needs and lifestyle. Ostomy appliances can be converted for daytime mobility by simply securing the ostomy bag to a belt at the waist.*

bypassing the bladder and urethra (Figure 2-19).

A **stoma** is the outer edge of an ostomy that opens onto the skin of the abdomen (Figure 2-20). Body wastes are eliminated through this opening. The stoma can be identified as the rounded pink opening with a raised gathered edge. Occasionally a colostomy may have two stomas opening onto the abdomen. But only one opening, the one connected to the active portion of the bowel, will excrete feces. Clients who have ostomies wear special collection devices referred to as ostomy bags or appliances, which are worn over their stomas to collect feces or urine (Figure 2-21).

There is a wide variety of ostomy equipment available at varying prices. When selecting equipment, the client should consider the fit, brand, type, size, and shape of the ostomy bag. He must also decide whether to use permanent or disposable bags, choose adhesives or special paste, and select from various assistive devices and belts. A nurse who has special training in ostomy care may consult with your client, using several ostomy products to determine which one works best for your client. There are many different ostomy products. Your nurse supervisor will give you instructions and direct you in the care plan for each client.

Clients have ostomies following surgery to repair damages to the colon or ureters. The colon or ureters may be damaged from diseases, accidents, or from the removal of a cancerous growth. Ostomies are temporary or permanent. Temporary ostomies require surgery to reconnect the bowel or ureter.

The ostomy bag must be emptied daily or when it is full. The client or family will discard a disposable ostomy bag and place a new bag over the stoma. A permanent bag must be cleaned before it is replaced. The bag will also need to be replaced if the seal or adhesive breaks free from the skin of the abdomen.

Cleaning a Permanent Ostomy Bag

You may have to assist your client with cleaning a permanent ostomy bag. If he cannot do this himself, you may need to clean the bag for him. Follow the directions from your nurse supervisor and the manufacturer's instructions with the ostomy bag. A general method for cleaning ostomy bags is to:

1. Follow the directions on the package. Or:
2. Use a general method:
   —Wear gloves.
   —Empty the ostomy bag and dispose of contents.
   —Rinse the bag with cool running water.
   —Make a solution of 1 part white vinegar and 3 parts water (some persons use full-strength white vinegar).
   —Pour the vinegar solution into the bag. Use this for cleaning the leg bag, bedside drainage bag, tubing, connectors, and bag.
   —Soak for 20–25 minutes.
   —Rinse with cool water.
   —Lay flat or hang to air-dry.
   —Lightly powder bag on all sides if it tends to stick. Do this only if the instructions permit.
   —Discard the vinegar solution and your gloves.
   —Wash your hands.

Maintaining Bowel Function with an Ostomy Device

A client who has a colostomy should have a bowel training program so fecal elimination is predictable and regular. The stool should be slightly soft, with form, not loose. Some clients have been instructed to irrigate their colostomies. This is similar to a cleansing enema. Check the client's irrigation procedures with your nurse supervisor.

Encourage your client, if he is able, to sit on the toilet or commode to change his ostomy bag (Figure 2-22). Many bags can be drained directly into the toilet bowl while the client sits on the seat. This makes the client more independent with self-care. It also places him in the usual room and position for performing activities related to bowel and bladder movements. Encourage your client to accept himself as a normal person.

• • •

Clients and families may have negative reactions to ostomies because of:

—a reluctance to deal with body waste.
—the appearance of the stoma as a change in body image. It may be difficult for a client viewing his own body or a family member viewing the client. Some clients or family members are very repelled by or express disgust about the ostomy and stoma. Do not force them, but inform your nurse supervisor about their strong reactions.
—embarrassment about the elimination process; for example, flatus or gas may be passed as well as feces.
—concerns about dying. Although not all ostomies are associated with cancerous conditions, many times they are. The client and family may have many fears or questions about cancer. Ask the nurse supervisor about a proper response to questions. Inform the nurse about questions or concerns expressed by the client or family.
—fear that the ostomy bag will break, leak, or have a bad odor. The ostomy nurse specialist can assist with the correct products and fit, which can make a great deal of difference in your client's adjustment.

You can assist by:

—discussing any of your concerns or negative reactions with the nurse supervisor before assisting your client with his ostomy.
—controlling any personal reactions you may have to the client's ostomy or body image.
—following directions carefully after supervision and direction from the nurse supervisor.
—wearing gloves and using aseptic techniques when assisting with care and changing the bag.
—assuring a safe, private location for your client's ostomy program.

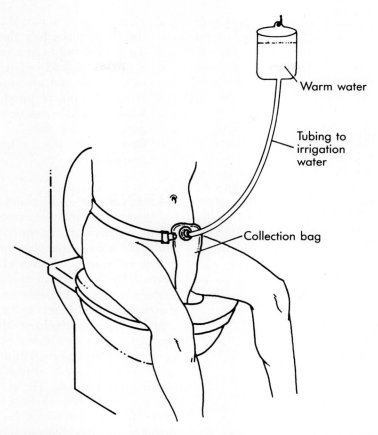

Warm water

Tubing to irrigation water

Collection bag

Figure 2-22. *If a client can safely balance himself on the toilet, he can irrigate his colostomy directly into the toilet.*

—assisting him to change the collection bag if he cannot perform this independently. It may be necessary to gather and assemble the equipment.

—assisting the client to irrigate the colostomy when directed by your nurse supervisor. Remember that only water that is safe to drink is safe to use for irrigations.

—preparing foods that follow the prescribed diet. The diet for a client with a colostomy differs from the diet for an ileostomy. Refer to the diets in the Appendix.

—keeping him clean, dry, and comfortable.

—preventing skin breakdown from appliances, cement or solvent, or tapes.

—disposing of body wastes and ostomy disposables as directed by the nurse supervisor.

Report to your nurse supervisor:

—skin breakdown or stoma ulcerations;

—bleeding from the stoma;

—diarrhea, constipation, impactions, or excessive flatus;

—complaints of discomfort or pain;

—difficulty with the ostomy appliances; or

—displays of continued upset or disgust with that ostomy lasting over time.

CARE DURING EMERGENCY SITUATIONS

The following section is devoted to emergency care for clients who may have emergency situations. These include fainting, burns, lost teeth, nosebleeds, seizures, episodes of choking, and ingestion of poisonous materials. See Chapter 11 for care of the client who may have a heart attack. Training and certification in cardiopulmonary resuscitation or CPR, using the American Heart Association protocol, is recommended for all home caregivers. See Chapter 9 for information on autonomic dysreflexia as a potential emergency situation for clients who have spinal cord injuries.

POTENTIAL FOR SUICIDE

If your client behaves in ways that may be early signs of potential suicide, you should immediately notify your nurse supervisor. Usually these signs are not obvious emergency signals, such as external bleeding. The signs may occur for other reasons or over a period of time. The best response you can give is to recognize them as potential warnings and report them. Potential signs are:

—changes in regular habits such as eating or sleeping. Usually there is a lack of interest in food and difficulty with sleeping or restlessness.

—increase in abuse of drugs or alcohol.

—decreased interest in associating with family or friends. He may seem to lose interest in everything.

—changes in personality.

—complaints about feeling poorly or increased complaints about health.

—if able, he may run away or hide.

—complaints of being bored with things.

—inability to pay attention or concentrate.

—giving things away.

—talking about suicide or death. He may make jokes about suicide.

—performing poorly in his work, school, or tasks.

If your client has these warning signs, *do not ignore them.* The nurse supervisor will evaluate your client's needs for assistance. A psychologist or other health professional may join the health team to work with your client. *Do not judge your client if he has these thoughts.* He may not see any way out of his situation. He may be depressed and have a hopeless outlook. These thoughts may be temporary until he works through his disability.

FAINTING

1. If the client says he is going to faint, ease him to the bed or down to the floor.

2. Place the person flat. If he has fallen to the floor, place him flat on the floor.
3. Turn his head to one side.
4. Recovery should begin within several seconds. Do not use smelling salts.
5. If he does not respond within several seconds, call the rescue squad or emergency medical unit.
6. Report to the nurse supervisor immediately.

BURNS

Burns are serious for your clients. **Always notify the nurse supervisor or call for emergency assistance when a client has been burned.** Do not attempt to judge the degree of the burn yourself. Burns can be deceptive. Burns may be more severe for the client with a neurological problem or an older person who has chronic conditions. For example, the person with a spinal cord injury has lost temperature regulators and may experience autonomic dysreflexia. He must avoid skin damage and infections that could arise from minor first degree burns. Persons who have diabetes may have skin problems and metabolic distress following burns.

Burns are classified by degrees.

First degree burns are red, with some swelling and mild pain. Common first degree burns are sunburn, hot liquids, or scalding with steam. *Immediately* apply ice or cold water for 5–10 minutes. Let the area rest. Repeat the ice or cold water if you cannot reach your supervisor. Do not keep ice or cold water on a burn longer than 5–10 minutes at a time. If the burned part is a hand or foot, place it under cold running water if possible; *but only if* you have been instructed that the client can tolerate this. **Do not** apply butter, oil, or cream ointments. Call the nurse supervisor.

Second degree burns are deeper burns than first degree burns. They penetrate through the protective outer layers of the skin, causing redness, blistering, and swelling. *Immediately* apply ice, immerse the area in cold water (if tolerated), or apply cold wet cloths for 5–10 minutes at a time. **Do not** apply any medication or other remedy. **Do not** break blisters. Blot the skin to dry and keep clean and away from other objects. Call the nurse supervisor immediately.

Third degree burns require emergency

medical attention. **Do not remove any charred clothing. Do not add water.** *Call the rescue squad immediately; notify the nurse supervisor.* In a third degree burn, all the skin layers are destroyed, giving a charred or white look to the skin. This type of burn is usually a result of flames, clothing catching on fire, electrical shocks, or direct burns from heating elements.

NOSEBLEEDS

Nosebleeds should be reported to the nurse supervisor. If you are alone with a client who has a nosebleed, you can do several things until assistance arrives. Stay calm and keep him calm. A client who has a nosebleed appears to be losing a great deal of blood. There is usually not as much blood lost as it may appear.

1. If possible, sit the client up with his head up straight, slightly tilted forward.
2. Apply steady pressure to both sides of his nose, just below the bridge of the nose. Do not squeeze the nostrils shut.
3. Apply cold compresses to the nose or to the nape of the neck.

LOST TEETH

If a client should accidentally dislodge or knock out a tooth, there are several things that can be done to try to save the tooth. A dentist may be able to reimplant the tooth. Most successful tooth reimplantation is done within a half-hour, but longer times are still successful, so the length of time is an important factor.

1. Do not touch the root of the tooth.
2. Do not clean the tooth.
3. Place the tooth in a cup of cool water or milk.
4. Call the nurse supervisor for assistance immediately. If the client or family is able, they may wish to contact their family dentist.

SEIZURES

Your nurse supervisor will instruct you about how to assist a client who may have seizures.

If a client should have a seizure, you can assist him by providing a safe environment and keeping a good description of what occurs. Generally, you will assist by protecting your client from injuring himself during the seizure.

Care for the Client Who May Have Seizures

- If there are instructions from the physician or nurse supervisor, follow them.
- If not, during a client's seizure you should:
  —help him to be lowered gently to the floor if he is standing or sitting when the seizure begins.
  —turn his head to one side.
  —clear the area of furniture or other items that might cut, burn, bruise, or otherwise injure him. Be sure he is not close to open stairways.
- **Do Not** force anything between his teeth or into his mouth. (You may have been instructed to do this in the past, but the training has changed.)
- **Do Not** give him anything to eat or drink.
- Loosen any tight or binding clothing or equipment.
- **Do Not** try to stop, control, or direct his movements during the seizure.
- If directed, place a pillow under his head. He may be too active to do this.
- Keep a record of what happened. Include the following information:
  a) What the client was doing just before the seizure.
  b) How long the seizure lasted. Time the seizure with a watch or clock if possible.
  c) What motions and actions occurred during the seizure in the order they occurred.
  d) Whether there was more than one seizure.
  e) What the client said and did following the seizure.
  f) Any injury or illness following the seizure.
- Report to the nurse supervisor immediately.

CHOKING

Read about preventing choking for clients who have difficulty eating and swallowing in this chapter. Recognize the universal distress signal that indicates a person is choking (Figure 2-23). Learn the steps of the Heimlich Maneuver. This is a technique that is used to dislodge pieces of food from a choking client's respiratory tract. Practice the Heimlich maneuver with your nurse supervisor. Post the instructions in the area where your client eats his meals.

If a client should begin to choke you can assist him in the following ways:

- Encourage him to cough out the food or foreign body. Do not attempt to do anything until he tries to expel the object. Do not slap him on the back.
- Find out if he can speak. If he can speak, leave him alone unless he becomes worse or is unable to speak. Only if instructed and directed by the nurse supervisor, try to assist him with coughing, using the method for quadriplegia-assisted coughing.
- If he cannot speak perform the following steps:
  - Stand behind your client and wrap your arms around his waist just under his rib cage. Form your hands as

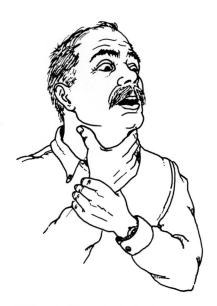

Figure 2-23. *A client who is choking because of an obstructed airway is unable to speak or cough. The client typically grasps his throat with one or both hands or may grasp his throat with one hand while pointing to his throat. This is recognized as a universal distress sign for choking.*

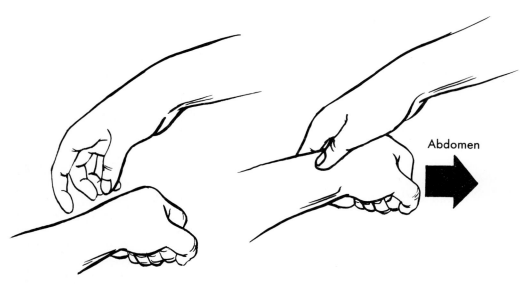

Figure 2-24. *The grasp of your hands and thumb are very important for effective abdominal thrusts. One hand is positioned into a fist; the thumb and index finger rest against the client. The other hand grasps and reinforces the fisted hand.*

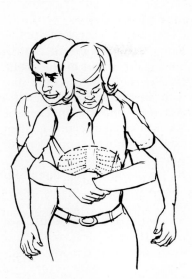 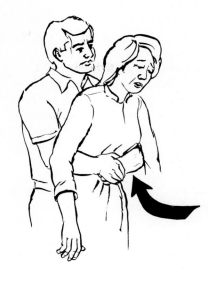

Figure 2-25. *Note the placement and position of your hands on the client's body during abdominal thrusts. Place your fist and hand just below the xiphoid process (end of the sternum) and in the midline of the abdomen. The client may be either standing or sitting. The maneuver may not be successful if the client is obese and is not suitable for pregnant clients. (Ask your nurse supervisor about chest thrusts for obese or pregnant clients and procedures for clients who become unconscious).*

shown in Figure 2-24. One hand is made into a fist. The other hand holds onto the fist. The thumb side of the fisted hand is placed at the center of the client's body above his waist and below his ribs (Figure 2-25).

- Push upwards and slightly inward against his body. Use quick and rapid thrusting pushes. You are attempting to launch whatever is obstructing his airway (Figure 2-26). Do Not push on his ribs or the xiphoid process of the sternum.
- Call the emergency unit or rescue squad and your nurse supervisor. Report what happened even if you are immediately successful in expelling the food or object.

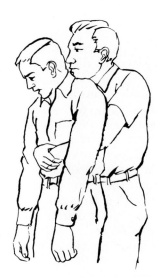

Figure 2-26. *Thrust your fist and hand together making upward, slightly inward movements; use quick thrusts. You are attempting to force air from the client's lungs and chest to dislodge the obstruction and launch it out of the airway. Continue the thrusts until the obstruction is removed, the client becomes unconscious, or the rescue squad arrives.*

When Contacting the Poison Control Center:

- Take whatever the person ingested, inhaled, injected, or absorbed with you to the telephone, if possible (if you know what it is). Be sure that you have the correct substance. If it is a commercial product, bring the label or other product information with you.
- Describe the client's behavior. Do not give him anything to eat or drink unless directed. If he vomits, save the emesis.
- Know the quantity of the substance taken, if possible.
- Know how long since the substance was taken, if possible.
- Know if the client is taking other medications.

- Know the age, weight (approximate), and health status of the client.
- *Do Not* use CPR or come into contact with the substance yourself until directed by the Poison Control Center. Use universal infection control precautions so as not to expose yourself to poisonous substances.
- Be prepared for the client to have convulsions, emesis, loss of consciousness, or shock.
- Stay with your client until assistance arrives. If he is alert, reassure him that assistance is on the way.
- Report to the nurse supervisor.

POISONING

Accidental poisoning happens more often than is commonly recognized. Children are particularly vulnerable to ingesting materials that are poisonous to them. However, you should broaden your thinking about poisoning. What is poison to one person may cause no reaction at all in another person. Because people have different tolerances to substances, it takes more of a substance to reach poisonous levels in some persons than in others. Some things are poisonous to all people. A person can be poisoned by swallowing a substance, breathing it in, absorbing it through the skin or mucous membranes, or taking it into the blood stream, as in an injection.

Each telephone directory lists the number of the area Poison Control Center. You should have this number written down where you can find it in an emergency. When someone has been poisoned, you must be ready to take the proper steps. This is often an emergency situation.

Do not attempt to treat anyone who has been poisoned without directions from the Poison Control Center. The exceptions to this are:

1) Remove the poison or cause of poisoning from the person. For example, if he has inhaled poison, remove it or him from the room. You can assist your client by having the correct information ready when you call the Center.
2) Lay the client down and turn his head to one side if he is unconscious so that he keeps a clear airway.
3) Call the rescue squad or emergency unit and the nurse supervisor.

HEAT REACTIONS

Older persons have difficulty adjusting to extreme changes in temperature. The older client may not tolerate winter cold or summer heat extremes. Heat reactions are more common among persons who have heart, lung, or kidney diseases, diabetes, circulatory problems, or weakened conditions. Some medications cause clients to become more heat sensitive. On hot, humid days you must be aware of your client's reaction to the heat.

If there is no air conditioning you can use a fan to circulate the air or a window fan to draw air through the room. Do not let the fan blow directly onto the client. You can also:

- Reduce strenuous activities. Plan exercises early in the morning or in the early evening when it is cooler.

- Bathe him with tepid, not cold, water. Bathe his hands, wrists, back of his neck, and behind his knees.
- Dress him in lightweight cotton clothing. Synthetic materials may cling to his body and keep the skin from breathing.
- Serve cool, light meals according to his diet plan.
- Maintain his fluid intake to help the body regulate its temperature.
- Avoid alcoholic drinks that cause body fluid loss.
- If he is able, go to an air conditioned library, shopping mall, theater, or visit his friend who has air conditioning.
- Be aware of the signs and symptoms of heat reactions.
- Notify your nurse supervisor about the client's reaction to heat.

Signs and Symptoms of Heat Reactions

Heat cramps are early signs of heat reaction. They are pains and spasm-like cramps in the legs, abdomen, and chest. You may give the client a half-glass of fluid every 15 minutes. If he does not feel better after 3 glasses (40–45 minutes) call for assistance.

- If he becomes worse, call the rescue squad and notify your nurse supervisor.
- If he becomes weakened and exhausted he may have **heat exhaustion.** Have him lie down. Loosen his clothing. Elevate his feet 8 inches unless you have instructions not to do this for the client. Do not give fluids if he vomits. He may have:
  —cool, clammy skin,
  —pale skin color,
  —nausea and vomiting,
  —weakness and dizziness,
  —cramping,
  —he may faint or collapse, or
  —his temperature may be normal. This is important. If his temperature begins to rise, he probably has heatstroke.
- **This is an emergency.** *Get help immediately before you attempt any assistance.*

Heatstroke may be the first symptom your client develops. He may not go through the other stages. He will have:

—high temperature;
—no evidence of sweating;
—hot, dry, red or flushed skin;
—heavy breathing;
—fast and rapid pulse; and
—he may lose consciousness

- *Get help immediately.* Ask the emergency medical unit or rescue squad to give you instructions for care until they arrive. Generally, you will be told:
- Do not give him fluids or stimulants.
- Lay him down and elevate his feet 8 inches.
- Keep cool air circulating through the room.
- Sponge him with tepid or cool water until help arrives.
- Watch closely to see that he does not cool down and become chilled.

The prevention of heat reactions is the best action.

SHOCK

There are a number of causes for a client going into shock. Shock often occurs in older persons after a fall. The body's circulatory system shuts down so the person cannot function. You must call for assistance immediately if you suspect your client is in shock.

The signs and symptoms of shock are:

—pale, cold, clammy skin.
—irregular respirations. He may breathe heavily and quickly.
—fast but weak pulse.
—weakness. He may collapse and faint.
—unresponsive, glassy-eyed look; he may have large pupils.
—may show bluish color around edges of his lips.
—possible nausea.
—if responsive, he may be anxious and restless.

You should:

- Call the rescue squad immediately and notify the nurse supervisor.
- Elevate his legs 8 inches unless instructed not to do so.
- Keep him warm if he is cold or trembling.
- Care for him according to the cause of the shock if appropriate. For example, if

he has fallen, keep him lying still. Do not attempt to move him or realign his body. Do not give him anything by mouth. If he is bleeding, follow the procedure for controlling bleeding. Stay with him and reassure him that help is on the way.

- Report what happened to the nurse supervisor.

HEMORRHAGE/BLEEDING

A client who has extensive, heavy blood loss or profuse bleeding that does not stop within several minutes may be hemorrhaging. The blood may be from any blood vessel. *This is an emergency situation.* His blood pressure will fall. He may become weak and unresponsive or go into shock. You should:

- Call the emergency unit or rescue squad. Notify your nurse supervisor. Call for help from anyone who may be at home to assist you.

- Immediately put pressure directly on the site of the bleeding. Use a clean cloth, towel, or bedlinen. Use whatever is available and clean. Use your hand if you have no other materials available.
- Put pressure on the bleeding site as you hold the cloth. Do not remove it.
- If the cloth soaks through with blood, put another cloth or material over the first one. Do not take one cloth off to add another.
- Continue to hold the cloth and keep pressure on the site until help arrives.
- If the bleeding is on an arm or leg, elevate it. Have the client lie down and elevate his feet if he appears to be in shock. Stay with him and keep pressure on the site of bleeding.
- Keep him warm. Do not give him anything by mouth. Follow instructions from the nurse supervisor or emergency squad.
- Report what happened to the nurse supervisor.

CHAPTER 3

Sensory and Communication Deficits

*O*BJECTIVES:

When you have studied this chapter and practiced the procedures it describes, you will be able to:

1. Define terms relating to sensory deficits and communication problems.
2. Identify the functions of the sensory system.
3. Describe the normal changes of senses that occur with aging.
4. Perform specific procedures to assist persons who have sensory losses or deficits.
5. Discuss the types of communication important in your care of any client.
6. Use techniques that promote clearer communication.
7. Work with clients who have impaired communications such as aphasia and memory loss.

*O*VERVIEW

Our senses enable us to see, hear, smell, taste, touch, and feel pain and temperature. We use our senses without thinking about them until one is diminished or lost. Some senses diminish as we grow older, causing such inconveniences as the need to use reading glasses. Sensory losses may also affect a person's lifestyle and health. For many of your clients, the normal sensory changes of aging will be compounded by sensory changes from trauma, breakdowns in the neurological system, or vascular problems. They will have sensory deficits in addition to or as part of their physical disabilities.

You will need to become comfortable working with people who experience sensory deficits (Table 3-1). You will need to be able to help them use the various aids that improve their senses, such as contact lenses, hearing aids, and mental stimulation techniques. You and your client can work together in many ways to make a rewarding difference in how he can view and sense his world. Think about your clients as you read this chapter. Think about what you can do to improve their sensory experiences as you care for them.

Table 3-1. Sensory Changes Normal in Aging:

Sensory Area	Normal Change with Aging
vision	—eyelids wrinkle and "bag" —side vision and night vision decrease —far-sightedness increases so that it becomes difficult to see things that are up close —yellow fatty deposits on "white of eye" develop —cataracts, glaucoma, corneal ulcers may develop —hand and eye coordination lessens.
hearing	—loss at higher frequencies, such as alarms, whistles, or higher musical notes; then general progressive loss —calcium deposits in middle ear may develop, causing hearing reduction —plugs of ear wax become more common, causing blockage of sounds until removed —deafness increases from various causes
smell, taste	—odors (gas, smoke, fumes) may not be detected —sweet and salt taste diminishes
touch	—sensitivity to cold increases
temperature	—temperature differences not readily detected
position	—senses of pressure, touch, and feeling lessen
place	—sense of body position decreases

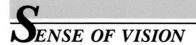

SENSE OF VISION

When a person's vision is impaired or lost, a part of his communication with the world is changed; it may even be shut off. The person with a severe visual deficit may have more difficulty interpreting the world. He cannot rely on non-verbal communication, facial expressions, and gestures to help understand meanings along with spoken words. This may cause frustration and insecurity. He must learn what things he can and cannot see and develop ways to cope with his disabilities. If he does not adapt to reduced vision, he may become withdrawn, depressed, angry, and bitter.

Many clients will have visual deficits following a stroke. One common deficit is **double vision.** Some may see several edges or repeated outlines for each figure or object. It may appear as if there are two of everything. One eyelid may droop (ptosis) due to nerve damage from the stroke or other nerve

palsys. These clients wear an eyepatch over one eye at a time. Every four hours the patch is moved to the other eye, then 4 hours later it will be moved back to cover the first eye, and so on. The eyepatch trains the muscles of both eyes to function fully. It also helps them understand and remember clear vision.

Another deficit that may follow a stroke is called **homonymous hemianopia.** This is blindness in one half of the field of vision for each eye. This visual deficit is like having a blind section cut out of the visual picture for both eyes while still being able to see all around that blind section. Functionally, the person does not see anything on one side of his field of vision, or he may not see things directly in front of him. Some persons see as if they had a drape over a part of their visual field. The person is not aware of what he does not see. He must be taught to pay attention to the areas where there is blindness.

You can simulate this condition by holding a card over half of each of your eyes. You cannot see your entire visual field. Try to eat a plate of food or put on your makeup. This is an approximation of what the client sees (Figure 3-2a).

For example, if he cannot see anything on the left side of his plate, he may not eat the food placed there. If he looks in the mirror, he will not see anything of the left side of his face and may forget to shave that part of his face. A client with this type of visual deficit is taught to turn his head during any activity where he must see what he is doing or where he is going. As he turns his head toward the affected side, he is able to see the entire plate or room. This is called **scanning.** He must learn to scan while he is eating, walking, or propelling his wheelchair. You will have to remind your client to scan until he learns to use this technique and becomes aware of what he is not seeing.

A diagram of the common visual deficit described above is shown with the complete visual field and anatomy. The visual deficit may occur after stroke (Figures 3-1 and 3-2b). Your nurse supervisor will assist you in identifying your client's visual deficit.

If your client is blind, the following suggestions will assist you in caring for him while maintaining his highest level of independence. Remember that a person can be "legally blind" and still have some vision. Be sensitive to your client and his needs and encourage self-care activities as long as they are safe for him.

WORKING WITH THE PERSON WHO HAS IMPAIRED VISION

Eating

Place foods separately on the plate. Identify and describe where foods are placed on the plate as if the plate were a clock face. For example, "the meat is at 1 o'clock, the carrots are at 9 o'clock" (Figure 3-3). Describe how foods are prepared and which items are intended to be finger foods. Pour liquids and set them and the utensils in the same place each time. It may be useful if you guide his hand to the beverages. Tell your client where hot foods are located.

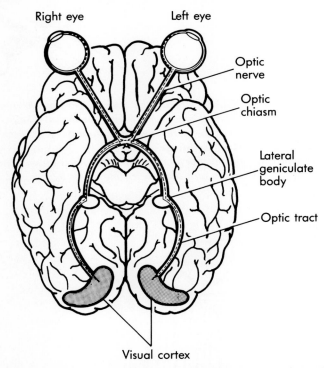

Figure 3-1. *Following a stroke, a client may have visual deficits similar to having a shade over part of his view. This literally "cuts off" a portion of what he sees on one side but affects the view with both eyes. Figure 3-2 further details how this occurs following a stroke.*

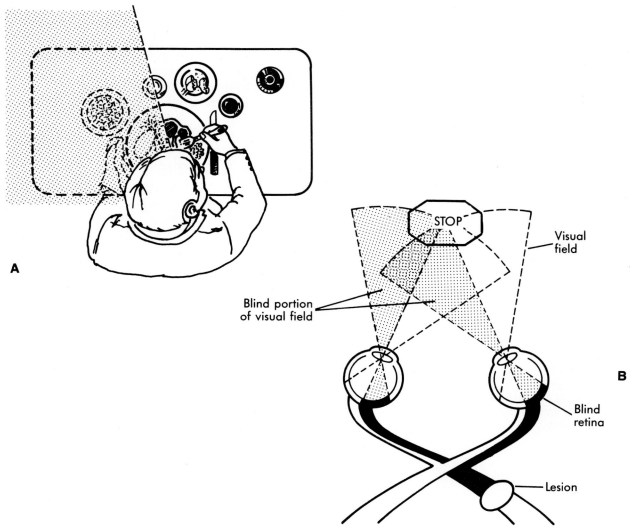

Figure 3-2.   **A,** *This cross sectional view details the pathways that govern sight from the visual cortex of the brain to the eyes. The optic nerves cross at the optic chiasm. Nerve fibers from the outer half of the right eye (at the retina) remain with the right hemisphere of the brain; fibers from the inner part of the eye cross over to the opposite left hemisphere. The reverse occurs for the left eye.*

  B, *Damage to a part of the brain affects the inner and outer optic nerve fibers causing visual field deficits. The type and degree of visual deficit differ for each client depending on the location and severity of the damage.*

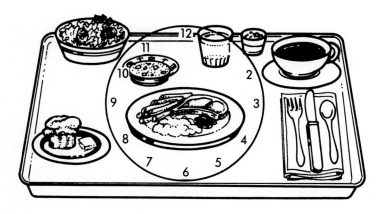

Figure 3-3.   *The concept of a clock helps a person with visual impairment to locate foods on his plate. For example, the chops are at 2 o'clock and the roll and butter are on a small plate at 8 o'clock.*

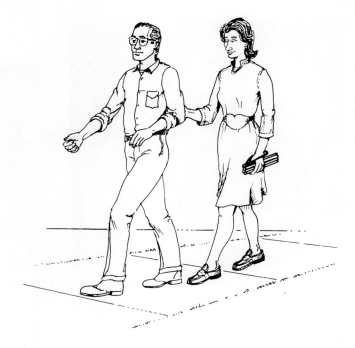

Figure 3-4. *Assist the client with visual impairment to walk so he has a sense of control and balance. Allow the client to take hold of your arm just above your elbow while you walk several steps ahead of him.*

Mobility

Allow your client to have as much control as possible. For example, when walking, walk one or two steps ahead of him, allowing him to hold onto your arm just above the elbow, rather than you holding onto him (Figure 3-4). Place his hand on the back or edge of the object before he begins to sit in a chair or car seat, or to move around an object.

Describe what is ahead and give a reference point. For example, when your client is going up or down stairs, count the number of stairs and alert him when he is at the last step. Likewise, give directions by starting from where your client is standing. Then describe specifically where he is to go from there and what landmarks he will cross: "From where you are, walk three steps until you reach the chair. Walk around the left side of the chair, and the refrigerator is four steps to the left. There is a cabinet directly across from the refrigerator."

Auditory

Talk to the person with a visual impairment in a normal tone of voice; do not shout. Use his name when you talk to him so he knows you are speaking to him and will expect a response from him. Tell your client when you come into a room and again when you leave, so he will not be startled or find himself talking to you when you are not there. If other people arrive or if you are in a group, introduce your client to everyone present.

Remember the importance of **touch** as a sign of caring and contact with the world. Use the person's other senses to assist him in enjoying the world. Let him smell the flowers and feel the texture of things. Describe events and places to him to include him further in what is going on about him.

If he enjoys talking books on tape, music, or other forms of recreational and educational materials, assist him in playing them. Ask the nurse or social worker and the family to look for materials with large type if your client has some vision (Figure 3-5). Discover your client's interest in and ability to use Braille materials. Keep your client stimulated so that he does not withdraw.

Mental

In addition to the stimulation just described, assist your client with keeping awareness and control in everyday activities for mental health. For example, if your client can use a touch tone phone, read him the number so

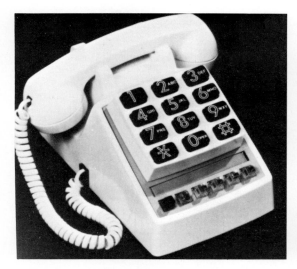

Figure 3-5. *Phones with large numbers can make dialing easier for the visually impaired person.*
Reprinted by permission of © Bissell Healthcare Corporation/Fred Sammons, Inc.

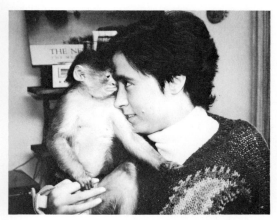

Figure 3-6. *Simian monkeys have proved to be ideal helpers for handicapped persons. Always obtain proper instruction from your supervising nurse when dealing with a client who has an animal assisting him.*
Courtesy of NJ Rehab Magazine.

he can dial by himself. Identify the worth of paper money and assist him in identifying coins. Fold paper money in different ways for each denomination. He will know the value of the money by the way it is folded. Most persons are able to identify different coins according to the size, weight, or finish on the edges. Let him pay for items and make change. Open mail and read it to your client, but only after he has been told the return address and decided for each piece whether it should be opened and read.

Safety

There is no substitute for safety in the home. Anticipate problems, but do not unnecessarily restrict your client. Watch for loose rugs, trailing cords or bedlinens, hot objects, projecting furniture, partly open doors or windows, sharp edges, or spills on the floor. Keep furniture and often-used items in the places your client expects them to be so he can use them safely. If he has a seeing-eye dog, know and follow the rules about behavior around the dog. Be sure that visitors also do not bother or distract the dog from doing its job. Some persons with severe disabilities have specially trained monkeys to assist them (Figure 3-6). Ask your nurse to give you specific instructions if you have a client with a monkey as a helper.

Special Techniques

If your client has contact lenses, follow your nurse's instructions about caring for the lenses. There are different procedures and rules about assisting clients with their contact lenses. Do not assist your client with contact lenses unless you are supervised and directed by your nurse supervisor. Figure 3-7 shows one way your client may have been instructed to remove his own **hard** contact lenses. Clients will have other instructions for extended-wear soft contact lenses.

Extended-Wear Soft Contact Lenses

A few clients may wear extended-wear soft contact lenses. These new soft lenses are advertised to be left in the wearer's eyes for 24 hours or longer, depending on the individual. As general rules:

● Clients should never leave contact lenses in their eyes for more than a week.
● Lenses should be left out overnight at least one night a week.
● Clients should wash their hands well before handling the lenses and should clean and disinfect the lenses as recommended by the physician and manufacturer.

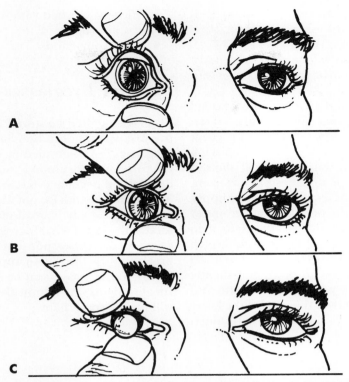

Figure 3-7. *Assisting a client to remove hard contact lens should only be done when he cannot do this himself and is always under the direction of the nurse supervisor. Wash your hands before and after the procedure. Do not perform this procedure over a carpet or basin where the lens could become lost.*

A, Assist him to gently separate his eyelids.

B, Assist him to bring his eyelids to the edge of the contact lens.

C, Gently press the lower eyelid margin under the contact lens to tilt the lens. The lens will slip off the surface of his eye as you assist him to bring both eyelids toward each other. Do not push in on the eye or press with any force. Place the lens in the proper storage container.

- Schedules for wear and use of lubricants are prescribed by the physician and must be followed closely.
- Notify the nurse supervisor if your client develops redness, itching, or swelling of his eyes, blurring or other visual disturbances, any pain, or scratchy or grainy sensations.
- If he can remove his own contacts, ask him to do so.

Assisting with Care of an Eye Prosthesis

An eye prosthesis may be referred to as an "artificial or glass eye." It is better to think of the eye prosthesis in the same manner as a lower limb prosthesis. It takes the place of an absent body part. Eye prostheses are cleaned

daily. Keeping the prosthesis and the eye area clean will prevent infection, provide good hygiene, and maintain the prosthesis. Your client may be able to remove, clean, and reinsert his eye prosthesis. Or your nurse supervisor will instruct you how to assist him. In eye prosthesis care you will generally:

- Wash your hands.
- Collect the cleaning solution, a towel, and bowl for washing. Some clients use a special cleaning solution and others use soap and water to clean their prostheses. Your client and nurse supervisor will direct you to the correct solution.
- If your client cannot remove his eye prosthesis, assist him by gently placing your fingers on his face just below his lower eyelid. Ask your client if this is the correct place for your fingers. Press in and up on the skin at the lower rim of

the prosthesis until it breaks loose. This will be like releasing an object from suction.

- The prosthesis will be released quickly. You will need to be ready to catch it with your hand.
- Wash the prosthesis with the selected solution and rinse it with warm water.
- Replace the prosthesis if your client needs your assistance. Before replacing it, wet it with water so it will slide in easier. Hold the prosthesis as it is to enter the eye socket. Begin at the upper eyelid. Place the prosthesis as far under the upper lid as it will fit. Hold it in place. Use your other hand to stretch the skin under the lower eyelid so it will pull the lower eyelid down and slightly outward. The prosthesis will slide into the eye socket over the edge of the lower eyelid. Ask your client if he is comfort-

able and satisfied with the prosthesis as it is inserted.
- Wash your hands.

Care for Eyeglasses

Eyeglasses should be stored in their protective case when not in use. Smeared or dirty eyeglasses can be cleaned by simply washing the lenses under running water, using a mild detergent if necessary to remove oily smears. Shake and blot dry. Do not wipe lenses or use an eyecloth. Only a small grain of grit can scratch the lens if wiped across the lens with a cloth. If the lenses pop out or the frames break, notify the nurse supervisor or the family so the glasses can be sent for repair. Ideally, clients who rely on glasses to function will have a spare pair.

*S*ENSE OF HEARING

There are four types of hearing loss: conductive, nerve or sensorineural, mixed, and central (Figure 3-8). There is also hearing loss from built-up earwax and from the normal reduction in hearing that may come with aging. If you suspect your client has a hearing deficit, report your observations to the nurse supervisor. Your client's physician may suggest a professional audiometric evaluation. No one should invest in a hearing aid before having a thorough examination to determine the cause of the hearing problem and whether a hearing aid could improve it.

Conductive hearing losses are caused by some obstruction of sound conduction in the middle or outer ear or by disease in the middle ear. Surgery or hearing aids may assist the person who has a conductive hearing loss. One common cause is otosclerosis, a buildup of calcified material in the middle ear that hinders sound transmission through the middle ear to the brain. Hearing aids amplify sounds for persons who have **conductive** hearing losses. A hearing aid does

not solve problems for all people with hearing deficits.

Hearing aids do not usually help persons who have **sensorineural** or nerve damage. A damaged nerve cannot carry clear information about sound to and from the brain. This client may hear sounds that are distorted or that affect certain levels or frequencies of sound. Sensorineural hearing losses may be mild or profoundly severe.

Clients who have both conductive and sensorineural deficits have a **mixed hearing loss.** This means that the hearing problems affect both the inner ear and the middle or outer ear. If the problem is severe, the person with this loss may have difficulties with hearing all but the loudest of voices and noises. He may hear sounds that he cannot identify. Some clients with mixed hearing loss may have improvement in some areas of hearing if they wear hearing aids. **Central** hearing loss occurs from damage to the central nervous system that results in damage to or impairment of the nerves in the brain or spinal cord.

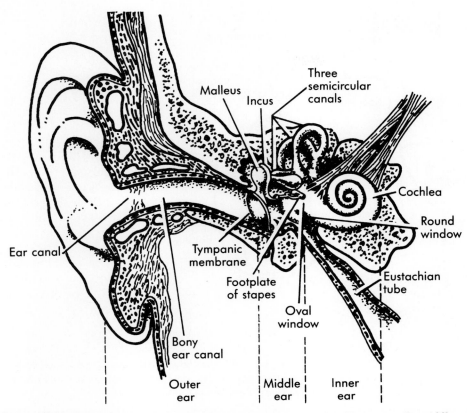

Figure 3-8. *The anatomy of the ear has three main areas: the external auditory area, the middle ear, and the inner ear. Obstructions, including ear wax, in the auditory canal or fluid in the Eustachian tube may reduce hearing. The middle ear contains three small bones (the incus, malleus, and stapes) that vibrate to assist in the transmission of sound during normal hearing. The bones may become stabilized by calcified deposits and produce conductive hearing losses. Inner ear deficits often involve sensorineural losses. These may affect a client's balance and produce ringing in the ears as well as hearing loss.*

SIGNS OF DIMINISHED HEARING

All clients may have some of these signs of diminished hearing at different times. Some may be concentrating on other things or hear but choose not to respond. If your client regularly has signs of diminished hearing, inform the nurse supervisor. For example, if he:

—requests the television or radio to be turned louder,

—does not look up when someone enters the room,

—does not respond to questions or conversations,

—responds inappropriately or with a sound-a-like word,

—"startles" at times as if surprised by a sound or person,

—speaks in louder than normal tones,

—does not respond consistently to normal household sounds such as clocks that chime, doorbells, or telephone bells, or

—asks you to speak louder or slower. Be sure you are speaking clearly and loud enough to be heard.

It is important to understand how a hearing aid helps your client to receive sounds. It does not "fix" hearing, but does make sounds louder, like an amplifier or loudspeaker. Many clients complain that their hearing aids seem to amplify all sounds. Some hearing aids can be adjusted to amplify only the frequencies the person cannot hear. The hearing aid may not amplify speech clearly if it is

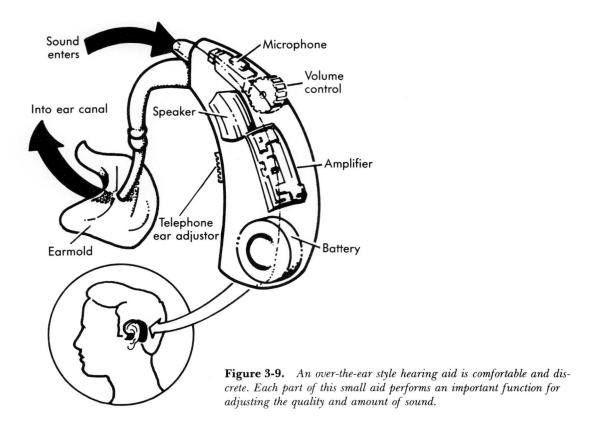

Figure 3-9. *An over-the-ear style hearing aid is comfortable and discrete. Each part of this small aid performs an important function for adjusting the quality and amount of sound.*

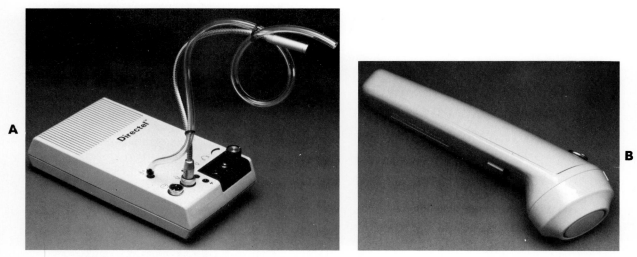

Figure 3-10. *Telecommunications devices for the disabled (TDD).*

A, *Persons with motion impairments can place, receive, and disconnect calls simply by blowing into a plastic tube on an instrument called a Directel. Calls are put through to a telephone operator, who then places the call. (Directel is a trademark of Bell Canada).*

B, *An electronic artificial larynx is used when a person has lost the use of the larynx. The client presses it against the throat and forms words with the mouth, and the unit produces electronic vibrations that stimulate the natural speaking voice.*

Courtesy AT&T.

turned up too high; it may whistle if not fitted properly, if the tubing connecting the hearing aid with the earmold is cracked, or if the earmold has become stiff and hard. It may amplify sounds at certain levels (decibels) but not pick up other sound levels adequately. Mechanical sounds or combined noises in large groups may be particularly annoying to the wearer.

Many persons attach a **stigma** to wearing a hearing aid. Sometimes they may choose to turn it off and on in various settings. Hearing aid designs have improved greatly in the past few years (Figure 3-9). Some models are so small that they fit right inside the ear and are the same color as the skin; others fit over the top of the ear. Other models are part of the frame of eyeglasses, which means that if the wearer's glasses are removed, he cannot hear.

Telephone receivers can be fitted with adjustable amplifier devices or even flashing lights for the severely impaired person. Telephones may also be fitted with Telecommunication Devices for the Disabled or TDD (Figure 3-10). When a call comes to a TDD the message is typed out by a typewriter so that it can be read rather than heard. The caller, as well as the receiver, must have a

---

Care of a Hearing Aid

- The hearing aid is an expensive piece of equipment.

- **Do** *not:*
  - place it under water,
  - drop it,
  - place it near heat (window sill in sun, radiator),
  - throw batteries away into fire (they may explode),
  - place it in high humidity (shower area, steam), or
  - pull on or use the tubing to disconnect it from the earmold.

- **Do:**
  - clean the earmold daily with soap and water, but without getting water into the tubing. Some aids can be easily detached from the tubing before cleaning. (Water will flow into the tubing if the earmold is tipped.)
  - check the hearing aid tubing and earmold to be sure they remain supple and soft. When they become hard and stiff, they should be replaced.
  - look for wax in the tubing. Use the special tool provided with the hearing aid to clean wax from the tubing. Use a slight turning motion to gently push the wax through the tubing. Be careful not to puncture or damage the tubing.
  - check for low or dead batteries. A wax plug in the tubing will shut off sound through the hearing aid, even if the batteries are new.
  - check your client's skin around and inside the ear for any irritation or excess earwax. **Never remove earwax** from your client's ear with a hairpin, cotton applicators, or any other object. Tell the nurse supervisor if your client has earwax buildup.

TDD. The telephone book lists a customer service number to call for current information about TDD services.

Television sets can be equipped with a device to show "closed captioned" programs. The closed caption briefly explains in writing the gist of what is happening on the television program. Some television programs open a small window in the upper right corner of the television screen. They feature an expert communicating the program in sign language for the non-hearing audience.

INSERTING THE HEARING AID

The following are instructions for in-ear and over-ear models:

1. Insert the battery, matching the + sign on the battery with the + sign on the hearing aid battery compartment. Close the sliding door to the battery compartment.
2. Set the switch to microphone (M) mark.
3. Turn volume control wheel to maximum, until the hearing aid whistles in your hand. This checks the battery. If there is no whistle, replace the battery.
4. Turn the volume to the low setting.
5. Insert the hearing aid mold into the ear canal first. Gently hold onto the outer edge of the person's ear, so that the rest of the earmold can be fitted into the curves of the ear. You may have to wiggle the outer ear gently and slightly push the earmold into place. The earmold is fitted exactly to the shape of the person's ear. It will fit right into place and will not stick out of the ear.
6. For over-the-ear models: Once the earmold is in place, loop the tubing and body of the hearing aid over the ear.
7. Slowly turn up the volume until your client says it is loud enough, or until the whistle starts. If the whistle starts, turn the volume down until it stops and check to see that the earmold is properly in place.
8. Your client may be able to hear you talk in a normal tone of voice. He should respond to you in his own normal tone of voice. If your client is not able to tell you what is comfortable, turn the volume halfway and observe how he responds for a while. Once the level is set, note the volume and use it for a landmark next time.

REMOVING THE HEARING AID

1. Turn down the volume and turn the hearing aid off.
2. Hold onto the earmold with your thumb and index finger.
3. Gently pull the entire hearing aid straight toward you.
4. Open the door to the battery compartment; leave the battery inside.
5. Wipe any wax off the earmold; do not use water.
6. Place the hearing aid in its box in a safe place.

CARING FOR THE CLIENT WHO HAS A HEARING LOSS

A person who has a hearing loss can become isolated from others, especially when he cannot understand what is going on in a conversation or respond appropriately to questions or comments. He cannot amuse himself and stay informed by watching television or listening to the radio, nor can he visit with friends on the telephone. Often a client becomes concerned that others are talking about him, which causes him to become depressed or angry at others. At other times, because he cannot respond, he may appear to be disinterested in what is happening, slow-witted, or hostile.

Do not allow yourself or others to treat your client as if he had any of these negative traits; do not allow him to become isolated; remind yourself and others about the communication lag. Remember that communication is very tiring for him—it is hard work with little return.

Some Things to Consider When Caring for a Client Who Has Hearing Loss:

- Do *not* yell or shout at your client.
- Learn about his hearing loss—know what he can and cannot do.
- Face him when you talk, looking directly at him.
- Use sign language, clear lip movements that are not exaggerated movements, hand gestures, and facial expressions.
- Speak slowly and distinctly, allowing him to lipread and to have time to think about the word meanings.
- Keep pencil and paper or other materials at hand for him to use.
- Talk close to, but not directly into, the better ear.
- Use assistive devices and aids, such as picture cards, lists, or possibly a computer.
- Reduce other noises in the environment.
- Do not cover your mouth with your hands or chew gum or food.
- Check the emergency plan in case of fire or other danger where he cannot hear the alarm.
- Remain patient.
- Treat the client like a responsible adult, not as if he were a child.
- Continue to communicate with him and keep him alert to the world about him.

OTHER SENSORY LOSSES

Smell and taste deficits usually accompany other sensory losses. Loss of taste may affect the client's appetite and food selection. Loss of smell can also affect appetite since taste and smell are closely linked. Smell deficits can be safety hazards if fumes, smoke, and other warning odors cannot be detected. Losses of sensation of touch and temperature are greater safety concerns for your client. For example, he may not respond to touching a hot object and may burn or injure himself without knowing he has done so.

DEFICITS IN SPEECH AND LANGUAGE COMMUNICATION

Disturbances in speech and language communication create some of the most difficult situations you will encounter in the home. Communication is more than speaking the same language. It is the ways in which we send messages to others and receive messages from them. We talk, write, and make facial, body, and hand gestures to others. Likewise, we receive messages by hearing, seeing, and understanding the messages others have sent to us. The brain is involved in all of these communication activities. Your client may have damage to parts of his brain, causing short circuits in how he sends and receives information.

This section discusses these basic aspects of speech and language communication:

Verbal and Non-verbal Communication
Formal and Informal Communication
Assigning Meanings to Communication
Tips for More Successful Communication
Some communication problems associated with specific disabilities and guidelines for your actions follow the discussion of these points (Figure 3-11).

VERBAL AND NON-VERBAL COMMUNICATION

We practice **verbal** (or oral) communication whenever we speak to one another. We use verbal communication in other forms when

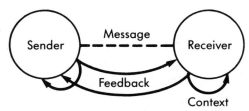

Figure 3-11. *The pattern of a completed communication is an exchange process. The sender transmits a message to the receiver. The receiver accepts the message, but compares it with his own understanding (context) before returning a response (feedback) to the sender. The sender verifies that the receiver understood the message as it was intended. This is an ideal model. Effective communication exchanges require skill and practice to avoid misunderstanding and error.*

we read or write information. We tell each other information, ask questions, give directions and orders, and describe our feelings through verbal communication. We also learn as children that there are certain ways to use verbal communication. For example, the words "please" and "thank" you are desirable additions to our verbal communication patterns. Many times we react differently to a phrase if a certain tone of voice is used or if "please" and "thank you" are included in the words. Try saying out loud, "Hand me that comb" with different voice tones. Then listen for differences when you add "please" to the sentence. The same verbal request can produce different reactions in what we hear. If we add different motions and facial expressions to our words, we add more meanings than what we actually say with words.

Non-verbal or unspoken communication is very important for us to recognize. Some non-verbal communication is referred to as body language, or the way we move our body to send messages. For example, if you move a step back and lean away from someone who is talking to you, your body has sent a message that there should be more distance between the two of you. If you yawn or begin to look about the room, you are using your body language to tell the person that you are losing interest in what he is saying or doing.

Be aware that you are communicating your attitudes about your client to him even without speaking them aloud. Ask your nurse supervisor if you have questions:

—about your attitudes toward caring for a person with disabilities,

—about certain tasks you perform for him, or

—about what your client can understand or do himself.

Some non-verbal communication means different things to people of different cultures or age groups. Be sure not to use non-verbal gestures or verbal expressions that are borrowed from other cultural groups until you are sure of their meanings to that group. If your client speaks a different language and you have no one to interpret for you, you must talk with your nurse supervisor. If the client and family agree, ask the nurse supervisor how to arrange for an interpreter for emergency assistance. Have a list of key words and phrases ready so that you can tend to your client's basic needs. Many agencies have interpreters who can prepare instructions in the client's language. Remember to include the family in planning the activity.

ASSIGNING MEANING TO COMMUNICATION

We cannot give any meaning to what we see and hear and touch until the brain tells us what it is. For example, a person can see a baseball game with his eyes, but he needs his brain to have a name for what he sees and to understand the rules of the game. We also know that the same words and actions can have different meanings for different people. For example, in some cultures it is not unusual for men to cry or hug one another, whereas in other cultures men consider these behaviors inappropriate.

Touch is a very important type of non-verbal communication for all people. Although some cultural groups do not like to be touched, this may change during an illness or when the person has disabilities. No one should be touched in places or ways that are offensive or painful to him. On the other hand, the older person frequently benefits from touching. The touch sensations of the skin tend to decrease as a person grows older, but his needs for affection, belonging, and reassurance may increase. Simply placing a hand on his arm as he talks to you, rubbing

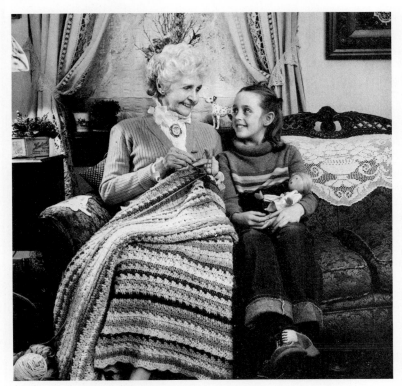

Figure 3-12.   *How you communicate nonverbally can be as important as what you say. For example, sitting close to someone may signal affection for that person.*
   Permission to reproduce this copyrighted material has been granted by the owner, Hollister Incorporated.

his back or arm as you give instructions, or gently patting his hand when he is upset or frustrated, can mean a great deal of support to your client (Figure 3-12). However, some people do not like to be touched. Learn how your client feels about touch and respect his wishes.

TIPS FOR CLEARER COMMUNICATION

We all think we communicate clearly, when, in fact, we often do not. These basic techniques may assist you to improve your communication skills:

1. **Introduce yourself to the person.** An introduction is important for several reasons. An introduction is the proper courtesy between newly met people in our society. Before you enter someone's home, it is natural and expected that you tell him who you are and why you are there. Secondly, many dif-

ferent caregivers enter a client's home and he needs to have a clear introduction to their purpose and job title. Additionally, if your client has sensory difficulties, he may not remember from one visit to another who you are and what you do. In these situations, you will have to introduce yourself at each visit.

2. **Establish the purpose of the communication.** Some communication is for conversation, some is for giving directions, and so forth. For example, if your are going to transfer your client from the bed to the commode, it will help if he understands that the purpose of the communication will be to give him directions about the transfer. You are telling him that he should be ready for information that has a specific purpose. He has to listen and remember this information in a different way than when you are talking to him about his menu selections or about the weather.

3. **Speak carefully.** Say the words slowly and clearly so that each one can be under-

stood. Do not mumble, run words together, or drop off at the end of the sentence. Be careful when using slang words or phrases that may be unknown to the person. Allow enough time for your client to comprehend questions and to answer. His answer may be slower when he is tired or upset. If his sensory intake is reduced he may have to think a while before remembering certain things. Frequently, your clients will be hard of hearing. Speak distinctly, slightly louder than usual, and move your lips to form the words while you are facing the person. Find out if he uses sign language for the deaf and lip reading.

4. **Be an active listener.** One of the hardest jobs we have is to listen instead of talking. Sometimes when we are supposed to be listening we are thinking about other things or even planning what we will say next ourselves. At times we even answer people before they have finished what they are saying. When these things happen to us, we are aware that the other person has not been listening. We become angry or frustrated because we have not gotten our message to the other person in the way we intended. It is especially difficult to be an active listener when working with a client who has communication disabilities.

5. **Practice listening.** Be patient and wait for the full message from your client. If you don't understand what is said, ask him to repeat it. If you don't understand what he means, ask him questions to check out the meaning. For example, "Is this the comb you wanted?" as you hold up the comb. Or "Are you telling me the belt is too tight?" Or "I do not understand; let's try to say it another way," or "Nod when I point to what you want, or what you mean." Being a good listener means doing whatever you can to be sure you receive the message your client intended to send to you. It is hard work, but very important work.

SPECIAL COMMUNICATION DEFICITS

Even when you practice good communication skills, it can be very difficult to work with a person who has brain damage and communication problems. We call these problems **deficits** because the person is deficient or lacking in certain communication abilities or skills in one or more ways. The most common types of deficits you will find are difficulties in speech and breakdowns in language. **The ability to speak and the use of language are two different things.**

You may have already learned that some of your clients are able to talk, but not to say what they intend, or that they can only repeat meaningless phrases. Others are not able to speak, but can understand what you say. Some clients may be able to speak clearly, but be unable to remember, or do, what they said. There are many combinations of speech and language deficits. To be able to work with your client, you must understand his abilities and deficits with speech and language and how they affect his behavior.

Persons with **speech** problems have difficulty moving the body parts and muscles that make the motions and sounds necessary for speech. Persons with **language** breakdowns cannot send and understand communications because of damage to the brain. Communication problems will be somewhat different for each person, depending on the areas of his brain that are damaged. Try to learn about your client's speech or language deficit and how you can help him communicate. Understanding his difficulty will help you to be more patient with him when he struggles for words or meanings.

COMMUNICATION DEFICITS AND THE BRAIN

The diagrams of the brain shown in Figure 3-13 are divided to show the right half of the brain and the left half of the brain. The drawings show the areas of the brain that are responsible for different speech and language functions. Remember that the nerve messages cross over from the brain to the other side of the body. This means that a person who has damage to the left side of the

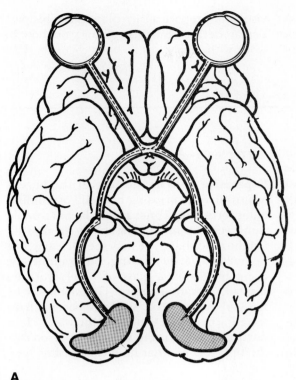

A

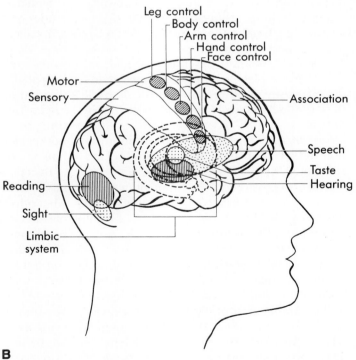

B

Figure 3-13. **A,** *The brain is divided into a right and a left half called hemispheres. The* **right** *hemisphere controls the* **left** *side of the body. The* **left** *hemisphere controls the* **right** *side of the body. Thus the client who has a stroke affecting the left hemisphere of his brain will have the right side of his body affected.*

   B, *Specialized areas located on each hemisphere of the brain control and direct certain body functions. Damage to a specialized area causes a deficit in that function; the damage following a stroke differs for each client. This illustrates why each client has individual deficits and strengths that cannot be approached only by the diagnosis.*

brain will have paralysis or paresis (weakness) on the right side of the body as well as various communication deficits. The nurse supervisor will prepare a care plan listing his particular deficits and instructing you how to work with him.

SPECIFIC DEFICITS

Persons who have strokes, traumatic brain injuries, some infectious diseases, multiple sclerosis, spinal cord injuries, tumors, and Parkinson's disease may have difficulties with communication. This section lists specific helping techniques for each type of communication deficit.

APHASIA

One common deficit following a stroke is called **aphasia.** It occurs most frequently in the person who has right hemiplegia (paralysis). Aphasia means the person has a loss of language that may or may not involve speech. For example, a person with aphasia may have difficulty with one or more of the following: reading, writing, recognizing people or objects, telling time, understanding what is being said, and arithmetic, spelling, and other problems. Aphasia is described as mild, severe, or complete according to how many deficits are involved. It may be difficult to tell that the person with mild aphasia has a deficit.

Severe aphasia can produce communication deficits that may disrupt daily life and functions. Aphasia may affect all language abilities so severely that a person cannot speak, read, or even recognize people. Complete or global aphasia is a total loss of communication; the person cannot speak, write, or even understand speech or writing.

Aphasia is categorized by the type of language skills that are affected. The three categories of aphasia are: expressive, receptive, and a combination of the first two, expressive-receptive aphasia. It is helpful to know what deficits are common to each type of aphasia so that you can anticipate some of your client's difficulties. Many times your client will know what he intends to say, but cannot make the speech and language happen. Or he may not realize that what he said doesn't make sense to you, so he doesn't understand why you don't respond to him. Some clients have no understanding of either intent or interpretation.

Types of Aphasia

Expressive aphasia means that the person has trouble "expressing himself" or sending out information. For example, he has trouble using words or may not be able to speak at all. On the other hand, he may speak clearly, but not mean what he is saying. For example, the client may want a glass of water, but says instead, "I want a comb." He may know he has said the incorrect word and become frustrated when he cannot obtain water. It is particularly confusing when the person says the opposite of what he means, using "yes" for "no."

Similarly, he may call people by wrong names or use known words put together into a nonsense order. Some of the people who have expressive aphasia can produce the words and thoughts they mean to say if they sing or chant them, but they cannot produce them in ordinary speech. It is very distressing for the client who wishes to ask for something or tell about something when he cannot speak. He may become very depressed or frustrated.

Receptive aphasia means that the person has trouble understanding or "taking in" what others are trying to say through speech or other communication. He cannot comprehend much of what is said or written; it may all be meaningless sounds or out-of-order communication. Or he may understand a word for a short time, but not be able to remember it or use it in a meaningful way. He may become increasingly isolated because he cannot relate to the world or what is happening. Because he cannot recognize things or people, it is difficult to have socialization. He cannot read or watch movies to entertain himself. The world is a confusion to him because he cannot receive information about it.

Try using picture boards, pointing to objects, or whatever means you, the family, and nurse supervisor or speech therapist can develop to help communicate with your client.

Table 3-2. Common Deficits with Aphasias

Expressive aphasia He may not be able to:	Receptive aphasia He may not be able to:

—write, count things,
—spell, speak sentences,
  tell time, use telephone,
—name objects, point to things,
—gesture properly, or
—use correct grammar.
	—recognize people, objects,
	—understand what is said,
	  understand what he reads,
	—realize his own location,
	—realize location of things, or
	—enjoy movies or TV.

Expressive aphasia

The person verbalizes "jargon"

or he produces *no words*

or he speaks unconnected
with his intentions and thoughts.

Receptive aphasia

The communication is not
accurately received.

Some clients will have been trained to respond to computerized learning programs, but these are not commonly found in home settings.

Expressive-receptive aphasia is a combination of the two types of aphasia. It usually is referred to as **global aphasia** because of the closed communication from within and from without. You will need specific guidance from your nurse about how to care for this client. Always be caring, use gentle touching, and be aware of your own level of frustration when working with these people.

Table 3-2 will help you remember the common deficits with expressive and receptive aphasias.

It is a frustrating situation for you, the family, and the client. He may become depressed, angry, withdrawn, or even suicidal. The entire family is affected by the client's loss of communication ability. For example, if the client was the major wage earner in the family or the person who managed the family finances, the financial and working structure of the family must be changed. If the person is a father, the family may begin to treat him as a child, rather than as a parent. His wife may have trouble seeing him in the role of her husband. Family roles and relationships change and this causes stress. Be patient, be alert, and try to understand as much as possible about your client's aphasia so you can help him to communicate.

Guidelines for Working with the Client Who Has an Aphasia

- Stand in front of the person so he can see your face.
- Speak clearly and slowly, use normal voice, never shout.
- Use short simple sentences and discuss one topic at a time.
- Add simple gestures to help explain what you are saying.
- Allow time for the person to respond—it may take him quite a while.
- Ask one question at a time to make sure he understands as you talk and to allow him to make choices and decisions.
- Try to use the same words for things you do regularly.
- Ask "yes" and "no" questions if these words are all he can use to communicate (be sure he does not have "yes" and "no" reversed).
- Do not treat him as if he were a child—he is an adult.
- Have several short conversations rather than one long one.
- Create a calm, quiet, unrushed environment for communication.
- Decrease stimuli, such as TV or other people in the room while talking.
- Stop briefly, wait a moment, and allow him to regain control if he cries, swears, or laughs out of order.
- Do not force your client to speak.
- Do not react to inappropriate actions or jumbled responses.

- Use communication aids appropriate for your client (Figure 3-14): (The nurse supervisor or speech therapist will identify these and direct you in their use.)
  —Flashcards or picture boards
  —Writing when speaking becomes frustrating
  —Computer programs for communication
  —Eyeblinks for "yes" or "no"
- Tell him what you are going to do with/for him.
- *Do Not talk about the person in front of him.* **Never** *assume he cannot understand you.*
- Continue to talk with a person who has receptive aphasia; he may be able to understand some of what you say and it is stimulating for him.
- Help him when he struggles for words with non-verbal prompts. For example, if he cannot say the word he means, ask him to show you the object or activity by pointing to a picture or similar prompt. Or ask him to give you one key word rather than have him try to complete a sentence or an entire thought.
- Don't take it personally or overreact when a client curses, even if he curses at you.
- Be patient, caring, and optimistic—keep your sense of humor.
- Don't say you understand your client when you don't.

DYSARTHRIA

Dysarthria may occur following a stroke. It affects speech production when muscles of the mouth, tongue, or throat become weakened or paralyzed following a stroke. The speech pathologist and the nurse will have specific instructions about how you are to work with this type of problem. You can expect that this person will drool when talking. He may slur his words and be difficult to understand. This person may be able to write or type out his messages. If so, once he has written the message, ask him to read it to you aloud. Listen carefully as he says the words while you are reading them. You may begin to understand him better if you practice this activity together.

Because of the weakened muscles he has

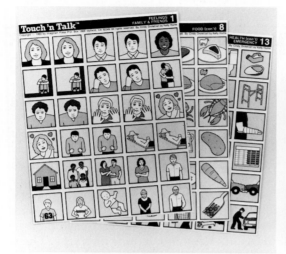

A

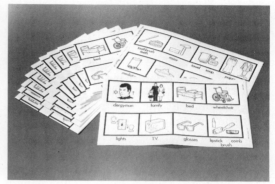

B

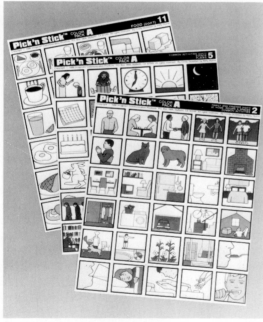

C

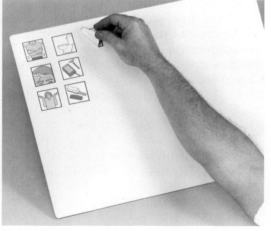

D

Figure 3-14.   *Many assistive devices for improving communication with clients who have aphasia can be made at home. Some clients may have computers and software packages available. Easy to use and excellent commercial products include these:*

    A, *Touch 'N Talk picture board.*
    B, *Identification picture board.*
    C, *Pick 'N Stick identification stickers.*
    D, *picture stickers.*
Reprinted by permission of © Bissell Healthcare Corporation/Fred Sammons, Inc.

loss of control and may have trouble chewing and swallowing his food. If your client has difficulty swallowing, **read about dysphagia** under nutrition in Chapter 2.

DEFICITS IN COMMUNICATING EMOTIONS FOLLOWING STROKE

Emotional changes affect the ways in which a person communicates with and relates to the world about him. Many types of emotional changes may occur following a stroke and your client may have little control over some of them. It is important for you to recognize and understand the emotional changes so that you can cope with the changes and continue to communicate with him. You can also explain some of these changes to others who might react negatively to your client's emotional changes. This section presents changes that lead to **depression, emotional lability, and confusion with memory loss.**

Depression occurs in many people following strokes. It is an emotional low period that lasts for a long time without a break. Everyone has low or sad days on occasion. When a low mood lasts for several days without an explainable cause, it can be depression. Report a client's long-lasting low mood or a change in behavior to a low mood to the nurse. Sometimes it may be difficult to decide which behaviors are caused by depression.

Some signs of depression you should be familiar with are:

—loss of energy;
—decreased appetite or increased, nervous appetite;
—irritability about many things;
—loss of interest in usual activities;
—avoiding people, less communication and more withdrawn;
—changes in sleep patterns—either sleeps all the time or cannot sleep;
—talking about being or feeling worthless, that life is over, or that he wishes he could die; and
—talking about suicide, hopelessness. This should *always be reported promptly* to the nurse and any family members who live with or are close to the client.

Emotional lability is a phrase that describes your client having inappropriate and sudden episodes of either laughing or crying. This behavior often occurs following a stroke and may or may not continue. He may begin to laugh or cry for no apparent reason. He may laugh when he should cry and vice versa. It is important to understand that the client has no control over these emotional episodes. The best thing for you to do is to wait until he stops laughing or crying. Then, without comment, continue what you and he were doing. If he is crying, offer him a tissue, and wait. For example, a client may be showing you a photograph of his family when he begins to cry uncontrollably. After the episode, he may express embarrassment about crying. You can reassure him that you understand and there is no stigma attached to his behavior.

Another technique that helps some clients is distraction. When he becomes labile, try to distract him. Ask your nurse supervisor to work with you so that your client can learn to distract himself. Otherwise you may briefly ignore the emotional lability by not calling attention to the behavior. Be sure that you *do not ignore your client as a person.* If you make a pattern of ignoring him, he may withdraw and become depressed.

It is more difficult to ignore a client who curses or repeats profanities over and over. This is something he has no control over because of damage that occurred during the stroke. Whenever your client curses or uses profanities, you must remember that they are not directed at you, even when he uses name-calling. This can be very difficult because we are all affected by what others say about us. Do not laugh at your client, or shame him, strike out at him, or become angry. Remember, he cannot control these episodes of unfortunate behavior, so ignore them. One thing you can do is to teach others about the cause of the inappropriate behavior so they do not respond negatively to the person.

Confusion with memory loss often occur together. A client who does not have other sensory or communication deficits can still be severely disabled if he is confused and cannot remember things.

Some signs of this type of deficit are:

—forgetfulness,
—short attention span,
—asking the same questions over and over,
—wandering about without knowing where he intends to go, and
—becoming unaware of what is going on around him.

Care for the Client Who Has Memory Loss

- Remind him who he is and who you are.
- Tell him where he is.
- Tell him what time of day it is and the date.
- Explain what is going on around him if he is confused.
- Be patient and kind.
- Be aware that he may wander off if not supervised.
- Keep him oriented to present reality.
- Help him to remember what has happened. For example, help him keep a diary, guest list, or daily log book.

The nurse supervisor will identify techniques from the following list that may work for you and your client. The nurse may conduct memory tests with your client as a part of the care plan.

TECHNIQUES FOR ORIENTATION TO PRESENT REALITY

- Have your client practice paying attention. The nurse can help you decide what to use for this and how long your client can pay attention.
- Use repeated words and directions.

- Work with associations between words and ideas, such as: Ruby loves to wear red . . . rubies are red.
- Keep items in a definite place to eliminate misplaced things.
- Develop a routine. For example, things to do before going to bed are: check front door, check stove, check alarm, and so forth.
- Develop safe ways to do daily tasks. Use props to remind him. For example, use a timer or put a pot in the room where he is so that the pot will help him remember the cooking in the kitchen.
- Develop a system to remember where things are hidden or put away. For example, paper money (green) is in a green can or $30.00 is in the 3rd drawer.
- Use time devices to keep daily reality. For example, use a large calendar to mark off each day. Show your client a clock and have him say the time.
- Correct him when he is wrong in a gentle way, but do not allow him to ramble on and pretend that he is somewhere else. Try to keep him focused on where he is and what is happening now. Keep him in the present.
- Give him any equipment he may need. This includes clean eyeglasses, dentures, hearing aid, braces, walker, canes, or slings.
- Talk to your client about current events or television programs he may watch, even if you are not sure how much he understands.
- Be patient and give reassurance when he fails something. Praise him for new accomplishments and promote self-care.
- Report to the nurse supervisor if he becomes:
  —anxious,
  —fearful,
  —nervous,
  —suspicious,
  —disinterested in life in general,
  —concerned about himself and his life, or
  —has mental, physical, or emotional changes.

See Chapter 11 for more information about Alzheimer's disease.

CHAPTER 4
Turning, Moving, and Positioning

OBJECTIVES

When you have studied this chapter and practiced the procedures it describes, you will be able to:

1. Define terms relating to mobility.
2. Recognize the role of mobility in maintaining functional abilities and overall well-being.
3. Use proper body mechanics whenever moving clients.
4. Protect your own health and safety when turning, moving, or positioning clients.
5. Position clients with disabilities correctly, using a variety of standard positions.
6. Assist clients toward achieving their maximum mobility.
7. Perform a variety of transfers with clients, using safe techniques and equipment.
8. Use mechanical lifts to move your clients.
9. Assist clients to ambulate, as directed.
10. Apply techniques of moving to the care of clients in areas such as bathing, travel, and household activities.

OVERVIEW

Activities that promote mobility are essential for your client's well-being. You are giving high-quality care when you keep your client moving, shifting his weight, and using proper turning and positioning. These are especially important when he cannot or will not move alone. The goals are to maintain the functional abilities and well-being that he has and to prevent further complications or disabilities.

There are two approaches to moving clients: the traditional method and the therapeutic approach method (often referred to as the Bobath Method). This chapter focuses on the traditional method because it is most familiar to nurses at this time. It is also a safe and useful method for all clients in the home setting. The traditional method teaches the client to use his unaffected functions and abilities to perform tasks. He is taught to work from his strengths.

The therapeutic approach or Bobath method has grown in popularity for treatment, especially in the rehabilitation of clients who have had strokes. It requires understanding the principles and practicing the techniques in a training session. Bobath methods are directed toward retraining clients to use their affected functions. Because learning and using traditional and Bobath principles simultaneously may be confusing, only a few basic Bobath movements are presented in this book.

You must read the section about Body Mechanics and practice using proper body mechanics under the direction of your nurse supervisor *before* working with a client. Body mechanics are essential to your own safety and safe mobility activities for your client. Think about proper body mechanics before and during every turning, moving, or positioning activity with your client. Body mechanics apply whether or not you are using equipment to assist with a mobility activity. The following sections describe the components of mobility activities for your client: body mechanics, positioning, turning and moving, transferring and ambulating.

BODY MECHANICS FOR MOVING CLIENTS

Millions of workers in our society have gone home with back injuries resulting from using improper lifting techniques; many more go home with tired, aching backs. Most of these injuries and backaches could be prevented if workers used proper body mechanics when lifting and correct posture to strengthen the muscles used during lifting.

You cannot avoid lifting when caring for a client in the home, but you can control how you lift. You must learn to think about **how** you are lifting as much as about **who** and **what** you are lifting. The proper positioning of the parts of your body during lifting is a skill you must learn just as you learn to position your clients' body parts. Then you must practice that skill regularly.

When you work with clients like those described in this book, you have a greater need to attend to proper body mechanics. Body mechanics are important because:

—the disabled client may not be able to help you during the lift,
—if you cannot complete the lift it becomes unsafe for you and your client,
—you are often alone in the client's home without others nearby to call for assistance, and
—the home may not have adjustable furniture or special equipment to assist you.

There are safe, efficient ways to move and lift clients and objects. Study the following information and apply it to your daily activities.

1. Draw an imaginary line from the top of your head down through the middle of your body. This is your *line of gravity*. A few inches below your waist, imagine a point on this line of gravity that is located in the center of your body. Compare your imaginary line and point with the drawing. This is your *center of*

gravity. Your feet, placed standing apart, form your *base of support* (Figure 4-1).

- Keep your center of gravity over your base of support.
  —Keep a straight back.
  —Keep your knees over your feet.
  —Stand in good, correct posture.
  —Sit in good posture, far back in the chair, feet on the floor. Avoid the "TV Slouch."
  —Carry objects in close to your line of gravity and your center of gravity.
  —Face the direction you are moving or lifting (Figure 4-2).
  —Turn with your entire body; do not twist.

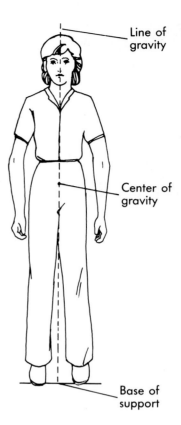

Figure 4-1. *Proper body mechanics keep your center of gravity over your base of support.*

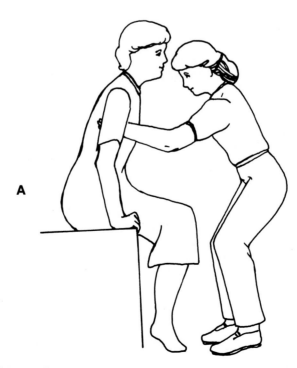

Figure 4-2. **A,** *Keep your knees over your feet and your back straight.*

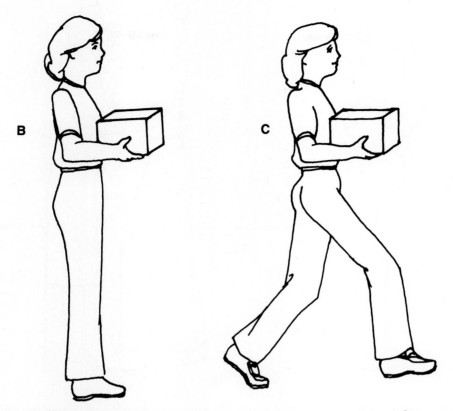

Figure 4-2, cont'd.   **B,** *Carry objects in close to your body.* **C,** *Face the direction you are moving or lifting; do not twist.*

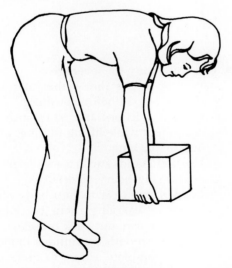

- Lower your center of gravity for more stability.
  —Bend at your hips and knees, not with your back (Figure 4-3).
  —Do not lean over to pick up or lift an object.
  —Use the large muscles of your legs to push against the floor as you rise or stand up.
  —Raise beds, tables, and stands to your best height for lifting or moving.
  —Do not carry or lift objects high enough so that you are working above your line of vision.

Figure 4-3.   *DO NOT strain to reach, or lift anything too heavy for yourself. Keep your back straight while bending your hips and knees. DO NOT use your back muscles to lift.*

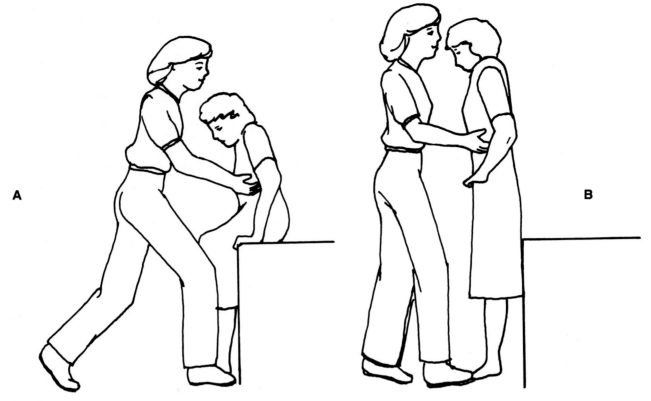

Figure 4-4. **A,** *Lower your center of gravity and widen your base of support.*
   B, *Use large leg and hip muscles to steady, balance, and lift. Shift weight between your forward and back feet for leverage.*

- Keep a wide base of support.
  - —A wide base of support can be established from front to back as well as from side to side.
  - —Use large leg and hip muscles to steady and balance and shift weight between forward and back feet, for leverage (Figure 4-4).
  - —Wide support allows you to move in more directions without twisting or bending.
  - —Moving things closer (pulling or sliding) to you before lifting, rather than straining to reach.

- Use your body for **leverage**
  - —Push or pull or slide rather than lift; choose to pull before pushing.
  - —Reduce friction and resistance to movement while lifting, sliding, pulling, or pushing.
  - —Use both hands and arms while lifting or carrying heavy objects.
  - —Keep objects close to your body while lifting or carrying them to reduce strain on arm and back muscles.
  - —Use one smooth continuous motion, as one complete action, to move objects from one point to another.
  - —Contract your abdominal and buttock muscles before you move or lift to ease strain on pelvis and back muscles and ligaments.
- Do not lift objects or people that are too heavy. Get help or use a mechanical lift.
- Think about every move you make.

General Rules for Moving and Positioning

- Use proper body mechanics.
- Check for safety such as locking bed and side rails.
- Know about your client before you move him; does he have:
  —areas with loss of sensation?
  —areas with pain or discomfort?
  —weakness or paralysis? where and to what extent?
  —dependent edema?
  —redness, sores, or infection of his skin?
  —difficulty breathing, respiratory equipment?
  —bowel or bladder incontinence, collection devices?
  —contractures, spasticity, or flaccid muscles?
  —special positioning requirements and schedule?
  —splints, braces, armboards, other devices?
- Know which positions and turns you can do alone and which require assistance.
- Keep the client in proper body alignment and provide necessary support.
- Protect your client from tendencies toward assuming any unusual positions. Examples include the natural force of gravity, which will pull the feet down and turn the legs out when a person lies supine. He may allow his disabled foot to droop downward, pointing the toes toward the ground. This may cause a permanent footdrop that will interfere with walking. Or a person with hemiplegia may have a tendency to dangle his affected arm over the side of the chair. Correct these positioning errors.

POSITIONS AND POSITIONING

This section describes correct procedures for positioning your client and aligning his body in commonly used positions. Try assuming these positions yourself or with a co-worker's guidance before positioning a client. You will be able to experience the differences that proper padding and alignment can make in positioning. Whenever you position your client, pay attention to movement and the placement, condition, and care of equipment. Attend to such items as drainage tubes and bags, external catheters, respiratory apparatus, ostomy bags, casts, and splints.

Prone

A client positioned prone lies on his stomach with his head turned to one side, preferably with no pillow (Figure 4-5). His arms are by his side, even with or just above the head and bent slightly at the elbows. His toes hang over the edge of the mattress with a small pad under his lower legs below the knee. Other padding can be placed under his shoulders if they fall forward, and also under the breast line. The spinal column must be in straight alignment. Observe your client regularly while he is in this position to be sure that prone positioning does not interfere with his breathing.

Semi-Prone

The person who is in prone position can be moved to semi-prone (Figure 4-6). Place him on one hip, without any twist to his spine. Bend his upper leg at the knee so it is in front of, but not resting on, his lower leg. Support it with a pillow. Extend his lower leg straight. Face your client toward his upper arm. Place his upper arm near his head, slightly bent at

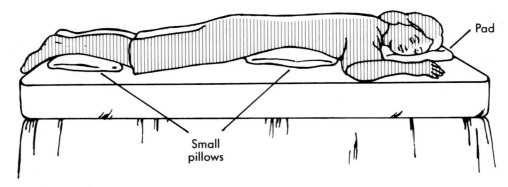

Pad

Small
pillows

Figure 4-5. *A client positioned prone. Check proper alignment and supportive pads or pillows.*

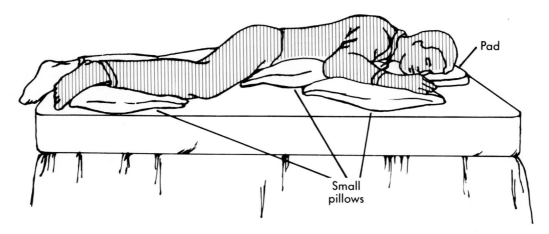

Pad

Small
pillows

Figure 4-6. *A client positioned semi-prone. Note the placement of pillows.*

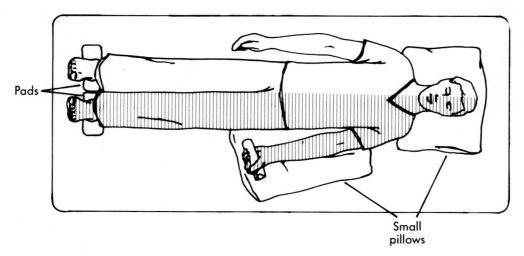

Pads

Small
pillows

Figure 4-7. *A client positioned supine. Attention to the details of positioning may prevent contractures, pressure areas, and other complications.*

the elbow, and supported on a pillow. The lower arm is extended behind him and along his side with the palm upwards. If he has a weakened or paralyzed arm, place that arm alongside his head. A pillow may be placed lengthwise from his lower rib cage to the upper abdomen.

Supine

A supine position places a person lying straight on his back with his arms and hands at his side (Figure 4-7). His legs and feet are extended and straight, not rolling in or out. Some clients use special rolled pillows called trochanter rolls, to keep their hips and thighs from turning inward or outward (Figure 4-8, a,b). If trochanter rolls are ordered for your client, be sure they extend from the client's knee to the top of his hip. Keep the bed flat except for a pillow under the client's head and shoulders.

Pad the client's elbows and heels to prevent skin breakdown, but avoid using a donut type of cushion. Do not use any cushioning that could cause uneven pressure on elbows or knees. Footboards benefit some persons, but may increase spasticity for others. Footboards are not recommended for every client. Alternatives for foot protection are discussed in Chapter 6. Prevent a client's feet from dropping or drooping with the toes pointed down. Do not allow the bedcovers to pull tightly across his toes. Instead use a bedcradle or box to support and lift the covers (Figure 4-9). A client may have difficulty extending his knee through the full range of motion. If so, do not place pillows under the thigh-knee area. Keep the knee straight.

A weakened or paralyzed arm or leg should be aligned and supported on a pillow. The palm of the affected hand is placed facing upward. The exception to this is the client who has an amputated limb. Do **not** place pillows under the hip, knee, or back and do

A

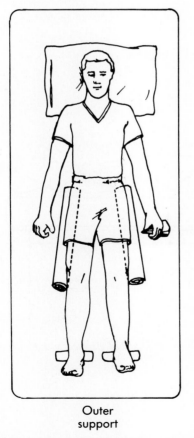

Outer
support

B

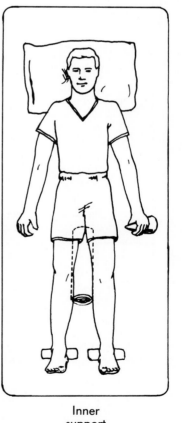

Inner
support

Figure 4-8. **A,** *Special rolled pads, called trochanter rolls, can be used to hold a client's hips and thighs in position so they do not roll inward or outward.*
  B, *Trochanter rolls extend from the top of the hip to below the knee.*

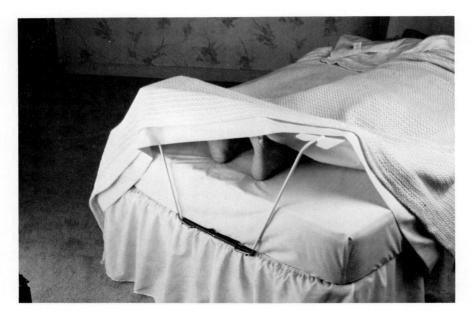

Figure 4-9. *Bed cradles can be used to keep the weight of bedcovers off the client's feet. Remember to position the client's feet flexed straight at the ankle, avoiding foot drop.*
  Reprinted by permission of © Bissell Healthcare Corporation/Fred Sammons, Inc.

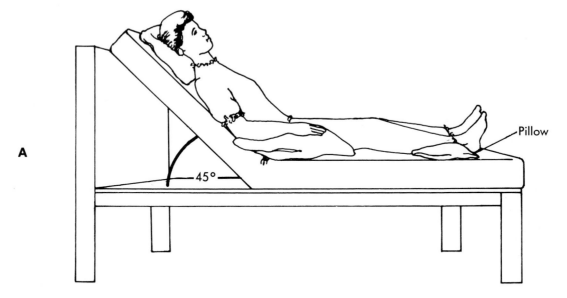

Figure 4-10. **A,** *An example of Fowler's position showing the head of the bed elevated to a 45-degree angle; it may be elevated to as much as a 60-degree angle.*

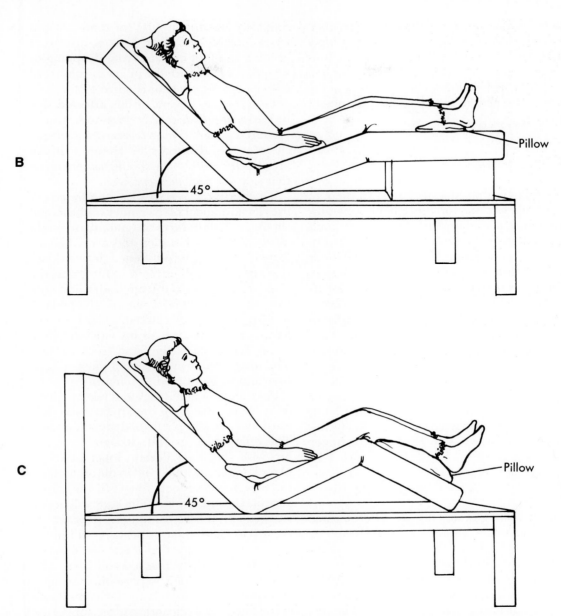

B

C

Figure 4-10, cont'd. **B,** *Fowler's position may include directions to flex the client's knees. Note the positions of the pillows under the legs and arms.*

 C, *Fowler's position may be ordered with the foot of the bed elevated as well as the head.*

not place pillows between the thighs of a person with a lower limb amputation. See Chapter 10 for special instructions about positioning clients who have had amputations.

Fowler's Position

Fowler's position is the same as supine except that the head of the bed is elevated to a 45-degree angle (sometimes as high as a 60-degree angle) (Figure 4-10 a). The client's arms are supported on pillows. Prevent your client from damaging his skin in this position. Whenever the head of his bed is elevated, he may slide and shear his skin on the bedclothes. This position is often recommended for persons with heart or respiratory problems and for those eating in bed. Your nurse supervisor will direct you when you are to use Fowler's position.

As a variation of Fowler's position, you may occasionally be instructed to elevate the foot of the bed (Figure 4-10 b). This is done for a client who has edema of the lower extremity. You may also need to flex his knee, using a knee gatch or a pillow under the back of his knees (Figure 4-10 c). If the foot of his bed cannot be elevated, read about elevating the foot of the bed on blocks in the Equipment Chapter.

Side-Lying

Side-lying is a position that allows a client to lie facing one way or the other. Generally, pillows are placed under his head and shoulder, under the upper leg and thigh, the upper arm and hand, and behind the lower back. There are some differences in side-lying positioning when the client has an affected side that is weakened or paralyzed.

The person who is *lying on his **unaffected** side* will use pillows under his head, upper arm and hand, upper leg and thigh, and foot (Figure 4-11). The entire length of the *affected* arm is supported on a pillow. The elbow is straight and the arm cannot drop or pull down his shoulder. His **affected** hand and wrist are supported with the palm facing either up or down. Use hand rolls or finger spreaders if they are ordered (Figure 4-12 a,b). Position your own arm and hand to test whether your palm naturally faces up or down.

If the client's leg and hip are *affected,* place them on a pillow, allowing a small amount of bending at his knee. Do not allow his foot to drop. Place a small pillow to support his upper back and to keep him from rolling back. Do not use the pillow if it causes him to arch his back or have a spastic response. The pillow at his back may cause a spastic response

similar to one that occurs for some persons when using a footboard. That is, instead of keeping the foot or back from dropping or sagging, contact with the pillow or footboard elicits a spastic reaction (Figure 4-13).

Do not place a client on his **affected** side unless *specifically directed* by your nurse supervisor. It is generally *not recommended* to place a client on his **affected** side. However, if you are directed to do so, he should *not* remain on that side for *more than one hour.*

The person who is *lying on his **affected** side* uses an additional pillow under his head and shoulder. This reduces the amount of weight on his affected shoulder and arm. The affected shoulder is positioned forward, including the shoulder blade. This places the affected arm fully out from under him onto the bed at a 45-degree angle with his body. A small pillow or pad is placed under his wrist, hand, and lower arm so his wrist does not bend. The palm of the hand faces upward. The **unaffected** arm rests on a pillow placed over and in front of the stomach.

Place a pillow at his back and rest him back on it. This helps keep the affected side forward and the rest of the body in alignment. The **affected** leg extends straight from the hip with the knee flexed. Small pads placed under the ankle and in the area where the toes meet the foot. They will keep pressure off the ankle bone. The pads will not be sufficient to relieve continuous pressure on the ankle. The nurse supervisor will direct you to use a device that elevates the entire heel off the bed, such as a cradle boot. The upper **unaffected** leg is positioned straight from the hip, but slightly forward and flexed at the knee. This leg and foot are supported on a pillow.

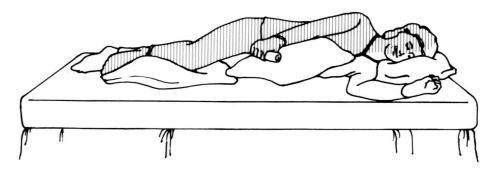

Figure 4-11.   *A client may be positioned side-lying on his **unaffected** side. His **affected** side must be supported in proper position and alignment.*

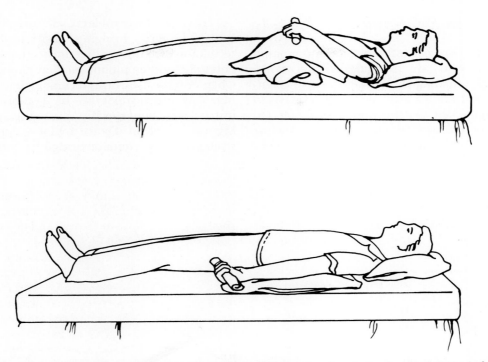

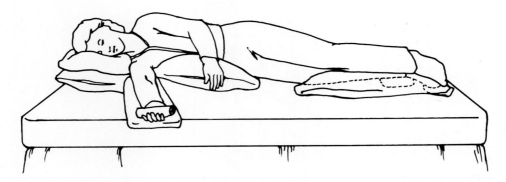

Figure 4-12.   *Hand rolls or cones are used to support the hand or wrist whether the client's palm is facing down or up.*

Figure 4-13.   *You may be directed to position a client side-lying on his **affected** side. If he has loss of sensation or other deficits, he may not be able to tell you if he has discomfort. Check positioning, alignment, and support carefully. Do not allow him to remain on his **affected** side for extended lengths of time.*

Position Bridging

This is a special technique for positioning persons who have disabilities. Pillows act like bridges, holding the body in proper alignment but not allowing certain body parts to touch the bed. One purpose of bridging is to keep pressure off sensitive skin areas, such as bony prominences or reddened areas, without creating other problems, such as contractures. The term "bridging" also refers to a technique used during dressing to enable clients to help when pulling on their pants. See Chapter 6 for use of this technique in dressing. Your nurse supervisor or therapist will instruct you about specific ways to use bridging for each client. Figure 4-14 a–c demonstrates the three common bridging positions.

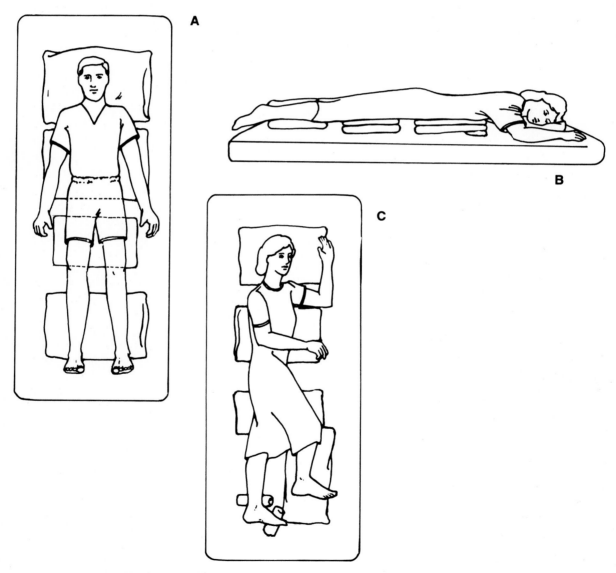

Figure 4-14.   **A,** *Bridging with pillows with the client in a supine position.*
   B, *Bridging with pillows with the client in a prone position.*
   C, *Bridging with pillows with the client in the side-lying position.*

TURNS AND TURNING

MOVING A CLIENT ON HIS BED

When clients spend increased amounts of time in bed, they may have problems with their basic functions. These include circulation and breathing, skin condition, and bowel and bladder function. Extended time in bed also produces mental sluggishness, dizziness, and reduced sensory responses. The amount of time spent in bed may be due to a physical cause. With disabling conditions, beds may also become places for clients to retreat and hide.

As a caregiver, you are aware of the problems your clients can develop simply from staying too long or too motionless in their beds. This section describes how to assist your client to turn in bed and to move in and out of his bed. Each client is turned or moved based on what he can or cannot do for himself and what special equipment or devices are available. Practice these techniques with your nurse supervisor. You should have practice and supervision for each exercise before performing it alone with a client.

Turning in Bed

There are three steps to think about for each move or turn. One step is the turning itself. The second step is the safety of both the client and yourself. The third step is the positioning of each body part after completing the turn.

Turning a Severely Dependent Client

One of the most difficult persons to move in bed is the person with a disability affecting all four limbs and the trunk, such as quadriplegia. The person with paraplegia can assist you in turning by using his arms and upper body. The person with quadriplegia, however, must be turned in bed frequently and regularly. Turning may be necessary as often as every two hours to avoid pressure areas.

Your nurse supervisor will direct you about the exact schedule for turning.

Establish the easiest and safest way for you and your client to make the turn before beginning the turn:

—review proper body mechanics,
—tell your client that you are going to turn him in a certain direction,
—listen to any instructions or concerns he may have to discuss,
—remove any jewelry that may cut or scratch him during the turn, and
—assist him to use a mirror to check any areas that are reddened as part of his morning or evening skin check after the turn.

Turning in Bed

The sequence of steps in Figure 4-15 a–e demonstrates how to turn your client when he is in his bed. Be sure to use proper body mechanics.

1. Lower the bed to a flat position and remove pillows. Raise and lock the siderails on the side the client will be facing after the turn. Siderails on the bed are necessary for safety and allow some clients to assist in the turns. You will be standing on the side of the bed opposite the siderails.
2. Remember that you must move the client's body without dragging it on the sheets. The bony areas of the body must be lifted when turning. Do not allow them to be dragged across the sheets as the skin will be sheared, causing sheet burns.
3. Place your hands under the person's lower body, under the buttocks and thighs, as illustrated in Figure 4-15 a. In a sliding motion, lift the person's lower body toward you. Repeat moving his legs and feet (Figure 4-15 b).
4. Stand by the upper portion of his body. Slide your hands under him at the shoulder level until you can reach his distant shoulder. Lift his shoulders and head toward you (Figure 4-15 c). This should place him closer to you so that he will be in the center of the bed when turned.
5. Raise the siderail, then walk around to

the other side of the bed. Lower that siderail. Place your hands as shown in Figure 4-15 d. Roll the client toward you. Place a small pillow under his head.

6. Check the position of his leg that is lying underneath so that it is in alignment with his hips and shoulders. Lift the top leg, flexing it at the hip and at the knee. This will position it slightly in front of his underneath leg. Support it with a pillow from mid-thigh to below his ankle and supporting his foot.

7. Position the client's lower arm with his elbow flexed and positioned out from under his body. The upper arm should come straight out from under his body. His forearm will be parallel with his body (Figure 4-15 e). Place a small pillow under the forearm, extending from above the flexed elbow to his fingers.

8. Make sure that the spinal column is straight and the hips are in alignment with the body. Position his head and shoulders with pillows so that he is comfortable. Look to see where pillows are needed to support his body.

9. The client can relieve weight from his dependent hip by rotating his upper leg back and letting the weight fall onto the dependent buttock. This position is recommended for clients who turn side to side frequently or who have areas of skin breakdown at the trochanter.

10. All resting splints, night splints, and other equipment should be checked to be sure they do not affect positioning or cause redness of the skin. Be sure that all drainage devices are free of constriction and properly affixed to the client. Move drainage devices from side to side as the client turns.

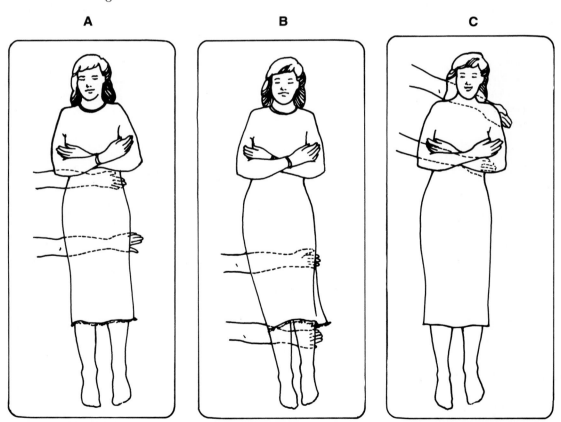

Figure 4-15. **A,** *Raise and lock the opposite siderail on the bed; lock the bed casters. Maintain good posture and use proper body mechanics. Begin by placing your hands under his buttocks and thighs as shown.*
  B, *Lift his lower body and legs toward you. Do not drag his skin across the sheets.*
  C, *Lift his upper body and head toward you.*

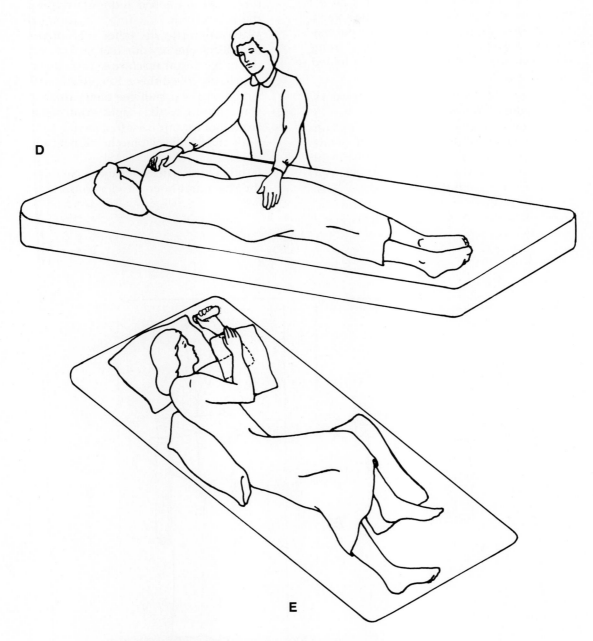

Figure 4-15, cont'd.   **D,** *Roll the client toward you.*
E, *Return the client to a proper position and alignment.*

Using a Turning Sheet to Turn a Severely Disabled Person

The turn just described is used for all severely disabled persons. If you cannot move or roll the person with your arms, you may want to use a turning sheet. This is a strong sheet (a draw sheet) or a smoothly folded straight sheet.

1. Place the sheet under the person as shown in Figure 4-16 a–b.
2. Allow enough of the sheet to extend on either side of the person. Roll the ends of the sheet into a handful. When you are ready to roll the client, you will need to have a good grip on the sheet rolls. Before turning him, raise the siderail on the side of the bed he will be facing when turned.
3. Stand on the side of the bed opposite the direction your client will face after the turn. Use the sheet to pull, bringing the person close to you. Do this before turning him to be sure he will end up in the center of the bed and not turn into the bedrails.
4. Walk around to the other side of the bed. Place one of your feet in front of the other as you reach over your client to grip the rolled sheet. Keep your back straight as you pull the sheet toward you, shifting your weight from your front foot to your back foot as you pull. Your client will roll onto his side facing you.
5. Position him as directed above. Smooth the sheet and linens under him.

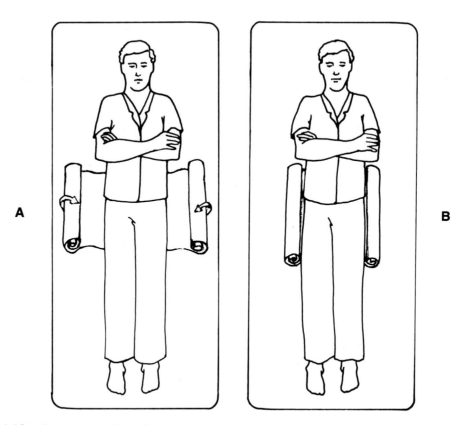

Figure 4-16.   **A,** *A turning sheet placed under the client's hips may assist you to move or turn him while he is in bed.*
    B, *Roll the ends of the turning sheet into tight rolls that can be used as handholds while turning the client.*

Pulling a Client up in Bed Using a Draw Sheet

Clients who are severely disabled may also be *moved up or down in the bed* using the rolled edges of a draw sheet as a lifting and pulling device.

- Use caution so that your client does not incur sheet burns or other skin damage.
- This type of move requires another person across the bed from you. Both of you stand facing the bed, then turn to face the direction of the head of the bed before you move.
- Keep the rolled draw sheet close in to your body, avoiding unnecessary reaching.
- Shift your weight from one foot to the other to give you leverage as you move the client up in bed.
- Remember to keep your back straight and your knees over your feet, pull with as little actual lifting as possible, and use large muscles to move the weight.
- Coordinate the steps of the move among the two movers and the client so that everyone works together with one continuous motion. Do not bump your client's head by moving him too far.

Turning Clients Who Have Some Abilities to Assist

Some clients can assist with turning and moving in bed by using overhead trapeze bars (Figure 4-17 a–b). They use the trapeze to pull up or to move sideways in bed. A client may have one paralyzed or affected side of

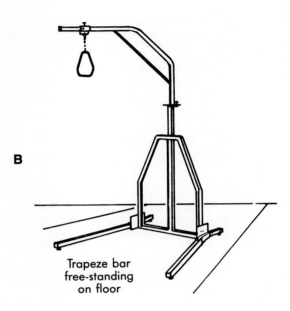

B

Trapeze bar
free-standing
on floor

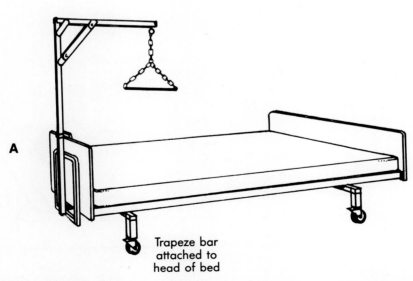

A

Trapeze bar
attached to
head of bed

Figure 4-17. *Clients who are able to use overhead trapeze bars can help to turn side-to-side, move up or down in bed, or get to a sitting position while in bed. Trapeze bars are attached to the head of the bed or an overhead bar (**A**) or may be free-standing floor models (**B**).*

his body. He can assist by using his **unaffected** arm with the trapeze to lift part of his body while you move his hips and shoulders. A person with a strong lower body can bend his knees, place his feet flat on the bed, and push to move up in bed or turn. You assist with his head, arms and upper body.

These clients can also reach the siderails or side of the mattress to help them pull and turn (Figure 4-18, a–b). To assist a client to turn toward his **affected** side, position his **affected** arm and hand toward the edge of the bed. Instruct him to reach the edge of the mattress with his **unaffected** hand. As he pulls himself toward the mattress edge, he pushes with his **unaffected** foot. Once turned, recheck the position of his **affected** arm and hand so they are not trapped under the weight of his body (Figure 4-18 a).

To assist a client to turn toward his **unaffected** side, place his **affected** hand and arm across his abdomen. Instruct him to grasp the edge of the mattress with his **unaffected** hand. Then he slides his **unaffected** leg under his **affected** leg. He uses the **unaffected** leg to slightly lift and move the **affected** leg toward the direction of his turn. Reposition his **affected** arm and leg. Straighten his shoulders toward the **unaffected** side (Figure 4-18 b).

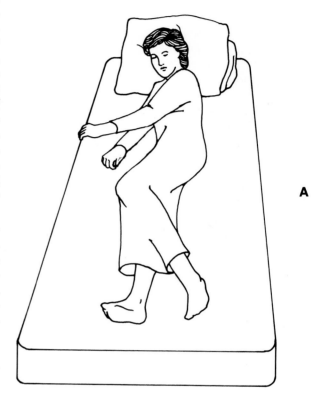

A

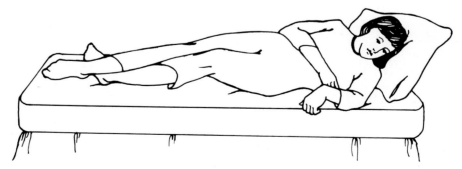

B

Figure 4-18. *Some clients are able to turn themselves in bed with minimal assistance. Encourage self-care whenever possible.* **A** *shows a client turning to his* **affected** *side;* **B** *shows a client turning to his* **unaffected** *side.*

Clients Who Have Pain When Turning and Moving

Some clients are restricted from turning and moving themselves because of pain or low tolerance to moving. Examples include clients who have chronic conditions like arthritis and Parkinson's disease. It is important to understand that people have different abilities and tolerances to turning and positioning at different times. Your client may do well at one time, but be able to do very little later the same day. Clients with arthritic conditions or Parkinson's disease are stiffer in the morning than in the afternoon. They can tell you how to help them without causing pain.

These clients can become totally dependent due to their pain. For example, they may be able to tolerate only a small pillow for positioning, for a short time, because of pain. At other times, they can assist and be positioned with pillows under each limb. An arthritic client may prefer to roll onto his stomach and then back himself out of bed. This works better if the bed is higher off the floor than usual. Some clients have had surgery to replace joints, such as hip replacement surgery. See Chapter 12 for information on hip replacement surgery. Check with the nurse supervisor or physical therapist for the safest way to move these clients until they are better able to assist you.

If you have a client who has pain, talk to your nurse supervisor about developing a schedule with your client. This client may be an older person or young and severely disabled. There are no general rules for moving these people. You must work together with your client under the direction of the nurse. Have the nurse supervisor check your turning and positioning procedures. Whenever possible, the nurse will include the client and the family in planning care. This helps everyone to work together for the best results. It will make your client feel less dependent if he can make some of the decisions about his care.

If turning is not tolerated well, you should ask the nurse about a different mattress for your client. There are many special mattresses designed to prevent pressure areas. Examples include air or gel Flotation mat-

tresses, eggcrate mattresses, Kodel pads, and others. Bedding is discussed in Chapter 6. If your client has a special mattress, you must be extremely careful about bowel and bladder care. All beds must be kept clean, dry, and free of wrinkles, sharp edges, and even scraps of paper.

Moving to a Sitting Position on the Bed

This is an in-the-bed sitting position with the *legs remaining in the bed.* It is important that clients sit up in bed because it helps them to change positions and to perform other activities such as dressing. Some people cannot get to a sitting position and remain sitting in bed unless they are supported by raising the head of the bed or with pillows. For example, clients with weakness on one side following stroke or clients with Parkinson's disease whose legs are rigid may not be able to sit this way without supports. Each person is very much an individual about what he can and cannot do.

Bed-Sitting for a Person with an Affected Side

This procedure is used for the client with an **unaffected** arm when he brings himself to a sitting position in bed (Figure 4-19). If your client can manage this move, it will be easier for others to assist him in turning and moving. If he has difficulty remembering, you may have to repeat the steps for him each time. Encourage him to do this for himself as much as he can.

1. Elevate the head of the bed slightly if it can be raised. If the bed cannot be raised, place extra pillows behind the person to lift him from the flat position. Too much height will work against the person (Figure 4-19 a).
2. Support and assist him if needed by placing one of your hands on his upper back. You will be able to support him if he starts to fall.

Have your client:
3. Cross his **affected** arm over the stomach.

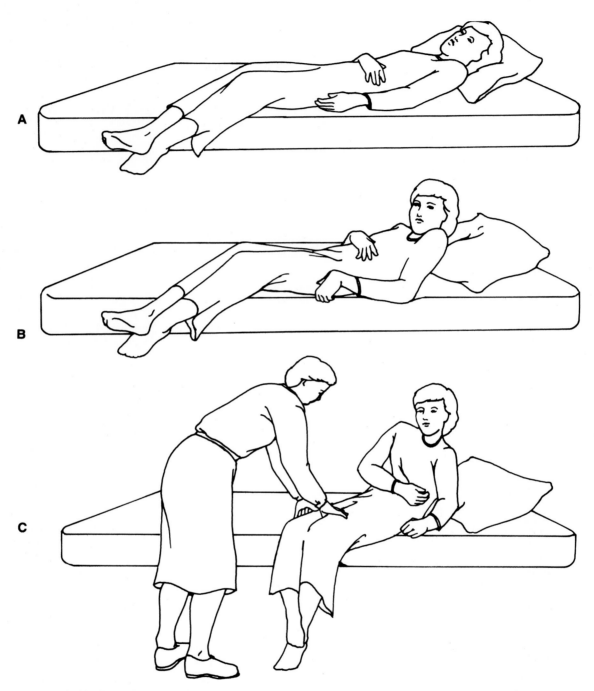

Figure 4-19. *Bed-sitting for the client with an **affected** side and requiring **minimal** assistance.*
    A, *The client places his **affected** arm across his abdomen.* **B** *and* **C,** *He slides his **unaffected** foot under his **affected** leg at the back of his ankle.* **D** *and* **E,** *He lifts both legs across the bed toward his **unaffected** side. Raising the head of the bed, if permissible, may assist him to sit.*

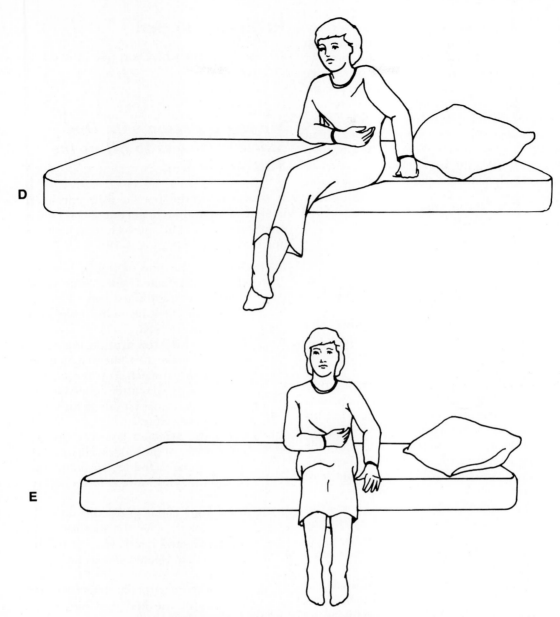

Figure 4-19, cont'd. *For legend see opposite page.*

4. Use his **unaffected** hand to grasp the mattress or siderail on the same side.
5. Pull forward onto his **unaffected** elbow.
6. Straighten the arm while lifting his head and shoulders forward until he is sitting.

You assist to:

7. Position his legs, arms, and hips. Use pillows to prop his **affected** arm and hand.

Some clients prefer to cross the **unaffected** arm over the **affected** side and grasp the mattress across their **affected** side. This is more difficult for the client.

Reverse these steps when your client returns to lie down in bed.

Short-Sitting in Bed in Preparation for Transfer for Persons with Spinal Cord Injuries

This procedure is the first step in preparing for a client with spinal cord injury to transfer from the bed to another seat. The transfer is usually to a wheelchair. Clients with spinal cord injury vary in their abilities to perform this procedure and to transfer. If your client can do these moves, he has probably also worked out his own methods. Any move or transfer should be in line with the procedure described below. Ask your nurse supervisor or the physical therapist to supervise and approve other procedures.

You must consider safety for your client and yourself. Know how much he can help himself during the movement. You need to work closely with the client, his family, and your nurse about how to move him. Your client may be able to tell you every step of the moves, but be unable to assist.

To Assist a Client to Short-Sit

1. Move the client's legs to the side of the bed while he is on his back. (Some clients do this after they are partially sitting.)
2. Have him sit up or assist him to a sitting position by raising the head of the bed. The client may not be able to bend his back far enough to reach his legs or not have enough arm strength to move his legs. Raising the head of the bed will also assist him to sit and provide support while you move his legs.
3. If he can assist, have him hold onto the side of the bed and pull himself forward. At the same time, you move his legs over the side of the bed. Then bend his knees.
4. He then needs to reach a steady balance point. For example, he may use his arms for balance by placing them in his lap, at his side, or behind him.
5. Lower the head of the bed so it is out of the way for the next step of transferring out of the bed.

Alternate Method

If your client cannot do this movement, you can try to have him assist you in another way.

You grasp his arms above the wrist with both hands. He also pulls as you pull him upright toward you. He may perform the same maneuver with a trapeze if he has one.

Returning to Bed

Reverse the steps when you put your client back into bed.

Moving a Person with One-Sided Weakness to Sit at the Side of the Bed

It is easier for the person with one-sided weakness or paralysis to get out of bed on the **unaffected** side. This allows him to assist as much as possible (Figure 4-19).

1. Stand at the side of the bed on the client's **unaffected** side. Your client will be moving toward you.
2. Have your client lie on his back in the middle of the bed.
3. Place the **affected** arm on top of his stomach. Make sure the arm stays in place on the stomach. You may need to remind him to pay attention to his arm if he is not aware of it due to his stroke or other condition.
4. Cross the **affected** leg over the **unaffected** leg at the ankles. He can then use his **unaffected** leg to lift the **affected** one and move it to the side of the bed.
5. Have your client grasp the siderails, the bedclothes, or the mattress with his **unaffected** hand. He will roll toward his **unaffected** side as he grasps and pulls.
6. Move his legs so that both feet are over the side of the bed. Let him do as much as possible.
7. Stand on his **affected** side, so that you can assist him to keep a steady sitting balance.
8. Make sure his **affected** arm is still in front of him and on his stomach.
9. Ask your client to pull up onto his **unaffected** elbow. Assist by holding the **affected** hand and arm in place, while rolling the **affected** shoulder forward. Do not pull or jerk. Use a firm, rolling motion.
10. Move his legs and feet so that both feet are as close to the floor as possible. This will let him pull against the bed for leverage.

11. Ask your client to straighten his **un-affected** arm (he is now on his **unaffected** elbow). When he does this, he will be able to reach a sitting position.

Lying Down after Sitting

To move your client from sitting to lying down, reverse the procedure (Figure 4-20). Be sure you know your client's abilities and preferred ways of moving.

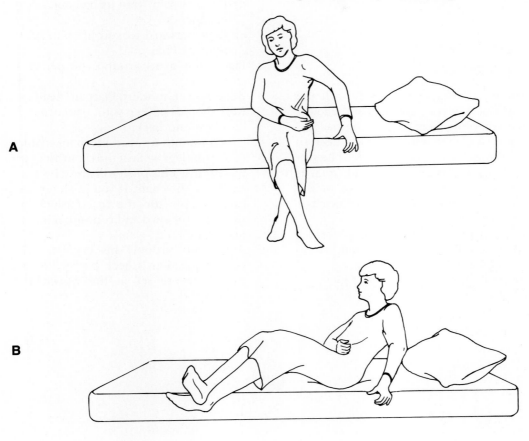

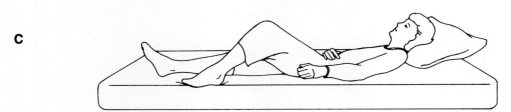

Figure 4-20. *Lying down from a sitting position for a client with an **affected** side.*

    A, *The client placed his **affected** hand and arm securely in his lap. His **unaffected** foot is behind his affected leg at the ankle. Check his position on the bed so he will arrive with his head on the pillow when he lies down.*

    B, *He uses his **unaffected** hand to grasp the edge of the mattress near his hips. As he bends his elbow, his upper body will lower onto the bed. At the same time, he lifts both legs using the **unaffected** leg, swinging them up onto the bed.*

    C, *Reposition his arm, hand, and body; uncross his legs.*

PULLING A CLIENT UP IN A CHAIR OR WHEELCHAIR

Two methods are suggested for this procedure.

Method 1—For one or two caregivers

1. Stand in front of the client with the lower part of your leg against the lower part of your client's leg. If he has slid down too far forward, you will need to have another person available. The second person, standing behind, guards against the client slipping out of the chair. Lock the brakes on a wheelchair or commode chair.

   Be prepared if you need to prevent a client from falling out of his chair. To do this: (Figure 4-21 a–c)
   a) Block his foot with your foot.
   b) Block his knee with your knee.
   c) Place your arms around his chest.
   d) Bend at your waist using good body mechanics.
   e) Rock forward as you lift him back into the chair.
2. Place your arms around the person's chest.
3. Bend him at his waist. Place his head on your shoulder. Keep your arms around his chest and back.
4. Give a smooth upward lift to his trunk.
5. Push your legs against the client's legs as you lift up. This push will move his seat back into the chair. If you push too far back, simply use the seat cushion to slide him forward and reposition him if necessary.
6. Align and support his body in the proper position. Check his legs to be sure they are set in the wheelchair footrests.

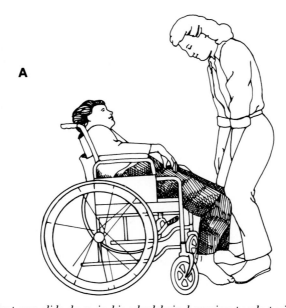

Figure 4-21. *A client may slide down in his wheelchair, becoming poorly positioned and in danger of falling. One or two caregivers may move him back into his chair using the following method. Practice with your nurse supervisor.*

   A, *Lock the wheelchair and swing away the footrests. Stand in front of your client with your knee and leg just below the knee against his knee and leg. Keep a wide base of support, one foot slightly ahead of the other for leverage. Place his feet flat on the floor.*

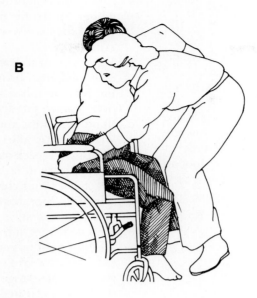

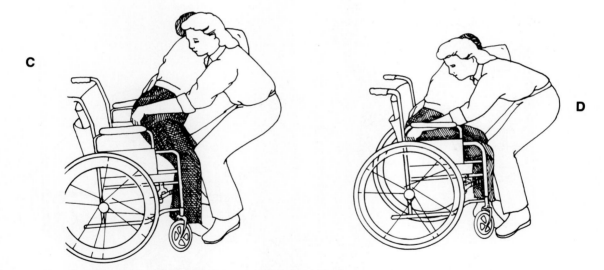

Figure 4-21, cont'd.   B, *Block him from sliding forward with your knees and legs. Place his head and arms over your shoulder as illustrated. Place your arms around his waist, under his arms, and your hand onto his lower back. The exact placement of your hands will vary according to your height and the client's size.*

   C, *Keep your back straight; use the muscles of your legs and buttocks. Lift as little as possible by using leverage to move him slightly forward and upward. Move smoothly, shifting your weight in a forward rocking motion.*

   D, *Finish the motion by shifting your weight and using leverage to rock him back into the chair. Keep your knees against his knees as you lower him down and back so he sits fully into the seat of the chair. DO NOT drop him down into the chair. Realign his position and supports.*

Method 2—Using Bobath principles, one caregiver

1. Place your client's feet flat on the floor, free of the wheelchair footrests.
2. Stand facing your client at his affected side.
3. Stand straddling his affected leg. Place your foot that is toward the outside wheel of the wheelchair (or arm of chair) forward. Keep your other foot on the floor. Place your inside knee against your client's affected knee (Figure 4-22 a).

4. Assist your client to fold his hands together in front of him. Have him straighten his elbows and reach with his arms.
5. Support him to lean over forward. His extended arms bring his hands toward his feet and his shoulders are positioned above his feet.
6. Bend your hips and knees. Keep your knee against the client's unaffected knee as you reach over your client's bent back (Figure 4-22 b).
7. Reach over your client and grasp either side of his hips, moving him toward the back of the seat.
8. Shift your weight from the front foot to the back foot as you move your client. Once your weight is on your back foot, put your knees together. Then press on the client's affected knee to push him back into the chair. Push him back into the seat. ***Do not lift him.***
9. Align and support him as necessary (Figure 4-22 c).

A

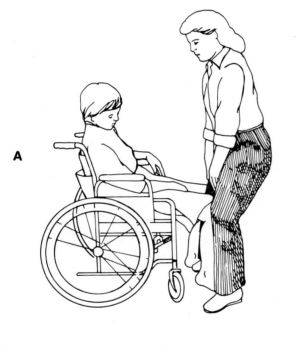

B

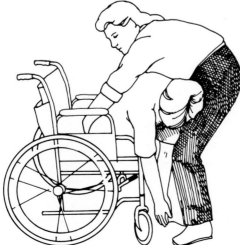

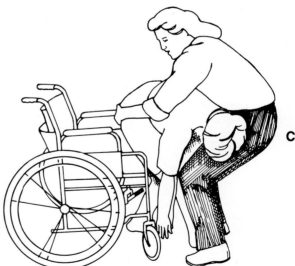

C

Figure 4-22. *For legend see opposite page.*

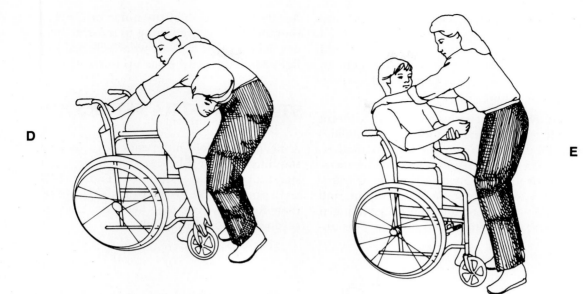

Figure 4-22. *An alternative (Bobath based) method for one caregiver to move a client up in a wheelchair or chair.*

*A, Lock the wheelchair brakes. Place your client's feet flat on the floor and stand facing his **affected** side (right side in this illustration). While straddling his **affected** leg at the knee, place your outside foot forward and your inside knee against his **affected** knee.*

B, Have your client place his hands with palms together; then straighten his arms at the elbows while leaning over to reach toward his feet. Support him carefully as he leans over, blocking him from sliding forward with your knees and legs. Bend your knees slightly as you support him.

C, Keep your back straight and use proper body mechanics. Reach over your client as shown, and grasp either side of his hips.

*D, Use your knee in a gentle, smooth motion to push against his **affected** knee, helping to push him toward the back of the wheelchair seat. Do not lift him; use leverage instead.*

*E, Reposition him in the chair with proper alignment and support. Encourage him to assist you as much as possible; he may be able to support his **affected** arm.*

TRANSFERS

The term **transfer** is used in rehabilitation to describe how persons with disabilities move from one point to another. Being able to transfer is an important step in independence and mobility for a disabled person. Remember that moving your client faster by yourself is not the goal. Keeping the client as independent as possible is one goal. Safety for your client and yourself is another goal.

The following list contains factors to consider before planning a transfer of any disabled person:

- What is your size, weight, and strength in relation to your client's?

- Does your client want to transfer?
- How aware or alert is your client? How much does he understand about what you are going to do together?
- Is your client able to assist you? How much and with what part of his body?
- Does your client need to wear a device to make the transfer? Is a long or short leg brace, a lower limb prosthesis, a sitting corset, or back brace needed for a safe transfer?
- Is a transfer belt available?
- Is the "landing" place prepared for the transfer from the bed? For example, is

the commode or wheelchair in place and locked?

● Have you decided on the easiest and safest transfer procedure for both of you? Can you review and see the steps in your mind?

Remember that each client is a bit different in what he can and cannot do. His abilities may be different from one time to another. You must be prepared for these differences. Read through the next section about transfers. Try to picture some of your clients and how they would fit into the transferring if you were doing them. Practice transfers un-der the supervision of the nurse or physical therapist before attempting to transfer a client. Never allow a client who feels dizzy or light-headed when he sits up to stand up.

STANDING TRANSFERS

A person is safely independent to make a standing transfer if he can walk, sit down, or stand up without assistance (Figure 4-23 a–f). Some people are safe once they are on their feet. However, they need assistance to sit down or stand up safely.

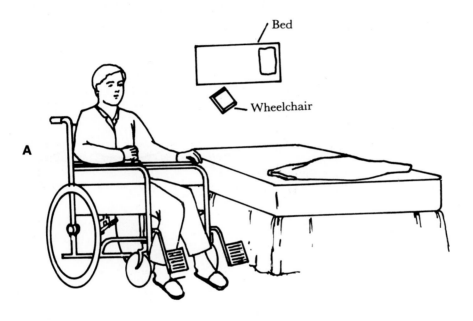

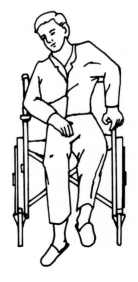

Figure 4-23.   *Independent standing transfer.*

A, *Lock brakes and lift footrests. Angle the wheel-chair close to the bed, facing the head of the bed, preferably on the client's **unaffected** side. Instruct client to place both his feet flat onto the floor.*

B, *Place his unaffected foot directly beneath the wheelchair seat. It will be slightly behind the **affected** foot. His **unaffected** hand is on the armrest and he sits to the front of the wheelchair seat.*

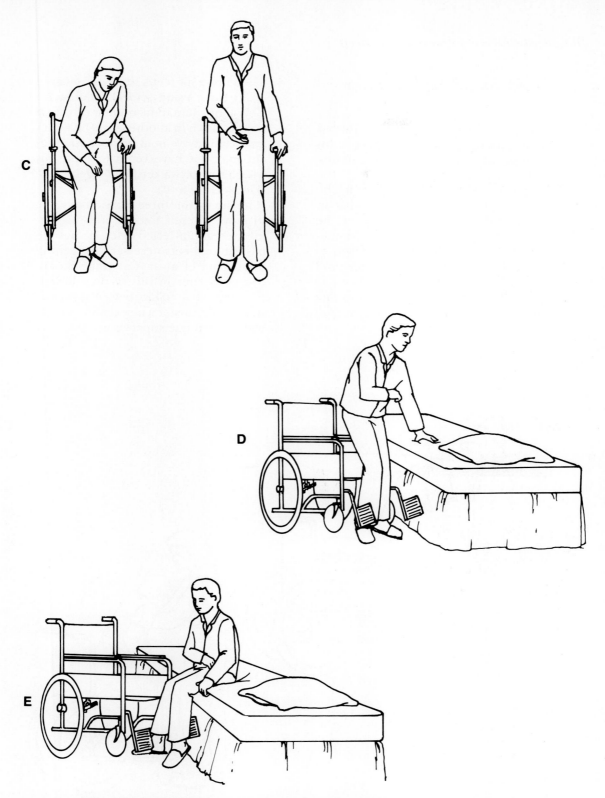

Figure 4-23, cont'd. **C,** *As he leans forward over his **unaffected** foot and pushes on the armrest, he will arise. His weight and balance depend on his **unaffected** arm and leg.*

   D, *The client continues to use the armrest and keeps his feet slightly apart for safety and balance. If he is tall, he may need adjustable height armrests in order to stand erect and reach the armrest to balance.*

   E, *The client uses his **unaffected** arm to balance and support himself on the edge of the bed. He will use short sidesteps to turn toward his **unaffected** side. When his back is to the bed, he can sit on the bed. Figure 4-16 illustrates lying down after sitting.*

Assisted Standing Transfer

1. To assist a client, stand on his **affected** side. This will allow him full use of his own strength and you will be standing out of his way.
2. You can hold onto the waist or belt if he is wearing slacks. Assist him with an upward movement as he rises. If he wears a long leg brace or an above-the-knee prosthesis, he may need you to assist him in keeping his balance until the brace or prosthesis is locked.
3. When this person transfers from one place to another he must first be in a *full upright position.*

4. Then move his feet a simple 45-degree or ¼ turn, using several small steps. This allows him to face a new direction or to sit down in another seat. This is an important movement because your client may not have room to move his wheelchair or walker from side to side (Figure 4-24 a–d).
5. If he can master these moves and is able to move himself toward both his unaffected and affected sides, he has the basic movements necessary for getting in and out of a car. Car transfers are discussed later in this section. Review the steps that follow before trying to stand and transfer a new client. Practice with your nurse supervisor.

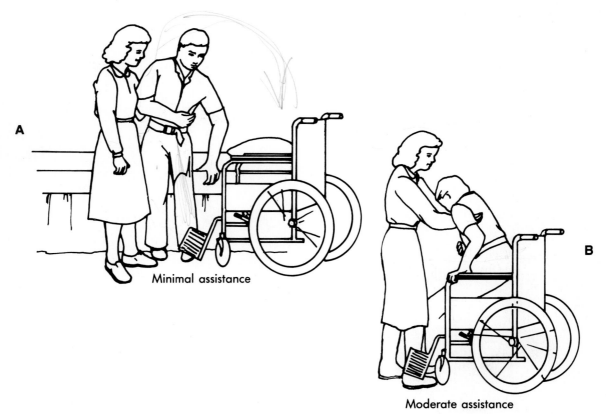

Figure 4-24.   *Three levels of assistance for standing transfers.*
   A, *Stand on the client's **affected** side when giving him minimal assistance. Use a transfer belt for safety.*
   B, *To offer moderate assistance, place your arms under his armpits. Extend your hands onto his back, and keep his head and weight over his knees until he can sit down. Do not lift with your back. Keep your feet apart and one foot slightly ahead of the other.*

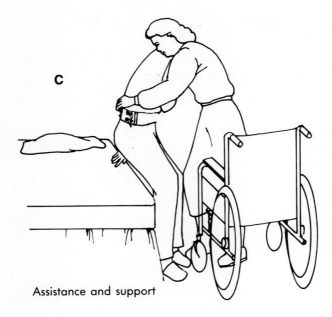

C

Assistance and support

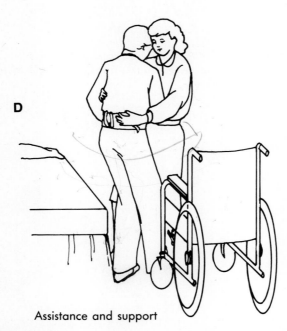

D

Assistance and support

Figure 4-24, cont'd. **C,** *When the client needs a great deal of assistance, you will have to balance, lift, and pivot him. Face your client and put your arms around his waist. Put your right knee against his* **affected** *knee to help brace it. Keep your other leg in a wide stance and slightly behind. He will bear weight on his* **unaffected** *leg. In one smooth movement, pull him forward and upward.*

D, *Pivot on your right leg and his* **unaffected** *leg. Turn toward his affected side and lower him to his wheelchair or bed.*

Moving out of Bed into a Chair

This move uses the same principles as the other transfers. Study the series of steps (Figure 4-25 a–c). Practice them under the direction of the nurse supervisor before assisting your client.

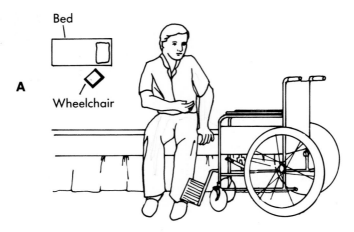

Figure 4-25.   *Standing transfer from bed to a chair, commode, or wheelchair*

   A, *Lock the brakes or casters and lift or swing away the footrests. Place the chair at an angle close to the bed or the client's **unaffected** side, as shown.*

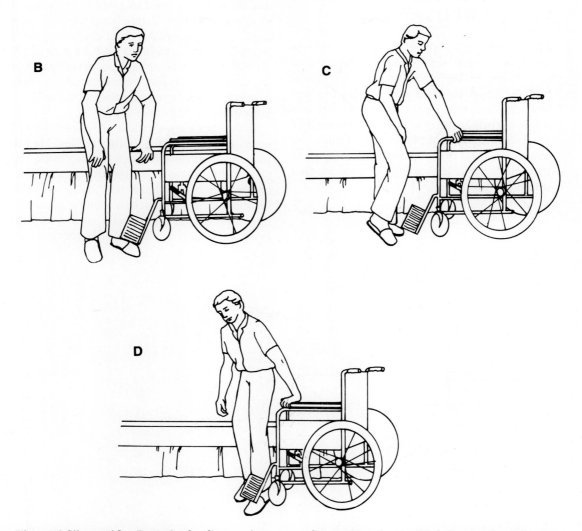

Figure 4-25, cont'd. **B,** *Assist the client to rise to a standing position, keeping his balance and weight supported on his **unaffected** side.*

C, *Instruct the client to turn on his **unaffected** foot while reaching for the chair armrest with his **unaffected** hand. He must keep his weight and balance over his **unaffected** side.*

D, *Once he has completed the turn, he may support himself with his hand on the armrest. Then he can ease himself into the chair; he should avoid dropping his weight into the chair.*

TRANSFERS FOR THE CLIENT WITH A LOWER LIMB AMPUTATION

Clients with either above- or below-the-knee amputations are able to do standing transfers. However, they must keep their balance. A client has both arms and one leg to assist him with balance. The transfer for this person is slightly different. He must remember not to hop on his foot as he moves. Unless the amputation was due to an accident, the other foot and leg may have medical problems that would be bothered by hopping.

The person with an amputated leg will position his residual foot slightly forward so that he will only need to pivot as he turns to sit. He will reach with one hand to the seat he is going to sit upon. An older client may need practice in order to build up his confidence. He will still tend to step out incorrectly on the leg that has been amputated. Study the picture below before moving the person with an amputated leg (Figure 4-26 a,b).

If the client is wearing a prosthesis, he will stand and pivot on his **unaffected** leg. He will move toward his **unaffected** side, using the arm and hand on that side for support. The opposite arm and hand will assist him with balance on the wheelchair arm or grab bar, but must not be his primary source of support and balance (Figure 4-27 a–c).

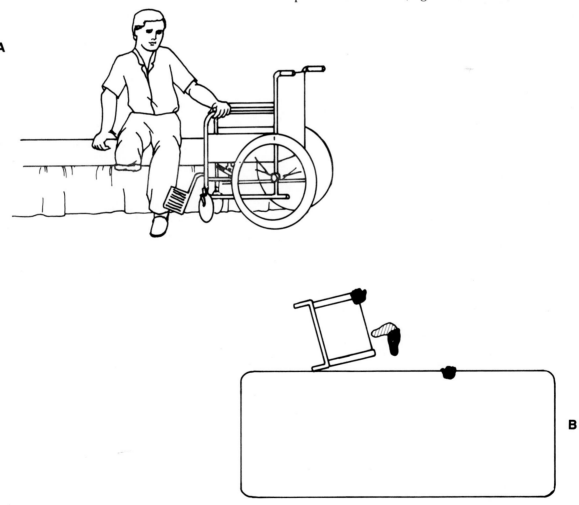

A

B

Figure 4-26. *Standing transfers adapted for the person with a lower limb amputation. Lock the brakes or casters and swing away the footrests. The client places his **residual** foot slightly forward to bear most of his weight. He pivots on his **residual** foot and leg as he changes position. He places his hand on the armrest ahead of his move, giving support and balance.*

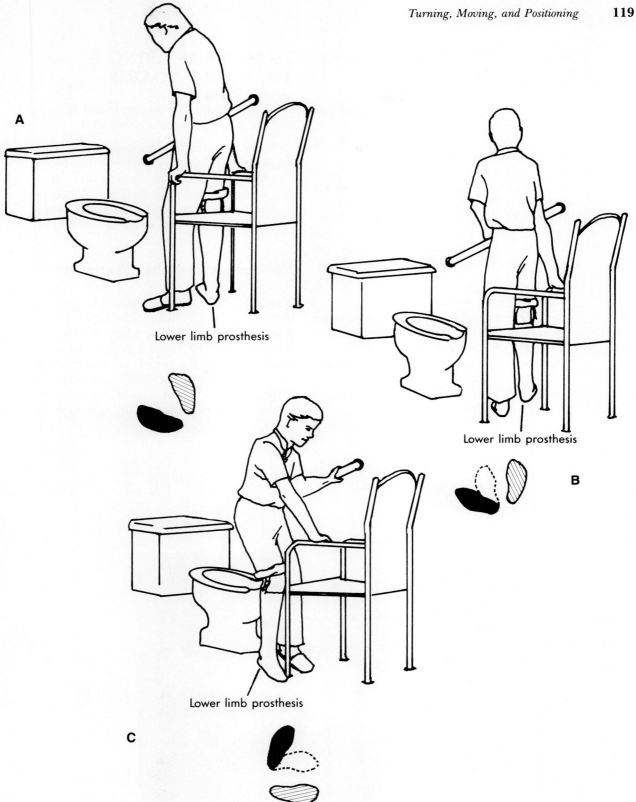

Figure 4-27.   *Pivot transfer for the client wearing a lower limb prosthesis.*

   A, *The client is shown wearing a lower limb prosthesis on his **affected** leg. Lock any braces or casters; lock the knee of the prosthesis if applicable.*

   B, *The client will pivot with his weight on his **residual** limb (his **unaffected** leg).*

   C, *His **residual** limb provides his main support and balance. Assist him as necessary for safety.*

SEMI- OR HALF-STANDING TRANSFER

The half-standing transfer can be done when you are moving your client alone. This is only done when the nurse supervisor has assessed the client's ability to make the transfer. This transfer should be easy to perform if your client is light in weight. Be sure your client is awake and alert. Remind him of the steps in the transfer. Tell him that you will do all the work. He will only be able to move over a few inches by himself. Study the steps below and practice the transfer before moving a client.

1. Move your client to the front of his chair or edge of the bed.
2. Place your hands either under his arms, around his chest, or grasp both sides of his waistband or transfer belt.
3. Use one continuous motion to transfer him:
   a) Begin with your back straight and knees slightly bent.
   b) Rock to get momentum and turn your client as you straighten your knees and turn.
   c) Turn the ¼ or half-turn necessary to place him on the seat.

TRANSFERS USING A TRANSFER BOARD

A transfer using a transfer board (Figure 4-28) is a way to move a client who:

—cannot perform a standing transfer;
—is too tall or too heavy for you to move;
—has multiple sclerosis and is too weak to stand, but can hold a sitting balance; or
—has spinal cord injury and can be maintained in a balanced sitting position.

Procedure for the Transfer

A wooden or fiberglass transfer board is placed under the client. The other end is positioned on the surface where the client is transferring. The client is assisted to move sideways across the board. He lifts his buttocks as he moves, performing a series of "little push-ups." (See Chapter 5 for information on the transfer board and how to make one.)

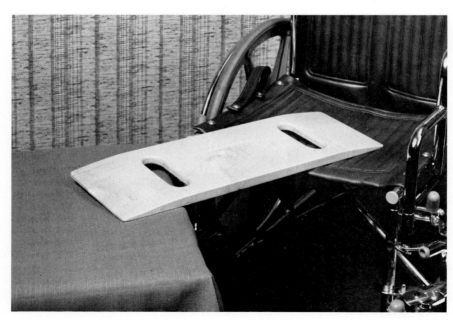

Figure 4-28.   *A transfer board may be used to assist clients to move from one seat to another. Reprinted by permission of © Bissell Healthcare Corporation/Fred Sammons, Inc.*

Transfer Board from Bed to Wheelchair

Some clients can get to and stay in a sitting position for a short time. You can assist these clients to transfer from bed to a wheelchair with the following procedure:

1. Position the wheelchair on the side of the bed where there is the most room. If your client has an affected side, try to place the wheelchair on the stronger side.
2. Lock the brakes, remove the armrest, and swing away or remove the footrest.
3. Set the transfer board on the end of the bed within reach. Match the height of the bed as closely as possible with the height of the wheelchair seat.
4. Bring your client to the edge of the bed, using the techniques described earlier in this chapter. His feet should be able to reach the floor securely or to step onto a sturdy wooden box or footstool.
5. Stand in front of him. Use your arm that is away from the wheelchair to tilt him toward the bed and away from the wheelchair. This will let you slide the transfer board under his thigh (on the same side as the wheelchair).
6. Reposition him upright so that he is sitting on one end of the transfer board and in good balance.
7. Point the other end of the transfer board toward the opposite corner of the wheelchair seat. The board will pass over the wheel and the end will rest on top of the wheelchair seat cushion.
8. Position your client for a successful transfer. How he is positioned depends upon his ability to balance himself.
   a) If he *cannot assist* in keeping his *balance:*
   —Position him with his head in front of his knees and his arms in his lap. He may rest his head on your shoulder to assist.
   —Use your knees against his knees to maintain a steady position and to keep his hips from sliding forward.
   —When you are ready to move him across the board, grasp a waistband, belt, or transfer belt on the wheelchair side with one hand.

—Use your hand on the side of the bed to balance his shoulder that is on the bed side.
—Move him across the board with a smooth movement. Keep his head and shoulders in front of his hips to prevent him from sliding to the floor.
   b) If he is *able to* maintain a *balance:*
—Place his hands on the transfer board on either side of where he is sitting.
—Rest his head on your shoulder as long as he does not block your line of vision with his head. Hold onto a belt, transfer belt, or his waistband with one hand. Hold his shoulder with your hand.
—Move him across the board until he reaches the wheelchair.
—Lean him forward and then help him slide back by pushing against his knees with yours. If he needs assistance, you can pull his hips back, using the transfer belt or waistband.
—Tilt him slightly away from the bed so you can remove the transfer board.
—Replace the armrest, reposition the footrests, and set up any other equipment. Lap trays, arm positioners, seatbelts, or belts may need to be adjusted or attached.

Transfer Board from Wheelchair to Bed

Before transferring a person from his wheelchair back to bed, set up the environment for the move:

• Remove equipment from the wheelchair, including the removable armrest and the footrest. Lock the wheelchair.
• Position the wheelchair at an angle to the bed. Use the same position as for getting out of bed. (For a person with hemiplegia, the wheelchair must be placed so he can transfer toward his affected side. His stronger arm and hand will be used for balance at the wheelchair. This is one of the few times that the person with hemiplegia moves toward his affected side using the traditional method.) The transfer back into bed will be more difficult if the bed is higher than the wheelchair seat.

- Remove the outer legrest or footrest so that you can get close to the person without reaching forward. This prevents back strain.

1. Lift and move the client's hips forward so that the hip next to the bed will be in front of the wheelchair tire.
2. Tilt your client away from the bed. This lets you place the transfer board under his thighs so it extends onto the bed.
3. Remove the transfer board once he is back on the bed. Position your client on the bed in the desired position (Figure 4-29 a–f).

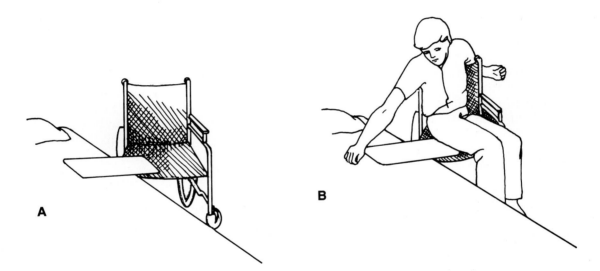

Figure 4-29.   *A client uses a transfer board to move from his wheelchair into bed. Allow him to do as much as possible for himself. The nurse supervisor or physical therapist will instruct you about the safest way to assist each client individually.*

*   **A,** *A client may use a transfer board to move from his wheelchair into bed. Note the position of the transfer board in front of the wheelchair tire and securely anchored over both the bed and wheelchair seat. Match the height of the bed and the wheelchair seat as closely as possible.*

*   **B,** *Lock the brakes, remove the armrests on the transfer side, and swing away the footrests. Use a transfer belt for safety. Assist the client to "tilt" to one side to place the transfer board under his buttocks; position him so he is balanced, as shown.*

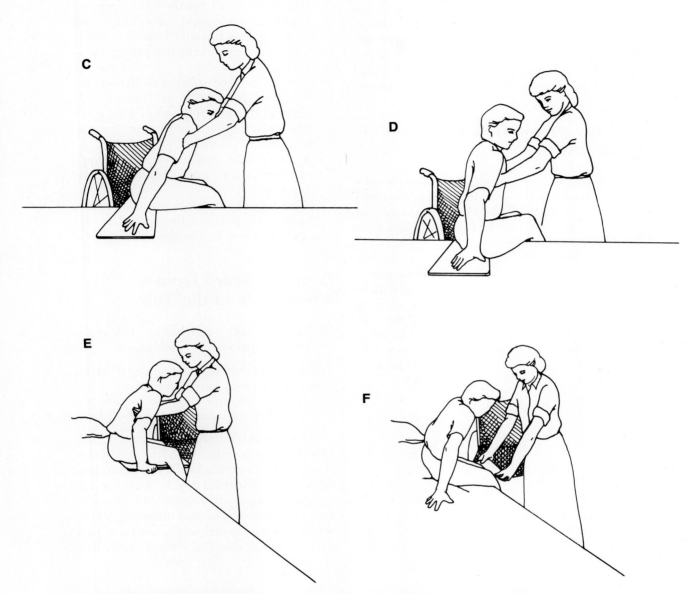

Figure 4-29, cont'd. **C,** *Stand in front of the client to assist and support him. He will use a series of "little pushups" to move across the board.*

D, *Do not allow him to slide or shear his skin during the transfer. The amount of assistance he will need will depend on his abilities, energy at the moment, and experience with transfers.*

E, *Once he is on the bed, assist him to move slightly backward and off the transfer board onto the bed. Continue to support him as necessary for balance and safety.*

F, *Assist him to "tilt" to one side and back so you can remove the transfer board. Reposition him in bed.*

Transfer Board from Bed to the Bedside Commode

The transfer from the bed to a commode chair uses essentially the same movements as from the bed to a wheelchair. There are some special factors to consider. A list of potential difficulties with suggestions for preventing or reducing them are listed below:

Some problems to guard against—

—The seat on a commode or toilet is not a solid covered seat. The person can easily drop a hip onto and his buttocks into the opening before he is securely seated on the commode.

—Your client will remove his underclothing before the transfer to use a commode. His bare skin will not move across the transfer board as easily as clothing. Skin can be damaged this way.

—There is no belt or waistband to grasp when your client is not wearing clothing. You do not have a handle while assisting him to transfer and to balance.

Some suggestions:

—Tilt your client toward the side of the commode away from the toilet opening. He will be leaning and this will allow him to lift up his hip and buttocks. Then move him again into the proper position.

—Use an elevated toilet seat, if possible.

—Fasten a draw sheet or transfer belt around the person's waist. This gives you something to hold onto for the transfer.

—Sprinkle baby powder on the person's skin and on the transfer board to reduce friction.

—Place a small towel on the transfer board under the person's buttocks. Use the towel to move him across the board.

Transfer Board from a Wheelchair to the Tub

A client may make a transfer to a tub bench (with a back support) in a bathtub if:

a) he is capable of making the transfer,
b) you are able to assist him, and
c) there is enough room for a safe approach to the bathtub in the wheelchair.

The approach must avoid all interference with the wheels of the wheelchair. The approach is not as great a problem when a commode chair with small casters is used to approach the bathtub. Practice this transfer under the direction of your nurse supervisor before moving your client. Figure 4-30 shows the correct approach to a bathtub transfer.

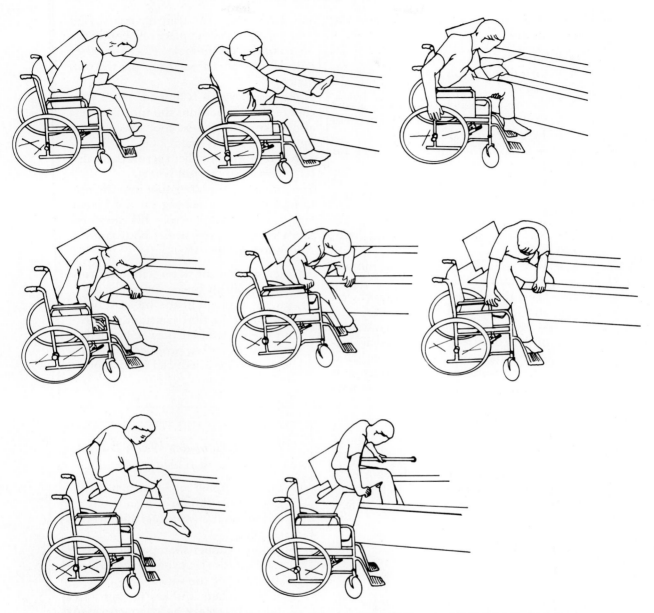

Figure 4-30. *A transfer board may also be used to move a client from a wheelchair onto a bathtub seat. Follow directions from the nurse supervisor or physical therapist carefully; safety is a priority and you may use a transfer belt. Read about the transfer in the accompanying text and about safety in Chapter 2. Study the illustrations and practice under the direction of the nurse supervisor or physical therapist before transferring your client.*

Using a Transfer Board to Move from a Wheelchair onto a Bathtub Seat

Before bringing your client into the bathroom:

- Be sure the tub is dry.
- Place a non-slip tub mat on the floor of the tub.
- Place the tub bench (with back) across the tub at the point where your client will transfer into the tub.
- Check the bathroom and tub area for any safety hazards.
- Remember that he does not have to sit facing the water faucets if there is a shampoo hose or shower head.

Step One Bring your client into the bathroom and:
  —Move the wheelchair or commode chair into position.
  —Lock the brakes. Move the armrest and footrests out of the way.
  —Move your client forward to the front of the chair seat. Make sure his balance is good and use a transfer belt if necessary. Be sure he understands what you are about to do together.

Step Two Powder the transfer board. Tilt your client so you can place one end of the board under his buttocks. Place the other end of the board securely on the tub bench.

Step Three If space is limited, place your client's closest foot into the tub. You may also place your closest foot into the tub onto the non-skid mat.

Step Four Move your client across the transfer board onto the tub bench.

Step Five Place his other foot into the tub. Complete his positioning on the bench. Use a safety strap across his chest for safety if he has poor upper body control. Add water to the tub.

Note: Monitor the water temperature and level at all times. Do not leave your client alone in the tub. Do not allow water to flow constantly onto your client's feet. He may be burned. Even cold water can produce burns in clients who have reduced circulation.

An alternate method for a tub transfer is placing both feet into the tub before performing a tub transfer (Figure 4-31 a–f).

Getting a Client out of the Tub

Be sure to dry your client as much as possible before beginning the transfer. Wet skin tends to stick to the transfer board. Powder the board and buttocks if this is helpful. Reverse the above procedure to transfer the client from the tub to the wheelchair or commode chair.

Things to Consider When Bathing a Client

—Place a rubber non-slip mat on the floor of the tub for you and your client to position your feet and prevent slipping.

—fasten a rubber shampoo hose to the tub faucet so that you can control the direction of the water.
  If your client dislikes having water fall on his face or head, attach a metal flexible shampoo hose to the overhead shower outlet.

—The bathroom sink or basin can also be used as a bathing place for clients who choose not to use the tub or shower. Position these clients at the bathroom basin with the materials they will need placed in front of them. They may walk or be wheeled up to the sink in a wheelchair or a wheeled commode. The kitchen sink may be too high, but can be used instead of the bathroom.

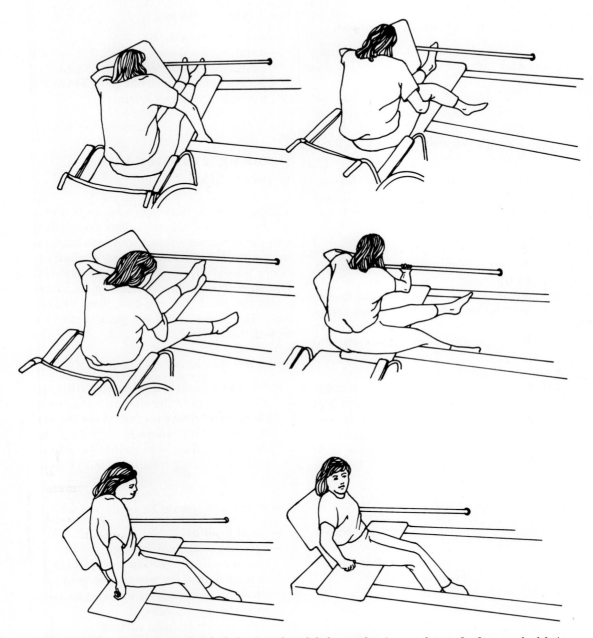

Figure 4-31.   *Some clients place both feet into the tub before performing a tub transfer from a wheelchair. All of the precautions about transfers, safety, and supervision apply in this transfer.*

STANDING TRANSFERS

Standing Transfer to the Tub Seat

Clients who may be able to make a standing transfer to a tub seat include clients who:

—can perform a rehabilitation standing transfer as described earlier in this chapter,

—can be wheeled in a wheelchair or wheeled commode chair into the tub area, or

—can walk with an assistive device such as a brace or prosthesis.

The nurse supervisor will discuss this procedure with you. Read about tub seats before attempting a standing transfer. When you and your client are prepared:

- Position the chair so that he can move with his stronger side toward the tub. Lock the chair.
- Stand at his weaker side to assist him to balance as he stands, turns, and sits on the tub seat.
- Remove the brace or prosthesis. Put it in a dry place.
- Move the chair out of the way.
- Instruct your client to steady himself with a wall grab bar as he lifts his legs one at a time into the tub. He should begin with his closer, stronger leg. Assist him as necessary for a safe move onto the tub seat.

Leaving the Tub Seat

- Instruct your client to step out onto a dry floor.
- Dry his feet and legs before donning his shoes, brace, or prosthesis.
- Reverse the process to return him to his chair and room.

Safety Considerations

Your client should:

—sit on the tub seat.

Your client should *not:*

—step into the tub, or

—stand in the shower or tub. He cannot wash his feet or legs without bending over or balancing on one foot. These are not safe activities for him.

Standing Transfer into a Shower Stall

A shower stall is more accessible than a tub. However it is a dangerous place for a client with physical limitations. Safety precautions are essential. For example, every surface becomes potentially wet, soapy, and slippery. The shower may have a door or a curtain across the front, but not have bars to hold onto. To ensure safety for your client in a shower stall:

Your *client* should be:

—able to make a sliding transfer from his wheelchair onto the shower seat as for a car transfer. Have him sit on the shower seat first. Then move his legs into the shower. Or the client should be able to make a standing transfer safely (Figure 4-32 a, b).

The *shower stall* should be equipped with:

—a wall grab bar,

—a shower seat high enough for him to return easily to a standing position or to slide back into his wheelchair, and

—enough room for you to stand to assist your client.

—floor mat or nonslip surface.

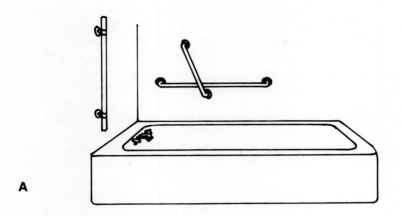

A

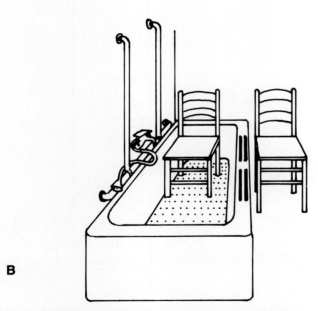

B

Figure 4-32.   **A,** *Grab bars are placed within reach for a seated or standing transfer into a tub. Grab bars must be firmly attached into the studwalls.*

   B, *A homemade shower seat, nonslip bath mat, and grab bars promote bathroom safety. The tub chair legs are cut to reduce the height of the chair so the seat is level with the chair placed outside the tub.*

TRANSFERS USING A MECHANICAL LIFT

Clients who are dependent are a special group of clients to keep mobile. You will not be able to move them using any of the methods already discussed. These people depend upon you to move them out of their beds at least once a day. You will need a mechanical lift and possibly a second person to assist you. A family member may be able to help. Your nurse supervisor will practice using the lift with you. She will direct you about using the procedure below and the need for assistance.

Placing the Sling Under the Client Who is in Bed

- Use the correct sling for your client.
- Place the sling under your client while he is still in bed (Figure 4-33).
- Turn your client onto one side.
- Position the sling with the top edge at your client's shoulders. The bottom edge should extend to at least mid-thigh. Request another sling if the sling does not cover this area of the client. Have the nurse supervisor check it.
- Extend one end of the sling that attaches to the lift to the edge of the bed.
- Roll the other length of the sling up against the client's back.
- Keep enough of the sling in the roll to pull through to the other side when he rolls over it. Turn the client over the roll.
- Straighten and smooth the sling under your client.

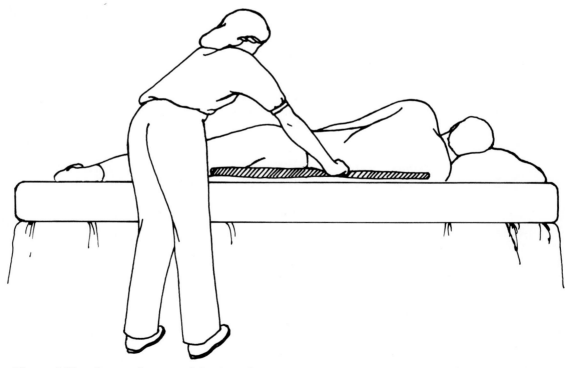

Figure 4-33. *Correct placement of the sling of a mechanical lift is important for a safe lift and transfer. The sling should extend from the client's shoulders to his mid-thigh and fit smoothly under him.*

Using the Mechanical Lift

- Inform your client about the lift and transfer.
- Place the sling under him or adjust the sling if it is already under him.
- Roll the lift to the bed.
- Roll the base under the bed.
- Secure the brakes on the casters before raising or lowering your client.
- Keep the legs of the lift spread open. This provides a wide base of support and prevents the lift from tipping.
- Lower the supporting arm of the lift.
- Raise the head of the bed slightly. If your nurse supervisor directs you that it is safe for your client you may elevate the bed under the person's knees if this assists him in the move. Be sure this is safe for your client. This will make it easier for you to connect the sling to the corresponding chains on the lift.
- Keep the chains untangled and evenly balanced. The shorter chains are placed near his shoulders to keep them raised higher than his hips. This will put the client in a sitting position when transferred. This creates easier positioning in the wheelchair or armchair.

- Connect the sling to the chains of the lift.
- The nurse supervisor will instruct you about which links in the chains you are to use for your client's lift. The chains will be marked for his shoulders and his hips. Generally, the hip chains are longer.
- Turn on the lift or crank the handle to lift your client. Lift only high enough to clear the bed safely (Figure 4-34).
- Roll the lift slowly until your client is positioned over the bed or seat.
- Stand beside your client as you move. Steady the sling with your hand. Do not allow your client to swing in the lift.
- Slowly and steadily lower the lift. Be careful not to bump your client.
- Be sure his legs do not hit the lift.
- Disconnect the chains and roll the lift away.
- Smooth the sling under your client.

A wraparound sling may be necessary if your client has spasticity or body tremors. A wraparound sling will keep your client safe while he is being moved even if he becomes very spastic or has tremors. Ask the family or your nurse supervisor to assist you.

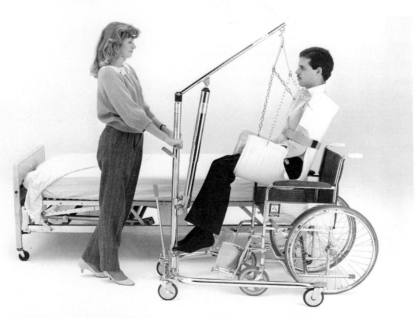

Figure 4-34.   *The mechanical lift can help to keep a client out of his bed. Note the use of an extra chest strap for support and safety.*
   Courtesy Ted Hoyer & Company, Inc.

TRANSFER INTO A CAR

Many disabled people feel that transferring into and out of a car is a very important step. A person who can manage this car transfer is able to be more mobile. He can go places in a car that he would not have access to otherwise. Some clients have special vans that carry wheelchairs. Specialized vans can be equipped with hydraulic lifts. The lift raises the client and chair as one into the rear portion of the van. Some are lifted into a position to drive.

The person who can manage a car transfer can sit in the regular front car seat for the ride. The wheelchair is loaded behind the front seat or in the trunk. When he arrives at his destination, he transfers from the car seat back into his own wheelchair.

The car transfer is essentially the same as the transfer from the wheelchair to sitting on the side of the bed. Practice this transfer with the nurse supervisor or the physical therapist. Use the car that the client will use in your practice. Figure 4-35 (a–d) demonstrates the movements in this transfer for a client who has an affected left side. Figure 4-36 (a–d) shows the same transfer for a client who has an affected right side.

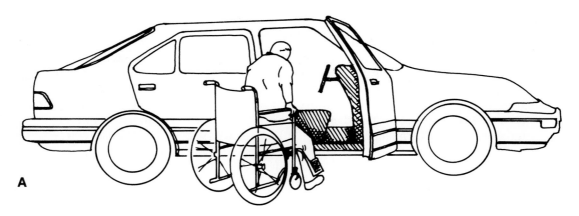

Figure 4-35. *Car transfer when the client's **left side is affected**.*

A, *Park the car either close to the curb or in a flat area away from the curb. Open the car door and lower the window on the passenger side. Position the wheelchair at an angle close to the front seat. Lock the brakes and swing the footrests out of the way.*

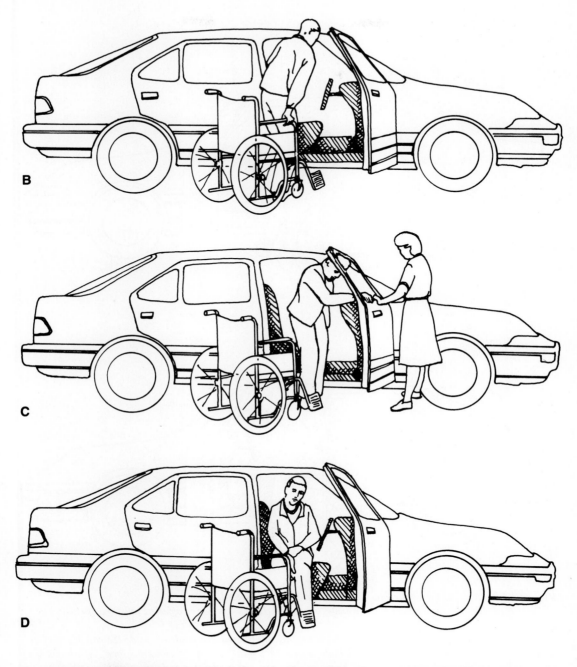

Figure 4-35, cont'd.   **B,** *Use the method for a standing transfer appropriate for your client. You may use a transfer belt. (Your nurse supervisor or physical therapist will direct you about the correct transfer method).*

   C, *Your client holds onto the open window frame of the car door. You stand outside and stabilize the car door. As he turns to sit, remind him that he must bend to avoid bumping his head.*

   D, *The client lifts his **affected** foot and leg into the car using his **unaffected** arm and hand. Once he is inside, close the car door before he arranges his position further. Fasten his seat belt when he is ready.*

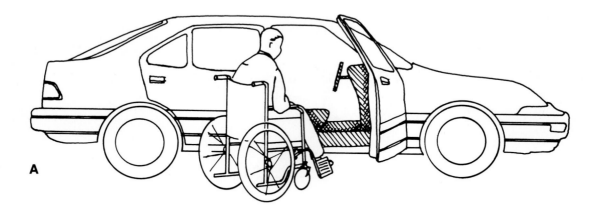

A

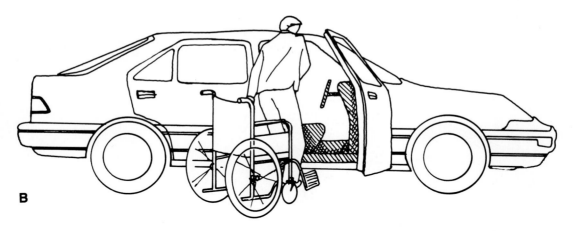

B

Figure 4-36.   *Car transfer when the client's **right side is affected.***
   A *to* **C,** *Follow the directions for the transfer when the client's left side is affected until the client moves onto the carseat.*

   D, *As the client moves onto the car seat, he places his **unaffected** arm and leg inside the car. He uses his **unaffected** arm and leg to lift his affected limbs into the car. Once inside, he closes the door, repositions himself, and fastens the seatbelt as he is able. Assist him as necessary to transfer and for safety.*

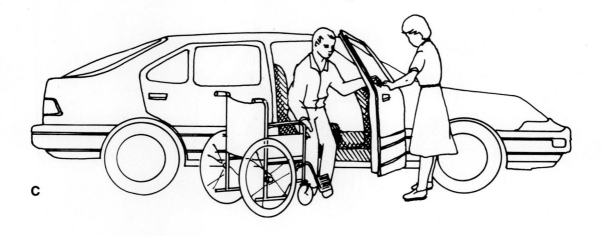

C

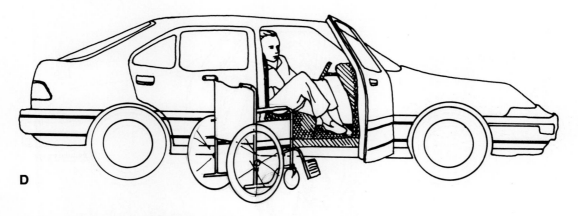

D

Figure 4-36, cont'd. *For legend see opposite page.*

Figures 4-37 (a–d) and 4-38 (a–d) show the reverse transfers from a car to a wheelchair.

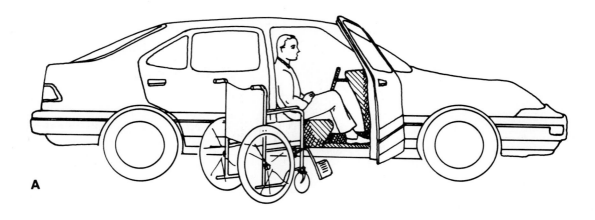

A

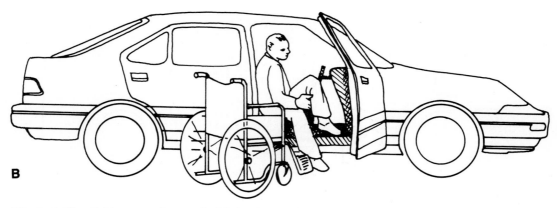

B

Figure 4-37. *Exiting a car into a wheelchair when the **left side is affected**.*
   A, *Park the car and arrange the wheelchair as for getting into the car.*
   B, *The client moves to outside edge of the seat, setting his **unaffected** leg out of car onto solid surface. He turns and lifts the **affected** leg out of car.*

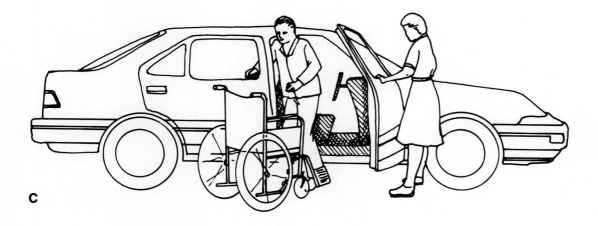

C

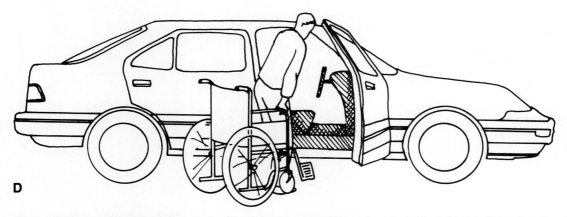

D

Figure 4-37, cont'd. **C,** *Sitting on the side of the seat, with his hand on the back of the seat, he pushes forward to a standing position. He places his **unaffected** arm on the closest wheelchair armrest.*

D, *The client moves his **unaffected** hand to the right armrest as he turns sitting into wheelchair. Unlock the brakes, back away from the car, and relock the brakes. Position the feet pedals, feet, and any other equipment.*

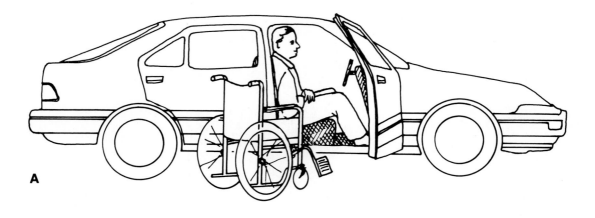

A

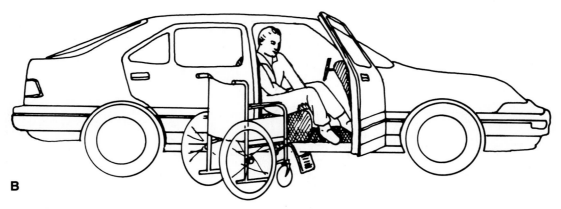

B

Figure 4-38.   *Exiting a car into a wheelchair when the* **right side is affected.**
     A *and* **B,** *Follow the directions in Figure 4-37.*
     C, *Sitting on the side of the seat, the client reaches forward to grasp the door. He pulls forward and upward. The driver maintains the position of the door.*

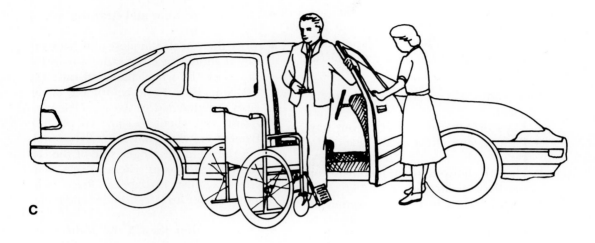

C

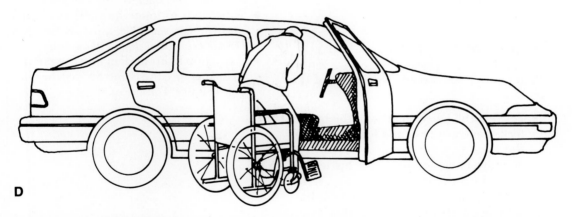

D

Figure 4-38, cont'd.   **D,** *The client will continue to hold on to the door as he turns and positions his back to the wheelchair. He then places his hand on the wheelchair armrest and sits down. Repositioning the chair is done as in Figure 4-38,* **D.**

Using a Transfer Board to Get into a Car

Your position for this transfer is the same as for a bed transfer. One problem will be the lack of space for you to stand between your client and the car door. Therefore, you must be sure your client moves far enough forward so that he does not rub his buttocks across the wheel of his wheelchair and the car door frame.

—Once your client has transferred into the car seat:
  ● Move the wheelchair out of your way.
  ● Position your client on the seat of the car.
  ● Place the bottoms of his feet firmly on the floor of the car.
  ● Keep both his feet straight so they do not roll over and cause his ankles to touch the floor. This small amount of poor positioning can cause a skin problem from the ankle rubbing on the floor of the car or from the heat on the floorboard of the car.
  ● Secure the seatbelt.

Getting out of a Car

When your client is ready to get out of the car:

  ● Position the wheelchair with the brakes locked and armrests and footrests out of the way.
  ● Turn your client and move his feet so they touch the ground.
  ● Place the transfer board under his buttocks and into the seat of the wheelchair. You may need to do this before you place his feet on the ground.
  ● Move him across from the car seat into the wheelchair.
  ● Secure him in proper position, reset the armrest and footrest. Secure the wheelchair seatbelt. Remember good body mechanics for all of your movements.

Standing Transfer into a Car

This transfer can be used with the client who is able to stand and balance during the process. It is similar to the standing transfers described earlier.

  ● Open the car door and clear the area of any hazards.
  ● Move the wheelchair close alongside the car. It should face the same way as the car. Lock the wheelchair and raise the footrests. Be sure no equipment or devices are attached to the wheelchair.
  ● Assist your client to stand in place in front of his wheelchair. He will be entering the right passenger side of the car.
  ● Stand facing your client. Place your knees against his knees. Place your hands under his left shoulder and on his right hip.
  ● Pivot together toward the right as he comes to a standing position. This will turn his back to the car seat.
  ● As he turns, instruct him to hold onto the arm of his wheelchair, the car door, and then the back of the car seat.
  ● Assist him to lower himself backwards into the car seat. He must **DUCK HIS HEAD** *before and during the seating.*
  ● Assist him to lift his feet into the car and to turn to face the front. Secure the seatbelt (Figure 4-39 a–e).

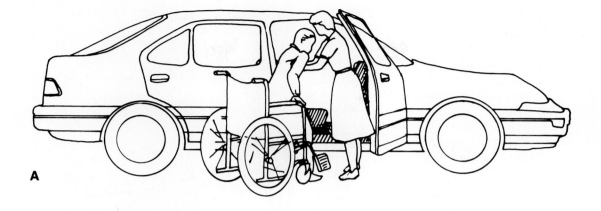

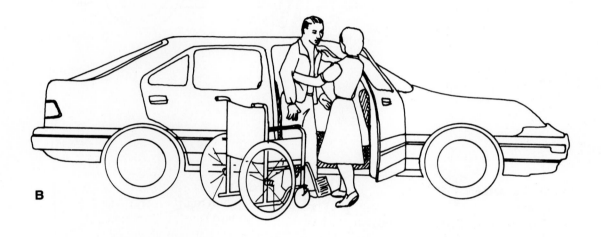

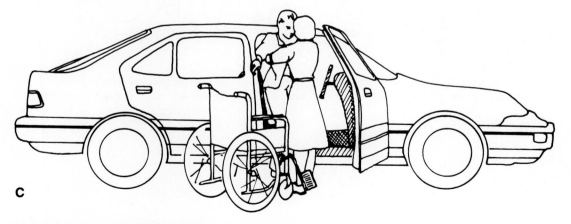

Figure 4-39. *Pivot transfer—assisting a client into a car.*

    A, *If assistance is needed, stand in front of client. Stand with your knees stabilizing his knees and your arm around his chest under his arms.*

    B, *When the client is standing, pivot back to the car seat.*

    C, *If possible, have the client hold the wheelchair armrest or door.*

Continued.

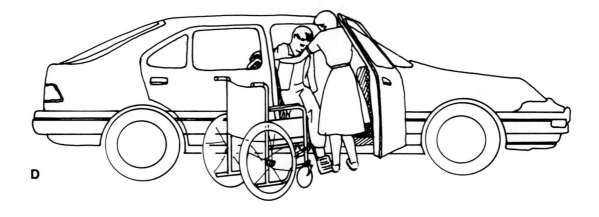

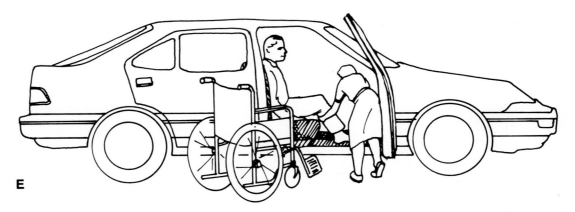

Figure 4-39, cont'd.   D, *Assist the client to sit by placing your hands on his shoulder to bend forward.*
E, *Position the client's feet in the car in proper position. Fasten the seat belt. Close and lock the car door.*

Avoid these potential difficulties:

- Do not let your client attempt to transfer without assistance. The exception is if he has been passed or certified as having learned the procedure successfully by the nurse supervisor or physical therapist.
- Do not let him "hang" on to your neck or arms.
- Do not let him sit on the arm of the wheelchair between the wheelchair seat and the carseat.
- Do not try to lift a client into a car, even with another person to assist you.
- Do not let him enter the car with his head first. Only let him back into the seat.
- Do not attempt this transfer until you have been instructed by the nurse supervisor or the physical therapist that this is a safe transfer.

Loading a Wheelchair into a Car

The wheelchair must be placed in the car after the transfer. This works better for a car with two doors. Many clients who have strong upper extremities can do this for themselves (Figure 4-40).

- Unlock the wheelchair brakes once your client has transferred.
- Fold the wheelchair. Pull it up on the middle of the seat upholstery and bring the armrests together.
- Fold the front car seat forward. Tip the wheelchair onto the back wheels and place the small front wheels into the car.
- Lift the back of the wheelchair with the handlebars as you roll it into the car behind the front seat.
- Position the large wheels in the footspace on the floor of the car and pull the front car seat into its upright position.

Reverse the process to *remove* the wheelchair from the car.

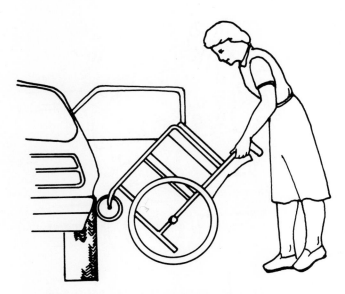

Figure 4-40. *Loading a folded wheelchair into a car.*

Loading a Wheelchair into a Car Trunk

If the wheelchair does not fit in the car, you may place it in the trunk (Figure 4-41). Before loading the wheelchair:

- Fold the chair as above.
- Remove all cushions, loose equipment, and footrests.
- Lock or unlock the brakes. This depends on whether it is easier to have the wheels stationary when lifting the chair.
- Lift the wheelchair by the front of the frame. Keep the back of the chair toward the edge of the car trunk.
- Lift the chair again to position it into the car trunk.

Sometimes wheelchairs cannot be loaded into cars. Carriers are available for the back bumper or car top. The carriers may be combined with a lift to place the wheelchair when the person cannot lift the chair or if it is a heavy wheelchair.

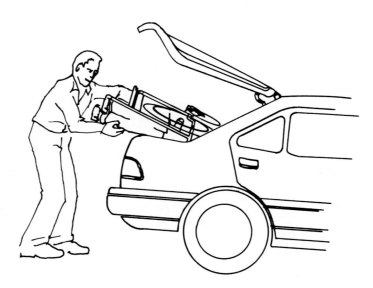

Figure 4-41. *Loading a wheelchair into the trunk of a car.*

CHAPTER *5*
Equipment for Clients with Disabilities

*O*BJECTIVES

When you have studied this chapter and practiced the procedures it describes, you will be able to:

1. Identify the pieces of equipment used by your client.
2. Know the basic parts, cleaning, and care requirements for your client's equipment.
3. Use the client's equipment properly and for his maximum safety.
4. Select the right equipment to assist your client, under your supervisor's direction.
5. Make simple equipment.
6. Contribute ideas about new and existing equipment that could assist you and your client.
7. Assist the family and other caregivers to use equipment properly.

*O*VERVIEW

This chapter covers equipment designed for persons with disabilities and its use in different rooms of the home. The chapter also contains plans for constructing inexpensive home equipment and purchase suggestions for the client and family. When caring for a person with a disability, you will use a variety of equipment. When working with any equipment for your client, it is important to remember the following points:

- Use equipment according to instructions provided in the manufacturers' instruction manuals and as directed by the nurse supervisor or therapists.
- Keep equipment clean and in good working order.
- Notify the family and nurse supervisor of needed repairs.
- **Never** use unsafe, poorly operating equipment.
- Observe all safety precautions.
- Listen to your client if he has concerns about his equipment.

Most equipment used by a person with a disability is either rented or purchased. It may surprise you to learn how much detail is involved in designing or fitting specialized equipment to meet a client's particular needs. For example, wheelchairs tend to look alike until you learn about the many options and features. Equipment is often donated to a client by someone who no longer needs the equipment. This does not mean it is safe or suitable for your client. Equipment is very costly, but unsafe equipment can cost you and your client. There are, however, some safe ways to "make-do," which are included in this chapter.

The most common equipment used in the home includes:

wheelchairs,
walkers,
canes, and crutches,
leg braces,
a variety of beds,
bedside commodes or toilets,
tub or shower benches,
raised toilet seats,
bars for the toilet and bath,
shower hoses,
commodes with wheels, and
mechanical lifts.

*E*QUIPMENT TO HELP CLIENTS MOVE

If your client is having physical therapy visits at home, the therapist will check the equipment and teach the client how to use it in the home. Many families are taught about the equipment before the person leaves the hospital. Others may have had the opportunity to visit their homes with the therapist prior to leaving the hospital. These home trial visits may be paid for by Medicare, Medicaid, or in some cases by private insurance companies. Also, some rehabilitation centers have private rooms or efficiency apartment units that are furnished and arranged in a home-like setting. The family or caretaker might spend several days working together with the client in the home unit. The nursing and therapy staff are available if necessary to answer any questions or supervise activities.

A client may wish to use his equipment before the therapist visits the home. If so, be sure to ask your client or family if he has been trained in the use of the equipment at the hospital or rehabilitation center. If he has not, discourage his using it until he has a home visit from the therapist. If you encounter difficulties with equipment or its use, contact the nurse supervisor before proceeding.

EQUIPMENT FOR WALKING

Do Not:

—use equipment if it does not appear safe or in good condition.

—attempt to assist your client to use stairs unless the nurse or therapist has given you specific instructions and has observed you practicing on the stairs with the client.

Do Check:

—to make sure there are solid, clean rubber tips on all feet of the equipment for walking.
—that all firm non-revolving handgrips are in good condition.
—the working order of any folding and locking parts.
—the area of the house the client must walk through. Look for anything that could cause him to trip, slip, or bump himself.
—the bathroom to be sure the client can support himself once he reaches the bathroom.
—for items that could become problems, such as throw rugs, water on floor, electrical cords, hanging materials, sharp projections from furniture or doors, or narrow passages.
—and report hazards and problems with the equipment or its use to the family as well as to the nurse or therapist.

The nurse supervisor or therapist may suggest ways to make the house safer and more accessible for walking equipment. For example, doors with lever-style handles are easier to open than round doorhandles that require a full grasp of the hand (Figure 5-1).

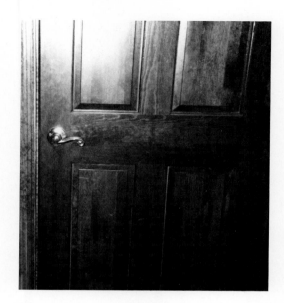

Figure 5-1. *Lever handled doors make it easier for clients to open doors.*

Replacement parts, such as rubber tips and hand grips for canes and walkers, can be purchased at local drug stores. Larger tips are preferable to those that are rounded or too small because they give a broader base of support. Folding equipment, such as some walkers, folds away and saves space. Clearing furniture and other materials from the room may enable your client to turn around if he needs more room. See Chapter 6 for more information on kitchen accessories, grooming, and dressing aids.

Walkers, Canes, and Crutches

If a client needs a walker, cane, or crutches, these are usually ordered for him and supplied to him before he leaves the hospital or rehabilitation center. Figure 5-2 shows the most commonly borrowed pieces of equipment. Although they appear simple, each one must be fitted for each client and checked carefully. If the equipment is not fitted, it can be unsafe and may work against

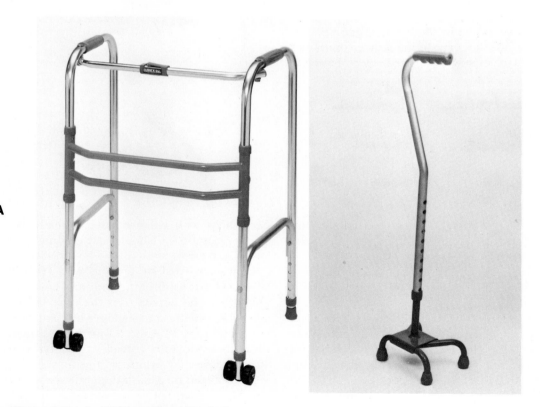

A

B

Figure 5-2. **A,** *Folding walker with wheels.*
B, *Adjustable cane with a base for added support.*

Continued.

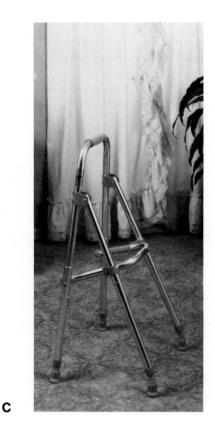

C

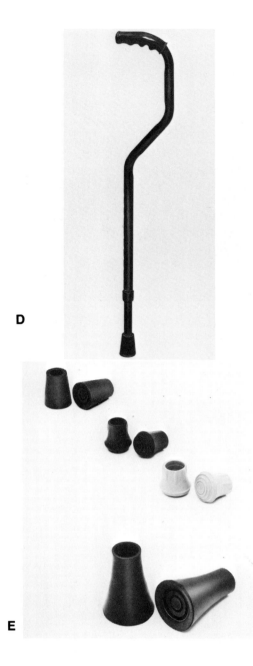

D

E

Figure 5-2. cont'd.   C, *Folding walk-cane.*
D, *Ortho cane.*
E, *Rubber tips for crutches and walkers.*
Courtesy of Lumex, Division of Lumex, Inc.

the client's success. Many clients have sore underarms from walking with ill-fitting crutches.

See Chapter 4 for more information about moving about using walkers, canes, or crutches.

A standard **walker** has four legs with rubber tips. The walker can be adjusted to fit the client's height. The walker is very stable, but its extended legs can catch on furniture in a crowded room. The client must be able to lift the walker slightly after each step. Persons who have weak legs and mild balance problems benefit from a walker. Persons who need help with balance but require extra safety precautions should use gliding and roller walkers.

Canes are used by persons who require support on one side of the body and have one able arm. The person uses the cane on the side where he has the stronger leg. Your client may begin by using a four-legged quad cane that provides a wide stable base of support. He may progress to using a single-legged cane as he gains independence. Occasionally persons with poor strength and balance, such as clients who have rheumatoid arthritis, will use two canes. Canes are made from wood or metal with rubber tips. They are measured to fit by height. Canes can be ordered fitted with special handgrips designed for persons whose arthritis affects the use of their hands.

Crutches are the least stable of the walking aids. They require good balance, good upper arm strength, and endurance. Crutches are made from wood or light-weight steel and have rubber tips. The underarm covers and handgrips should be padded. The handgrips and underarm braces are adjusted to fit the person and to accommodate his swing through as he walks (Figure 5-3).

Crutches are fitted to the person by his height (Figure 5-4). Generally, crutches are 16″ shorter than the user. If crutches have not been fitted, you can make a simple check on the fit. Have your client stand with his feet together. Mark 5″ to the front and 5″ to the side of his foot. Put the tip of the crutch on the marks with the crutch under his arm. Approximately 3 fingers should fit between his armpit and the top of the crutch. If your client has difficulty with his crutches, report the situation to the nurse supervisor. The physical therapist is responsible for exactly measuring and adjusting crutches.

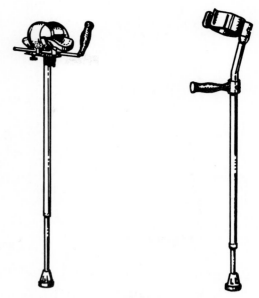

Figure 5-4. **A,** *Platform walking crutch.* **B,** *Loftstrand forearm crutch.*

There are a number of crutches styled for special uses. Lofstrand crutches, for example, are multipurpose crutches that combine the weight bearing assistance of a crutch with added wrist and forearm support.

Leg Braces

Many clients are trained to wear **long or short leg braces.** Leg braces enable a person to walk safely, to have additional support in standing and walking, and to make transfers easier. Each leg brace is designed for an individual's size and needs. Braces give support, but they should not be uncomfortable, cause pressure, or rub or chafe the skin. Your client should maintain a proper posture when using braces. Figure 5-5 shows the difference between long and short leg braces.

Braces are made of metal with cuffs, laces, or leather straps or Velcro fasteners to hold the brace in place. A short leg brace has a cuff around the calf of the leg. A long leg brace has both a calf and a thigh cuff. Cuffs are fitted to the person's leg. The brace, cuffs, and shoes will not fit if a person gains or loses weight (20–30 lb.) or a child grows. The size changes can cause pressure areas on the skin, loose brace attachment, and falls.

Another type of bracing is a plastic long or short leg brace that fits inside the shoe (Figure 5-6). These are becoming more popular.

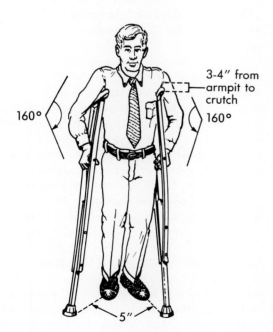

160°   160°

3-4″ from armpit to crutch

5″

Figure 5-3. *To measure the proper height of a crutch, place the tip of the crutch 5 inches to the side and in front of each foot. The top should come within 3 to 4 inches of the client's armpit.*

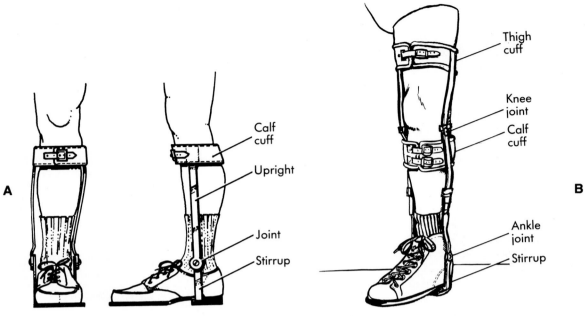

Figure 5-5. **A,** *Short leg brace.*
B, *Long leg brace.*

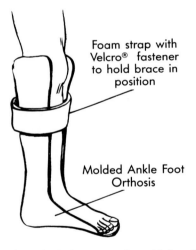

Figure 5-6. *Plastic braces can be molded to the client's foot and leg and can be either long or short.*

The client and his family are taught to put on the brace before inserting it into the shoe. Because the brace is plastic, it will bend on pressure. The plastic will break if the brace is bent too much. This brace is held together at the top of the brace with a Velcro strap. Remove lint, fuzz, and threads from the Velcro hooks so that it will hold securely.

The person who uses the short plastic brace can usually attach and care for the brace himself. He needs supportive shoes that are in good condition. The shoe without the brace has a liner inserted to take up the room that the brace uses in the other shoe. This lets the client buy a single pair of shoes. The client or family can replace lost or damaged liners.

A client who has weakness at his knee or hip may need a long leg brace. Braces are made with knee joints that lock so that the joint does not bend. These are used when a client requires solid support to stand and walk. A short leg brace is used when a client needs support to keep his foot, ankle, and knee in proper alignment. A molded ankle foot orthosis (MAFO) is used to control toe pick up or poor foot placement that occurs when a client has weakness in his ankle.

Care and Storage of Braces

Some braces are heavier than others to accommodate the person's age, activity level, or safety needs. Most braces have moveable joints, usually at the knee and ankle. Some are fixed at the ankle or shoe. The knee joint in most braces is equipped with a lock designed so the client can lock and unlock the joint. A locking knee joint allows the person to lock himself securely in a standing position and unlock to bend his knee for comfortable sitting. The brace metal is usually built into the shoe on either side of the heel. The joint is part of the brace metal, not part of the shoe attachment.

Screws secure the metal parts of the brace at the knee and ankle joints. The brace will come apart if these screws become loosened or lost. If parts of the brace do fall off, keep them for repairs. Notify your client, his family, or the nurse supervisor immediately when brace parts are loose, worn, or missing. Do not let your client use a brace that is not in excellent operating condition.

Braces are expensive and must be cared for properly. Braces can be twisted or bent if not properly stored.

- When a brace is not being worn, prop it carefully against a wall or inside a closet. Some clients will have a special brace storage bag.
- If the brace is placed on the floor or table, it should be laid out straight.
- Other objects should not be placed on top of the brace.
- The metal should be wiped with a soft cloth.
- Look for any rust or corrosion if the brace is not stainless steel. Look for wear of the metal such as:
  —chips, nicks, or gouges in the metal;
  —scrapes or dull, rubbed areas; or
  —changes in the actual shape of the metal piece from the original shape

Shoes for Braces

Proper shoes are essential for safe and useful leg braces. The shoe itself should be a sturdy well-supported leather shoe with a leather sole and rubber heel or a prescribed surgical shoe that is custom-fitted. Surgical shoes are made from special leathers, with inner supports or linings and built-in ankle supports. The shoe may have a hard or soft toe box. The long laces (54–72 inches) can be tied securely. The nurse supervisor or therapist will show you how to work with shoes that have leather straps or buckles.

Check shoes for:

—broken laces (replaced at shoe repair or department stores).

—worn or damaged soles and heels. These can cause the person's leg to move out of position.

—loosened parts, breaks in stitching, or worn or torn leather.

—excessive perspiration, producing odors and deterioration of leather. The client should wear cotton socks to absorb perspiration if it is a problem, especially in hot weather.

Shoes that are soiled and stained should be cleaned with saddle soap. Orthotic or prosthetic shops often repair shoes as well as braces.

WHEELCHAIRS

Wheelchairs are designed in a wide variety of sizes and shapes to fit the person and meet the needs of his particular disability. For many clients the purchase or rental of a wheelchair is covered by Medicare, Medicaid, or private insurance. These wheelchairs may be in good condition, however, they are not always the correct size or type for the person. Tell the nurse supervisor if you, the family, or your client encounter problems. Wheelchairs can be exchanged. Other clients must buy their own wheelchairs. Brand new wheelchairs carry warranties in the event of problems. Figure 5-7 shows the parts of a wheelchair.

The upholstered seat of the wheelchair should fit exactly into its space in the chair frame. The seat should not sag toward the center as if it were a hammock. A poorly fitted seat can cause poor posture and alignment, irritation to the skin, and difficulty propelling the chair (Figure 5-8). The seat should extend no more or less than 2 inches on either side from the person sitting in the chair. It should also be two to three inches shorter than the length of his upper leg. It should never reach the back of the person's bent knee. The person sitting in the chair seat should be able to securely place his foot flat on the floor when he is not moving.

Some wheelchairs have removable, desk, full-length or adjustable-height armrests. Adjustable-height armrests allow the client to sit in a proper position. The arms of most

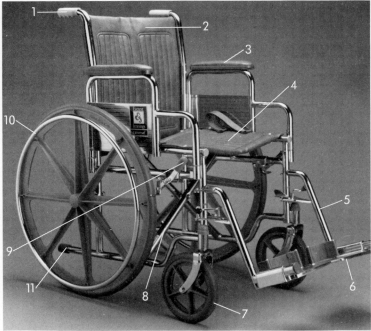

1. Handgrips/push handles
2. Back upholstery
3. Armrests
4. Seat upholstery
5. Front rigging
6. Footplate
7. Casters
8. Crossbraces (Serial number)
9. Wheel locks
10. Wheel and handrim
11. Tipping lever

Figure 5-7. *A wheelchair has many parts. Some parts are removable and many are adjustable; others can be locked into place.*

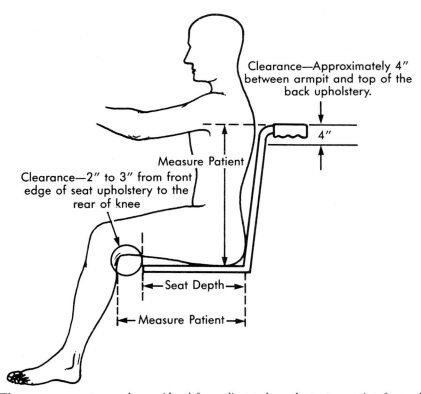

Clearance—Approximately 4" between armpit and top of the back upholstery.

4"

Measure Patient

Clearance—2" to 3" from front edge of seat upholstery to the rear of knee

Seat Depth

Measure Patient

Figure 5-8. *These measurements must be considered for a client to have the proper seating for a wheelchair.*

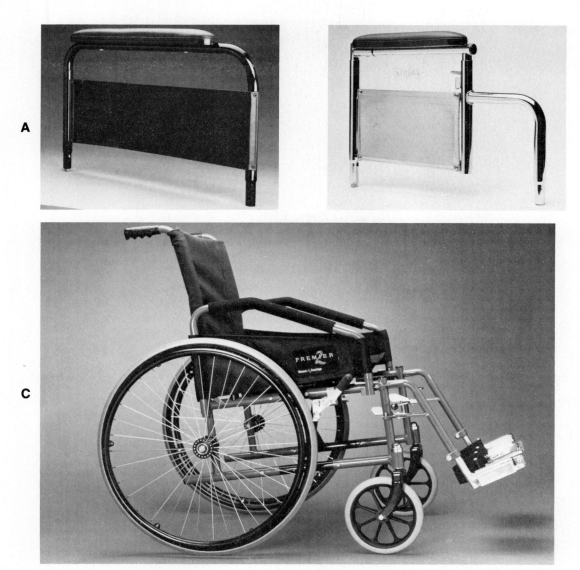

A

B

C

Figure 5-9. **A,** *Full-length wheelchair arm.*
B, *Adjustable desk arm.*
C, *Lightweight wheelchair with slanted arm rests.*
Courtesy of Everest & Jennings, Inc.

wheelchairs supplied by Medicare coverage have non-removable desk or full-length armrests. Removable armrests are helpful for clients who use a seated transfer to move from their wheelchairs to their beds, commodes, tubs, or cars. Some clients must be lifted out of their wheelchairs. Removable armrests are helpful in that the person does not have to be lifted over the chair arms. This prevents back strain for you and keeps the client from potentially having his buttocks, back, or extremities shear on the chair arms as he is lifted over them.

The desirable height for the arms is the distance from the person's bent elbow to the wheelchair seat, plus 1 inch. This is an important measurement. The correct armrest height assists the client to maintain good posture, be comfortable, and perform weight-shifting exercises. The new light-weight wheelchairs may have slanted armrests that are not strong enough to support weight shifts. Figure 5-9 shows different types of wheelchair armrests.

Footrests are also available in several versions. Standard footrests are attached to the

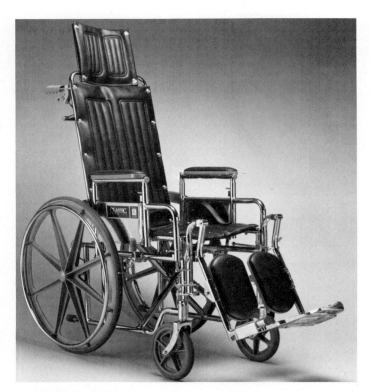

Figure 5-10. *High-backed wheelchair with elevated leg rests, adjustable back, and headrest extension. Courtesy of Everest & Jennings, Inc.*

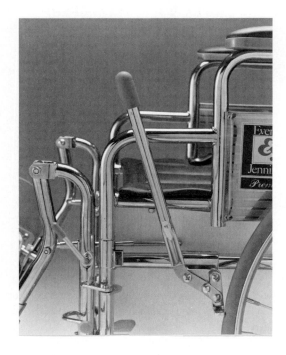

Figure 5-11. *Wheelchair brake and extension handle. Courtesy of Everest & Jennings, Inc.*

wheelchair. They are adjusted so that the client's thigh is slightly elevated above the front edge of the seat. The bottom of the footrest with the footplate attached must clear the floor so the wheelchair can move. The length of the footrest and footplate should be the same as the length of the person's leg from the bend of the knee to the heel of the foot with the foot flat.

Adjust the footrest and footplate by loosening the bolt on the side. Then push in or pull out on the footplate to fit the person and retighten the bolts. The footplate flips up so the person can step out of the chair onto the floor or sit down in the chair. Be sure the footplates are firmly up before the person gets in or out of the chair.

Legrest styles include those that swing and detach, swing but remain attached, and elevate. These styles make it easier to enter and exit the chair and allow the chair to be moved closer to other objects. Some footplates are fitted with loops at the heel and/or toe to help hold the feet in place. Elevating legrests are used to reduce swelling and promote circulation in the client's feet and legs (Figure 5-10). They will help to prevent or reduce knee contractures.

Safety precautions for footrests are as follows:

- *Do not* allow your client to step onto or stand on the footrest.
- *Do not* let a heavy metal footrest fall back onto the client or you.

Wheelchairs come equipped with **brakes** on both sides (Figure 5-11). Be sure both brakes are securely locked before you attempt to move or transfer your client. Long brake extensions can help some clients to reach and to operate the brakes. Check for flat tires if both brakes are on but do not secure. If the brake is loose or placed too far away from the tire it will not lock. A lever brake may bend more easily than a toggle brake.

Report any wheelchair problems to the nurse supervisor. The family or client may need to call the rental agency for a repair or replacement. Many problems can be corrected with a simple brake adjustment, using a screwdriver and a drop of 3-in-1 oil. Using a chair with unsafe brakes can injure you or your client.

Wheelchair wheels have spokes similar to those of bicycle wheels. Loose, missing, or damaged spokes can cause difficulty moving the chair and locking the brakes. Wheels have two rims. One supports the spokes and the other is used by the client to propel the chair. Handrims may have a variety of attachments designed to assist the client in propelling the chair (Figure 5-12). The small wheels under the chair are casters and help to stabilize and guide the chair.

The standard semireclining wheelchair has a back that reclines to 30 degrees. Wheelchairs are also available with full reclining backs, which recline to full horizontal positions, and backs that have varying extended heights or hook-on extenders or headrests to raise their height (Figure 5-13). Custom-made supports for correct positioning may be substituted by some clients.

Other wheelchair parts are the tipping lever to assist with curbs and stairs, and the skirtguard, which keeps clothing from becoming tangled in the wheels and spokes. Anti-tipping levers are added to the back or front of a wheelchair. They prevent the wheelchair from tipping too far forward or backward. The tipping levers are used most often for clients who are very tall persons, have heavy upper bodies, move about in their wheelchairs or are extremely agitated, are wearing Halo vest tractions, or have bilateral leg amputations.

Clients have a number of accessories for their wheelchairs. These range from bags for carrying personal items to sophisticated equipment specific to their needs. Equipment companies make special trays that fit under and behind wheelchairs. These trays hold equipment such as oxygen machines, mechanical ventilators, or suction equipment. Cushions and sheepskins are other wheelchair supplies that are important to your client. See Chapter 6 about seating.

Basic Wheelchair Care

All moveable parts of the chair benefit from a drop of 3-in-1 oil on occasion. Parts that slide together are not oiled. If these parts stick, paraffin can be rubbed on them to ease sliding. The seat, back, armrests, and footrests should be cleaned as frequently as necessary.

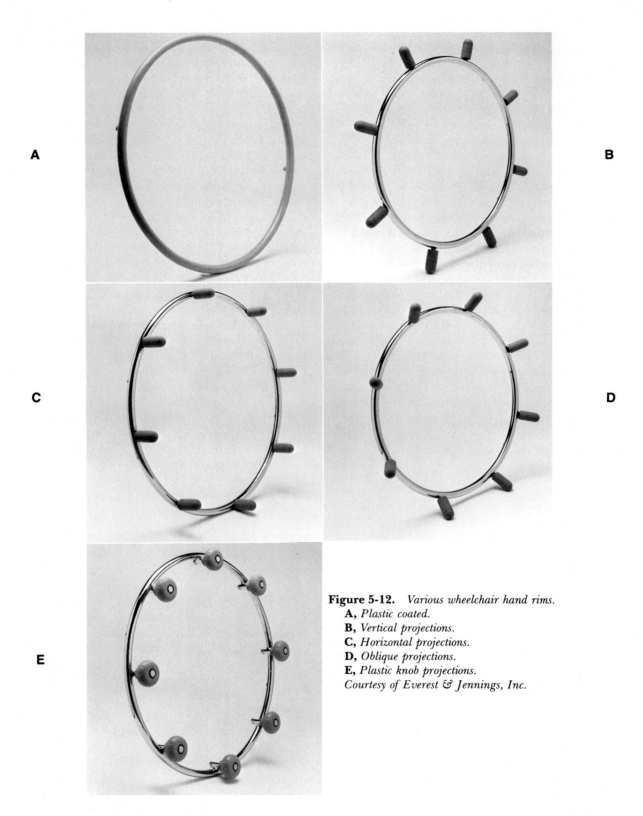

Figure 5-12.   *Various wheelchair hand rims.*
   A, *Plastic coated.*
   B, *Vertical projections.*
   C, *Horizontal projections.*
   D, *Oblique projections.*
   E, *Plastic knob projections.*
   Courtesy of Everest & Jennings, Inc.

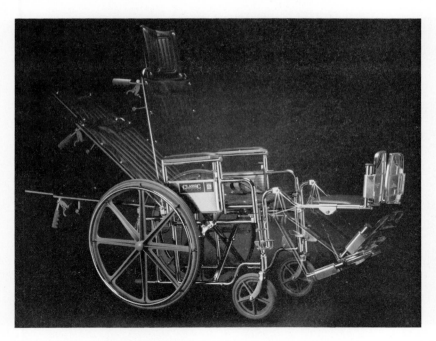

Figure 5-13. *Wheelchair with high back that adjusts to recline to 30 degrees and full recline. Note that the leg rests elevate to support positioning.*
Courtesy of Everest & Jennings, Inc.

Use mild detergent, rinse with water, and dry. Keep the wheels and casters free of dirt and materials like hair, string, and lint that will clog the wheels.

Specialty and Motorized Wheelchairs

A person with severe disabilities usually has a wheelchair fitted with special features, including a motor. Customized and motorized wheelchairs may have many parts that differ from a standard wheelchair (Figure 5-14). Some motorized chairs have a simple hand control called a "joy stick." They can be operated at several speeds. Chin or mouth controls and even head controls are available for clients who cannot use their hands. The client who has very limited head control but is fully alert and aware may choose a "Puff and Sipp" control that is breath-operated. The client simply sips or puffs on a straw-like device to activate and move the wheelchair in a variety of directions. A client must be trained in the use of this specialized wheelchair. It requires specialized maintenance as well.

Medicare and Medicaid reimbursements and increased private insurance coverage are making these chairs available to more people who need them. Customized wheelchairs are larger than a standard wheelchair. They are designed to maintain the person's head and body in a position that will prevent pain, maintain good posture, and promote the best mobility. The wheelchair may be the only means of mobility when the client is out of bed. Most of these chairs are equipped with a solid padded vinyl-covered seat and back. All parts, straps, and other pieces must be kept together, maintained in clean condition, and used as directed.

A motorized wheelchair will have one to two batteries in a box behind the chair (Figure 5-15). Wires run from the batteries to the motor and to the control box. The battery box has a cover that should be kept on to keep the batteries clean. You or the family will be instructed in the care of the batteries by the therapist.

Remove the caps from the batteries once a week to check the level of the water. If the water is low, carefully add distilled water until you can see the water level just below the opening. Wipe any spilled water with a paper

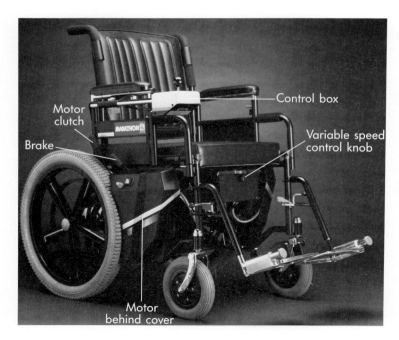

Figure 5-14.   *Parts of a motorized wheelchair.*
Courtesy of Everest & Jennings, Inc.

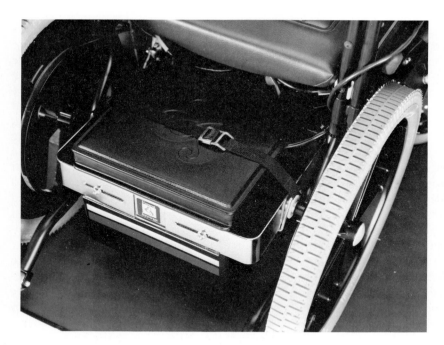

Figure 5-15   *A battery box for a motorized wheelchair can hold either one or two batteries and fits under and behind the wheelchair seat.*
Courtesy of Everest & Jennings, Inc.

towel or rag and discard it. Replace the caps and the cover. Reconnect any wires that are loose or not connected. If you are not sure, check with the nurse supervisor or therapist.

The control box has an on/off switch. Turn the switch off whenever you move your client. If possible, he should transfer from the side of the wheelchair opposite the control box. Keep the control box clean; watch for spilled liquids or food. The nurse supervisor or family member should call the vendor that services the wheelchair about any problems with the control box.

If the chair is used a great deal during the day, the batteries will need to be recharged every night after the client is in bed, using a special battery charger (Figure 5-16). Do not charge the chair in his bedroom. There are fumes released from the battery as it charges. This is also contrary to most fire codes.

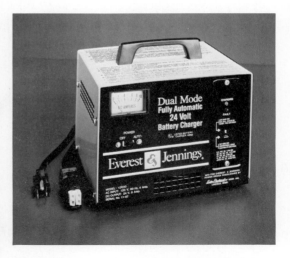

Figure 5-16. *A motorized wheelchair battery charger is designed for use with gel or water-filled batteries.*
Courtesy of Everest & Jennings, Inc.

Recharging Wheelchair Batteries

- Connect the charger with the wheelchair plug that is labeled charger.
- Plug the charger into a household outlet.
- *Check the instructions for **each** client's wheelchair:* Do the instructions state that the power to the hand control unit be turned "on" at this point in the recharging cycle? Not all wheelchairs have this requirement.
- Complete the recharging cycle.
- Remove the plug from the wall socket before disconnecting the wheelchair plug from the charger.

This is an expensive and complex piece of equipment. If repairs are needed, the nurse supervisor, client, or family should contact the equipment vendor. The chair may have to be taken out of the home and often the client is not able to get out of bed until the chair is returned. Many vendors will supply a "loaner" chair if one is requested.

Battery Charger

The motorized wheelchair has two handles near the wheels. One handle controls the brakes as on other wheelchairs. The other handle pulls the belts tight so that the motor will move the chair. The belts run around two wheels so that the chair can be pushed when the belts are loose. It will only move by the motorized control when the belts are tightened. Some motorized chairs and batteries weigh over 200 pounds. They are difficult to move if not kept in good condition. Newer light-weight wheelchair models are becoming popular for many reasons. The lighter weight is clearly one reason.

A three-wheeled scooter is available for clients who have fairly good sitting balance, but poor ability or inability to walk (Figure 5-17). A scooter is not as bulky as a standard motorized wheelchair. It has special adaptations for moving easily about the home, especially in the kitchen. Scooters are battery operated and need the same care and maintenance as motorized wheelchairs. Clients who have chronic respiratory diseases, cardiac insufficiency, arthritis, multiple sclerosis, or Parkinson's disease are examples of persons who may benefit from access to scooters.

Wheelchair Attachments

Armboards

A simple **armboard** can be attached to a wheelchair armrest (Figure 5-18). Arm-

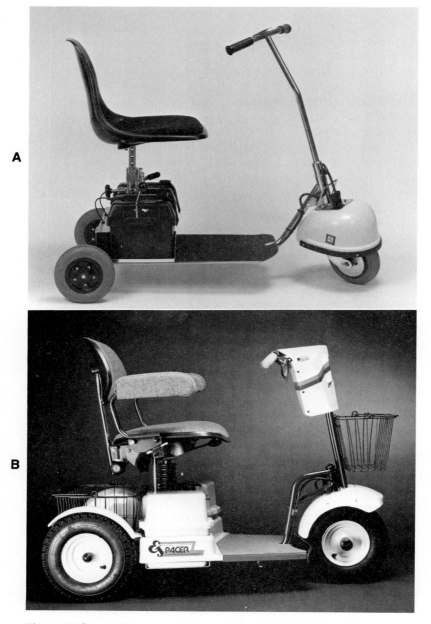

Figure 5-17.   A, *Scooters provide excellent mobility for clients with good seating balance.* **B,** *Three-wheeled scooter with swivel seat and armrests. Courtesy of Everest & Jennings, Inc.*

boards are used for persons who have one weakened side. Such clients include those who have had a stroke or brain injury or have one of the neuromuscular dystrophies or multiple sclerosis. The armboard is used on the *weakened* side to:

—support a weakened arm in proper position,

—hold up a weak or painful shoulder, or
—elevate a swollen hand (Figure 5-19).

Armboards can be purchased through any wheelchair or supply company. If insurance does not cover the cost, a family member can make one at home with a small investment in materials and equipment. The occupational

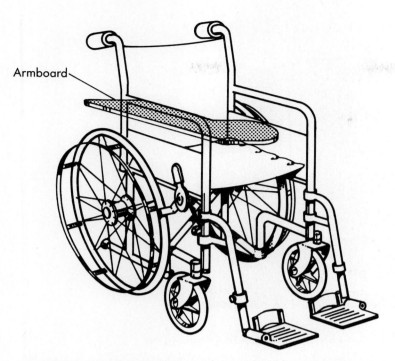

Armboard

Figure 5-18.   *Armboards can be attached to the arm of a wheelchair to support a client's arm on his **affected** side.*

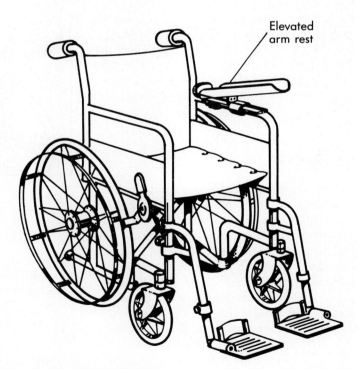

Elevated
arm rest

Figure 5-19.   *An elevated arm rest may be ordered for a client whose **affected** hand becomes swollen.*

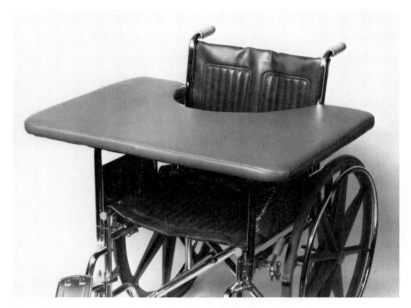

Figure 5-20.   *Padded lapboards are available commercially.*
Reprinted by permission of © Bissell Healthcare Corporation/Fred Sammons, Inc.

therapist or nurse can offer assistance and approve the final product.

An armboard is cut to fit over the wheelchair armrest. It should extend over the sides far enough to provide additional support for the person's arm, but not to intrude on his sitting space. The surface of the plywood board is covered and padded to protect the skin. The armboard should fit snugly on the armrest and not rock back and forth. However, it must be easily removable for transfers out of the wheelchair.

Lapboards

A wheelchair **lapboard** is an item that can be purchased or easily made at home. Homemade lapboards are fashioned from wood products. Commercially made lapboards may be purchased that are padded for extra comfort (Figure 5-20). Clear lucite lapboards may also be purchased. These allow the client to see what is occurring below the board, on his lap, and around his feet. Clear lapboards may also be more cosmetically acceptable to clients because they are not as obvious. One style rests across the top of the skirtguards under the wheelchair arms. It extends across the person's lap as he sits in the wheelchair.

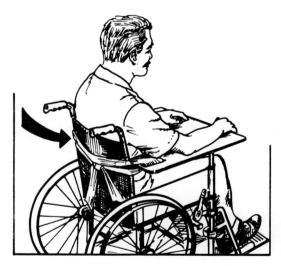

Figure 5-21.   *A lapboard can be secured with straps behind the wheelchair.*

Another style rests on top of the wheelchair armrests and extends over the wheelchair sides and the front. The lapboard is secured to the wheelchair with straps that tie behind the back of the chair (Figure 5-21). A lapboard:

—provides support for the client who has weakness in one or both arms or shoulders,

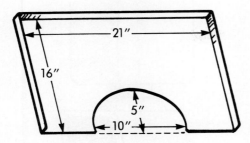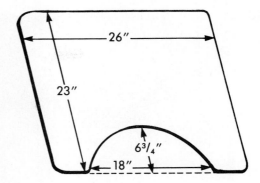

Figure 5-22

—serves as a tabletop for food or books,
—provides a work area, and
—provides a place to carry things from one place to another while propelling the wheelchair.

A wheelchair to be fitted with a lapboard should have removable armrests or desk arms that can be turned around to fit backwards as a supporting frame. A family member may want to make a lapboard at home. The nurse supervisor or therapist will approve the final product for the client.

Suggested Plans for Making a Home-Made Lapboard

● Measure the wheelchair to determine the exact dimensions for the lapboard.
● Check the amount of room between the board and the lap of the person sitting in the wheelchair. This is especially important if the client is heavy.
● Select the lapboard materials. The board can be made of plywood that has been sanded smooth and varnished. A strip of quarter-round or molding glued across the front and side edges of the board creates a ledge to keep things from sliding or rolling off the edge.

EQUIPMENT FOR CARE IN THE HOME

BEDROOM EQUIPMENT

A proper bed serves many purposes for a person whose disability causes him to use the bed as a piece of equipment, not merely a place to sleep. A proper bed will assist the client to move while in bed. The bed may be a rented hospital bed, purchased bed, or the person's own bed. Whatever the type, the mattress must give firm support in the middle as well as on the sides. A bedboard or piece of plywood inserted under the mattress will help to firm up a mattress (Figure 5-23). However, it will not solve the problem of a sagging, soft mattress.

The mattress should have a waterproof cover, preferably one that encases the entire mattress. Hospital beds have waterproof mattresses. A piece of plastic or a heavy duty trashbag can protect the mattress in a temporary situation. These covers must be kept wrinkle-free to prevent skin problems. Clients may have a wide variety of bedding, much of which is discussed in Chapter 6.

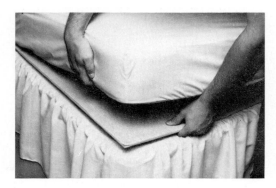

Figure 5-23. *A bedboard can be made out of plywood to firm up a mattress.*
Reprinted by permission of © Bissell Healthcare Corporation/Fred Sammons, Inc.

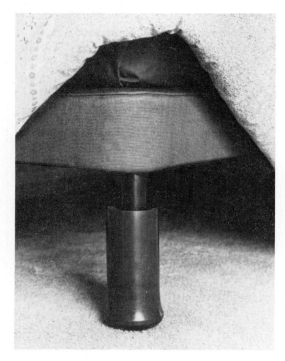

Figure 5-25. *Bed extenders can be used to elevate two or four corners of a bed. Commercial bed extenders such as this one are made of plastic.*
Reprinted by permission of © Bissell Healthcare Corporation/Fred Sammons, Inc.

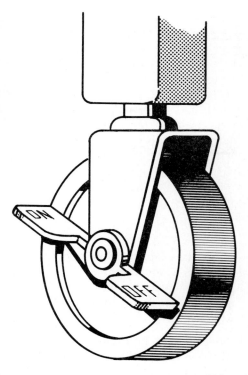

Figure 5-24. *Caster brake locks keep a bed stationary.*
Courtesy Ted Hoyer and Company, Inc.

giver may make transfers more difficult. For this reason, consider using a hospital bed that has either hand cranks or electrical adjusters to raise and lower the bed.

The bed legs have **casters** with brake locks to keep the bed from moving about the room (Figure 5-24). Keep the casters locked unless you are moving the bed. The casters can be removed if the bed is too high, but then the bed cannot be moved. Wooden blocks about 4–6″ high under the bed legs can help you reach without straining your back. The blocks will also prevent the bed from being moved. Be sure the blocks are large and stable enough to support and balance the bed safely. Bed extenders that are made commercially will also serve the same purpose (Figure 5-25).

Safety Siderails

Many beds come equipped with **siderails** that slide up and down. However, many clients resist siderails because they make them "feel like children." Siderails must be securely locked in place to prevent falls. If side-

When caring for someone who is in bed, consider your posture and safety as well as the client's. One consideration is the height of the bed. There are varying heights of mattresses, boxsprings, and beds. The mattress height should be higher than your lower back. The bed height that assists the care-

rails are stiff, add a drop of 3-in-1 oil at the lock. If no rails are available, ask the nurse supervisor to instruct about using household furniture in the place of siderails. This will only be an option if your client is not overly active. Portable siderails such as those used for youth beds can be inserted between the mattress and box springs. If the person is restless and requires siderails for safety, pad the siderails with blankets, towels, or thin pillows. This prevents the client from being bruised by the railings. Inform the nurse supervisor if a client requires siderails.

Trapeze Bars

A client may have a **trapeze bar** attached to the bed so that he can lift his body weight off the bed, using one or both hands. This maneuver is useful when you are turning the person, adjusting the linens, or providing the bedpan. The trapeze bar must be firmly attached to the bed and stationary during use. Swing or lift it out of your way when you are working at the bedside. A standing floor

model is usable when the bed has no headboard. This needs to be kept in proper position to be safely used.

Bedside Commodes

A **bedside chair commode** is used for toileting by a client who can get out of bed, but who cannot get to a bathroom. Always encourage your client to use a commode if it is available. Discourage use of a bedpan. Moving to the commode and sitting upright will assist him to empty his bladder more efficiently and completely.

A bedside commode is basically a toilet seat built into some type of supportive frame (Figure 5-26). Test the commode to be sure it is braced for support and will not tip when the person moves to and from it. Adjust the commode legs to the height where he can sit with his feet flat on the floor. Folding commodes have armrests that will swing or drop out of the way for easier transfers. Keep the armrests clean and oiled (Figure 5-27).

An important part of a bedside commode is the seat. Seats are available with open or closed fronts and are made from hard or soft materials. Check wooden seats for splinters that may develop over time. The family may

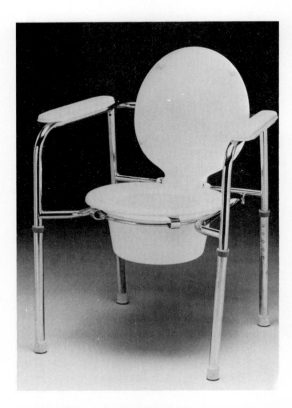

Figure 5-26. *Adjustable-height bedside commode with removable bucket to permit using over the toilet. Courtesy of Everest & Jennings, Inc.*

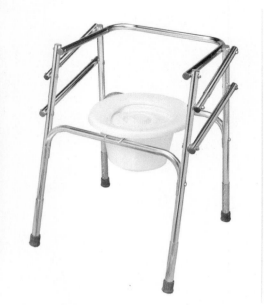

Figure 5-27. *Adjustable-height folding commode with removable bucket. Courtesy of Lumex, Division of Lumex, Inc.*

need to sand, refinish, or replace the seat. Check soft seats for cracks or splits in the plastic covering. Use tape or plastic patches to repair the damage or replace the seat. Tell the family or nurse supervisor about needed repairs. All seats must be kept clean with soap and water, or with other solutions as directed.

Most commodes have a plastic bucket that slides under the seat to catch the wastes. Consider lining the bucket with a small plastic bag. This is especially helpful with bowel movements because they can be taken directly in the bag to the toilet. This saves extra cleaning and keeps the plastic bucket from absorbing odors.

Commode Chairs with Wheels

Some commode chairs have small wheels and must be pushed from place to place (Figure 5-28). Others have large rear wheels, like wheelchair wheels. These may be self-propelled if the client is able to wheel them. For safety, these chairs must have brakes on at least one front wheel and one rear wheel on opposite sides of the chair. This is necessary so the chair is not able to move around in a circular motion. The chairs may have hard or soft seats, armrests, backrests, and footrests. Some styles have high backs or fully reclining backs. They are checked and cleaned as other bedside commodes.

- You can use this chair to wheel your client into the bathroom if:
  —he can sit and balance on the commode chair,
  —there is a clear passage to the bathroom, and
  —he can be safely moved.
- You are responsible to:
  —assist the person to transfer to the commode chair,
  —wheel him into the bathroom on the chair,

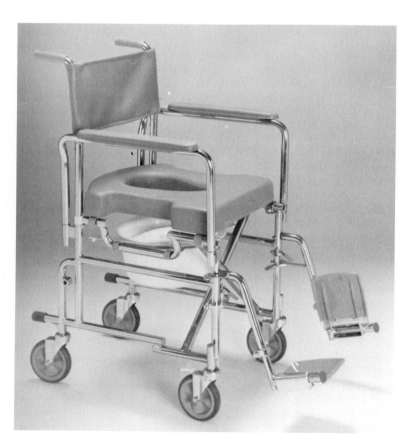

Figure 5-28.   *Commode chair with wheels and underseat bucket. Courtesy of Everest & Jennings, Inc.*

—remove the plastic bucket from under the commode chair,

—raise the bathroom toilet seat,

—wheel the person still on the commode chair to sit directly over the toilet,

—lock the brakes on the commode chair, and

—provide for his safety at all times.

Overbed Tables

The **overbed table** is used to assist the person who takes meals in bed. It can be lowered to fit in front of the wheelchair or to hold water and supplies for bathing. The table may be used for holding assistive devices while the client is reading or answering the telephone, or for holding remote control devices for operating televisions. If a bedside table is not available, a cardtable will hold supplies at the bedside. A sturdy box can be cut out and used as an in-bed tray if necessary.

BATHROOM EQUIPMENT

The bathroom is the room in the home where most accidents happen, to both able-bodied and disabled persons. Take up loose floor rugs and wipe up water whenever you and your client use the bathroom. Do not use electrical appliances such as hairdryers, razors, or radios, around water. Be sure your client does not drop appliances such as electric toothbrushes, into the water.

Toilets

Most home toilet seats are 16″ from the floor. This is lower than a standard kitchen chair. Some clients have difficulty standing up and sitting down at regular toilet height. An elevated toilet seat with adjustable height armrests may assist him to stand. Elevated toilet seats must be securely attached to the toilet and not move (Figure 5-29).

Rails for alongside the toilet are available in many styles and sizes. Rails fasten over the toilet and under the back of the seat (Figure 5-30). Some are attached in front of the toilet and others are attached to the bolts that hold the toilet seat. They are easy to move from

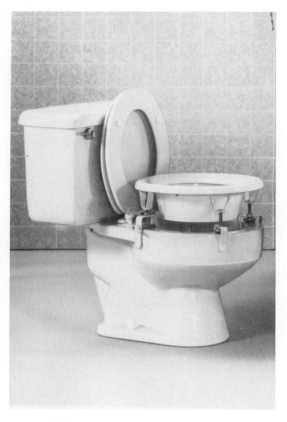

Figure 5-29.   *Elevated toilet seat.*
Courtesy of Lumex, Division of Lumex, Inc.

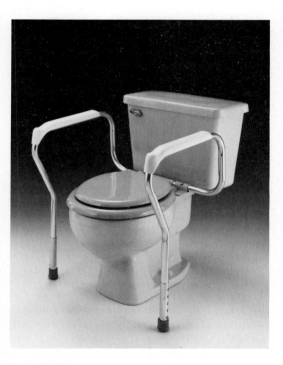

Figure 5-30.   *Adjustable toilet safety rails.*
Courtesy of Lumex, Division of Lumex, Inc.

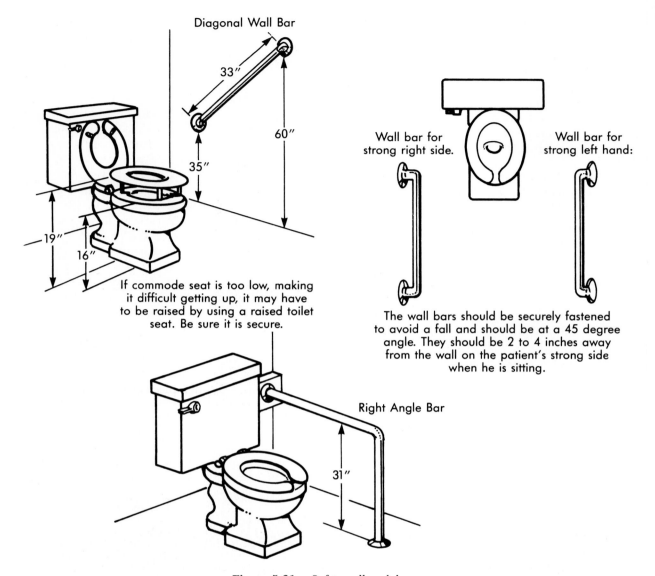

Diagonal Wall Bar

33″

60″

35″

19″

16″

If commode seat is too low, making it difficult getting up, it may have to be raised by using a raised toilet seat. Be sure it is secure.

Wall bar for strong right side.

Wall bar for strong left hand:

The wall bars should be securely fastened to avoid a fall and should be at a 45 degree angle. They should be 2 to 4 inches away from the wall on the patient's strong side when he is sitting.

Right Angle Bar

31″

Figure 5-31. *Safety wall grab bars.*

place to place. They have few moveable parts. Rails with legs to the floor should have rubber tips on the legs. The tips should be in good condition and not cracked or dried. The tips prevent the rails from moving when they have to hold a person's weight. Wash rails with soap and water.

Bars may be fastened to the wall or set in the floor (Figure 5-31). They assist a person to rise and move from one place to another with support. Bars must be permanently and securely fastened directly into the 2×4 wooden wall studs. Doorknobs and towel racks glued to the wall or into the tiles are *not* safe. Even a bathroom sink may pull loose if

your client uses it to pull up from the toilet. The bars should be made of rust proof or plastic-coated metal.

Tubs

A bathtub can be a dangerous piece of equipment because it is hard, potentially slippery, and contains water that may be very hot or too cold. Also, your client's body may be wet and slippery as he is going in and out of the tub. *Always test the water temperature before your client enters the tub.* Another safety rule is that no client should enter a tub beyond a point where he can easily and safely get himself out. Following this safety rule, a person with a disability may not be able to get into the tub at all. However, he can use other equipment to sit on and shower rather than soak and bathe in the tub.

Bath Aids

Benches and seats that allow a person to sit in the tub or shower are very popular. They are available in a wide range of prices, sizes, and heights, including adjustable heights (Figure 5-32). Few persons should use a bath seat without a back. A person who can walk to the tub himself may use a seat or bench height of 15″ with a back. Larger benches extend the full width of the tub and measure 16″ or more in seat depth with adjustable legs. The larger seat will work better when you must move and bathe the client.

Many benches have padded seats that must be kept smooth, without tears or splits, to prevent cutting or scratching your client. If the seat is split or torn, check to see if the entire seat (or parts of it) must be replaced. This type of seat may become slippery when it is wet and soapy. The bench legs are adjustable with rubber tips on the ends for stability. Rubber tips can be purchased at the same store that supplies the seats. To prolong its

wear, the bench should be taken apart, washed, and dried to remove soap and hard-water residues.

Rubber mats must be placed in the bottom of the tub to give you and the client safe footing in the tub. Place the mat under the tub seat and the bench. Use it whenever you have to step into the tub to assist or move your client. Rubber tub mats are cleaned with soap and water. They should be laid over the tub edge or bench to dry when not in use.

A shower hose makes showering easier for the person who is using a tub bench or chair. The shower hose attaches directly to the tub spout. A rubber shower hose is inexpensive and can be purchased at discount or hardware stores. Metal shampoo hoses are more expensive, but can be permanently installed.

If there is no tub equipment, a wooden or chrome kitchen chair can be used if the legs have rubber tips. The family may choose to cut the chair legs down 2 inches to make the chair low enough for easy use. The family member covers the seat with oil cloth or vinyl stretched over a 1-inch piece of foam to provide a softer seat. A higher seat may cause the person to slide off once he is wet and soapy. If possible, the family member should apply marine varnish or outdoor paint to cover the wooden part of the chair.

Other helpful aids for the bath include bath mitts (Figure 5-33) and soap bags made

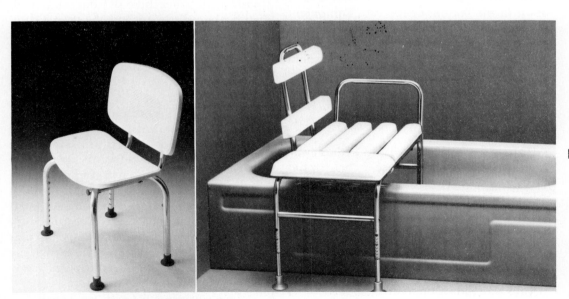

A

B

Figure 5-32. **A,** *Adjustable-height tub bench.*
B, *Padded adjustable transfer tub bench.*
Courtesy of Lumex, Division of Lumex, Inc.

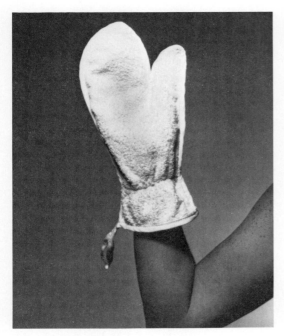

Figure 5-33. *Bath mitt.*
Reprinted by permission of © Bissell Healthcare Corporation/Fred Sammons, Inc.

from a dish cloth with a bias binding string. If the person drops the soap or has difficulty holding the soap while bathing, he can pull it back by the string. Other supplies and holders can be attached with suction cups to the tub or tile.

Your client may be unable to manage to sit down in the bottom of the tub. Equipment and procedures may be needed so that he can do so safely. First practice a transfer into the tub while he is clothed, including shoes and a transfer belt for his waist. He should be able to hold onto a grab bar. Concentrate on practicing sitting down into the tub. Hold onto his belt to stabilize and guide him. Use proper body mechanics.

If the toilet is more than 2–4 inches away from the tub, you may place a chair at the outside of the tub as a safe "landing place." A rubber tub mat and a grab bar anchored to the wooden studs in the wall, not a towel bar, are essential. The grab bar must be strong enough and securely attached. It must support the weight of a person as he moves down to the bottom of the tub.

Tubs with sliding doors are very difficult to enter unless the person can stand and step into the tub with two strong legs. It is easier and safer to have the family remove the doors and store them out of the room. The tub is then open for a semi or full seated transfer into the tub. The family may install a curtain on a tension rod for privacy.

Stall Showers

Showerheads and controls are tested before the client enters the shower. Automatic temperature controls, if affordable for the client, help prevent accidental burns. Single-action faucets with lever type handles are easiest to operate.

Most equipment used for a tub is also used for a stall shower:

—a bench or chair 18–19″ high with or without a back,
—a stationary commode chair with legs lowered to make up for the height of the shower floor, or
—a chrome kitchen chair modified by the family as described earlier.

Specialized Equipment for Moving Clients

Lifts and Slings

Many persons cannot transfer from the bed to the wheelchair with or without assistance. In the hospital, the nursing staff uses a **mechanical lift** to get these persons out of bed. Lifts for home use are made by several companies. Medicare or Medicaid usually will rent or purchase a lift for a person who needs one. A lift will ensure your safety while moving a person who is very heavy or one who cannot assist you.

If your client has been moved using a lift, he may know about its care and use. Have your nurse supervisor direct you through the move with your client before trying to move him alone at home. Listen to your client if he can instruct you about the use of the lift. But be sure he suggests safe procedures. Clients who use mechanical lifts are likely to be very heavy or have multiple sclerosis, muscular dystrophy, hemiplegia with both sides of the body affected, high level quadriplegia, cerebral palsy, or severe brain injury.

Before you use a lift with your client:

● Practice first with your nurse supervisor.
● Discuss the steps in the move with your client.

- Check the room or yard for safety hazards.
- Use two people for a transfer until everyone has practiced and is competent with the procedure.
- After you use a lift, ask your client what went well and what he would suggest changing about the move. Discuss any changes with the nurse supervisor before performing them.

Mechanical lifts are available in manual or electrical versions. Most lifts have parts similar to those in Figure 5-34. The lift has four casters with one brake on each side. The hand crank has a hydraulic unit filled with oil.

The sling under the person's body supports his trunk and, if necessary, his head.

The safest style sling is made from one long piece of material that connects to the lift with chains. When you crank the lift handle it causes the hydraulic unit to raise or lower the sling. Once the person is seated, the chains swing away with the lift. The sling remains under the person. Figure 5-35 illustrates the placement of the sling under the body and support of the shoulders and upper legs.

An electric lift operates on the same principle as a hand-cranked lift. Simply turn the switch on or off to operate the electric lift. Electrical outdoor lifts are installed in many homes or apartments to give clients access outside the house. Do not use an **outdoor lift** if you have any questions about its condition or if the client tells you it is not operating properly. Report any suspected problems to the family and the nurse supervisor. They

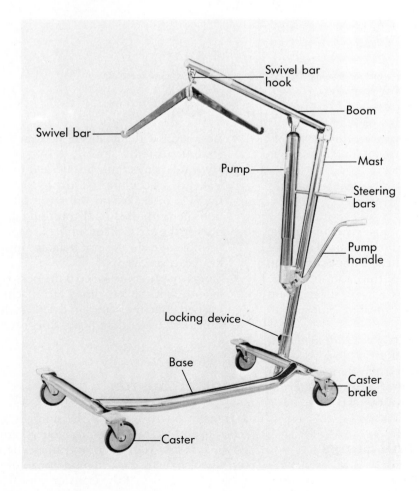

Figure 5-34. *Hydraulic lift with adjustable base. Courtesy Ted Hoyer and Company, Inc.*

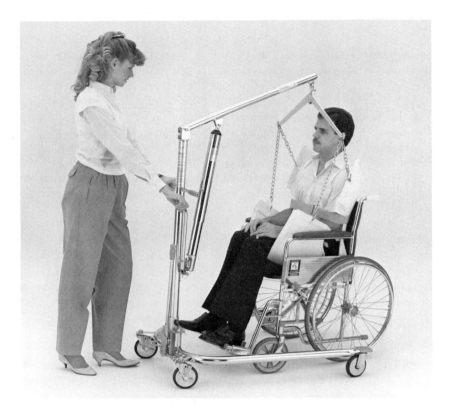

Figure 5-35.   *Proper alignment for moving a patient in a sling with a mechanical lift. Courtesy Ted Hoyer and Company, Inc.*

will notify the equipment vendor or supply company.

Specialty Lifts

A mechanical lift is available for use at the bathtub. This special lift can be used to move your client from the wheelchair or commode directly to the bottom of the bathtub (Figure 5-36 a, b). This lift has a nylon sling. Nylon remains strong after repeated exposure to water and dries quickly.

Other specialized lifts are designed to lift a person into and out of a car (Figure 5-37). One style has a low top frame designed to lift a person into and out of a car. Another attaches across the top of the car.

Care of Lifts and Slings

- Casters must be kept clean and oiled. Keep casters free of dust or threads and clean off any spilled foods or liquids.

- Do not allow the chains to become tangled or twisted.
- Hydraulic units must be checked for oil leakage. Check for oil drops on the floor. If oil leaks you will see it on the floor beneath the lift. If you find oil, **do not** use the lift. Call for service as soon as possible and do not use it again until it has been serviced.
- Slings may become soiled if the person is incontinent. Soiled slings are machine washed, but must be air dried. Nylon slings dry faster than heavy duty canvas slings.

Transfer Boards

A transfer board is one of the simplest and most useful pieces of equipment (Figure 5-38). It assists your client to transfer from the wheelchair to the commode or to other places. Proper use of the transfer board and methods of transfer are taught in rehabilitation centers. If your client has been taught to

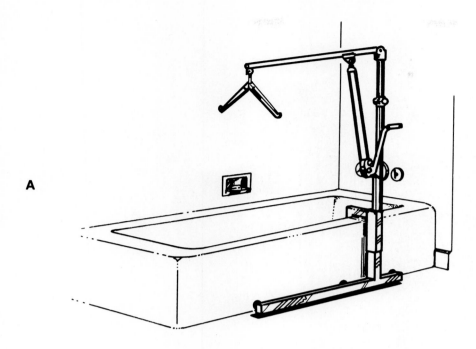

A

Figure 5-36.   **A,** *Tub lift for sling.*
B, *Tub lift with seat.*
Courtesy Ted Hoyer and Company, Inc.

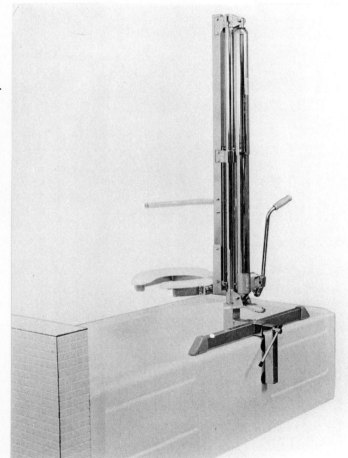

B

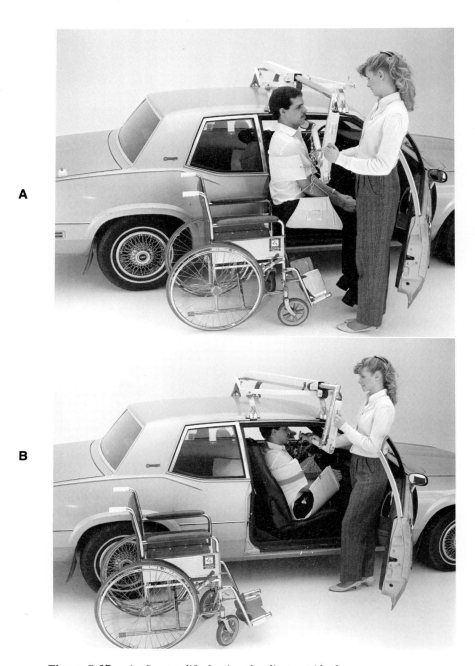

Figure 5-37.   **A,** *Car top lift showing the client outside the car.*
B, *Car top lift showing the client inside the car.*
Courtesy Ted Hoyer and Company, Inc.

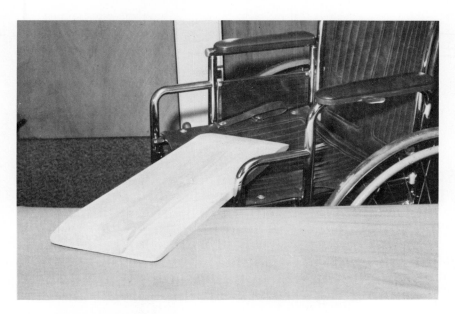

Figure 5-38.   *Transfer board.*
Reprinted by permission of © Bissell Healthcare Corporation/Fred Sammons, Inc.

use a transfer board he will have found the easiest way to transfer. He must have a strong upper body, especially his arms, and reasonably good balance if he is to use the transfer board safely and independently. Clients who have quadriplegia can use a transfer board to transfer with different amounts of assistance, even if they are fully dependent.

The techniques for using a transfer board are discussed in Chapter 4. A client should not actually slide on the transfer board. Instead, he uses a series of small push-ups along the board. Your role is to assist the client to complete a safe transfer without any skin damage from transferring. You must also be sure he has proper body position after the transfer is made.

Transfer boards are made in different sizes for different uses. Standard thickness is ³/₈-inch made from solid hard wood, such as maple or birch. Plywood is not usable because the layers will splinter and may warp. Transfer boards may be made at home by the family, in a local wood shop, or purchased through commercial vendors. Commercially made transfer boards may be made from plywood, nylon, or hardboard. They may have various sizes and shapes.

Figure 5-39 (on p. 176) illustrates the di-

mensions that are to be used when making a transfer board. The family should always consult with the nurse supervisor when making a transfer board.

Making a Transfer Board

Transfer Board Dimensions:
  bed transfer board—10 × 25 inches
  bed/car transfer board—10 × 30 or 36 inches
  transfer boards for large and heavy persons—12 × 30 or 36 inches
Steps for a family member or volunteer to make a transfer board:
- Taper 4 inches back on both ends of the board, leaving ¹/₁₆ inch at the ends.
- Bevel the sides in 1 inch.
- Sand the wood smooth.
- Finish with varnish.
- Wax the board with hard-finish wax such as a gym floor wax.
- Keep the board polished with furniture polish so the person can easily transfer across the board.

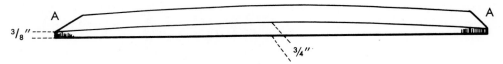

Figure 5-39.   *Measurements for making a transfer board.*

OTHER SPECIAL EQUIPMENT

Hand and Wrist Splints

Hand and wrist **splints** are appliances that are prepared and specially fitted for a client by the occupational therapist. There are several styles of splints but each one is carefully modified to fit each client (Figure 5-40).

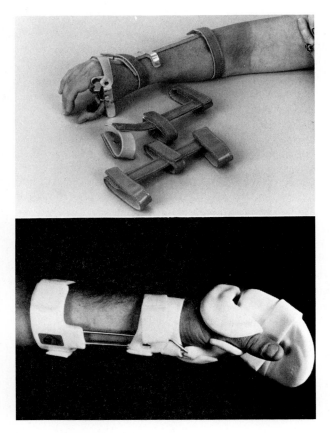

Figure 5-40.   *Wrist supports to maintain normal positioning and to permit hand function. Reprinted by permission of © Bissell Healthcare Corporation/Fred Sammons, Inc.*

The basic reasons for a client to wear wrist and arm splints are:

—to correct various problems related to the disability,
—to help and support weakened muscles,
—to keep the joint from moving,
—to hold the hand and wrist in a particular position,
—to prevent hand or wrist drop or contractures, or
—to provide enough wrist support to propel a wheelchair or to hold a special spoon for feeding himself.

It is your responsibility to

—care for the splint as directed by the nurse supervisor or occupational therapist,
—help the client properly apply the splint as directed by the nurse supervisor or occupational therapist,
—apply the splint at the scheduled times of day or night (some splints are worn only at night), and
—observe the skin for irritation, redness, or early detection of breakdown.

Foot and Ankle Supports

Foot and ankle positioners are used to prevent contractures of the ankle or foot drop (Figure 5-41). These positioners may be used only at night or over 24 hours if the client is in bed. A soft liner protects all skin areas of the foot and ankle within the supports.

Supports are made from plastic parts joined with screws or from rigid foam. The liners may become soiled and dirty from perspiration. Liners can be washed with mild soap and water.

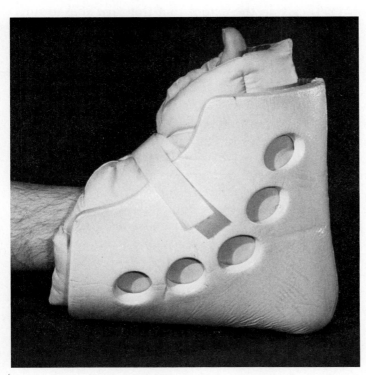

Figure 5-41. *Foot and ankle positioner with removable liner.*
Reprinted by permission of © Bissell Healthcare Corporation/Fred Sammons, Inc.

CHAPTER *6*

Activities of Daily Living and Assistive Devices

*O*BJECTIVES

When you have studied this chapter and practiced the procedures it describes, you will be able to:

1. Identify types of assistive devices available for persons with disabilities.
2. Assist clients and families to use assistive devices.
3. Assist clients with activities of daily living, including dressing, eating, and grooming.
4. Assist clients with activities to maintain independence in daily living, including proper seating and ambulation.
5. Encourage clients to perform self-care to the extent that they are able to do so.

*O*VERVIEW

Activities of daily living are the activities that individuals perform in their personal care. This chapter describes the activities of eating, dressing, grooming, and personal hygiene. It also discusses the array of assistive devices suitable for each activity. Each client's functional abilities and degree of independence in performing activities of daily living will differ. Self-care for your client does not mean that your client will be able to perform all care for himself. It does mean that he may direct the care, perform parts of the care, use assistive devices or aids to perform the care, or require varying levels of assistance from you.

There are many assistive devices and aids available for persons with disabilities. Some of these can be purchased at local stores, others must be ordered from specialty vendors, and still others can be easily made at home. This chapter describes assistive devices from all of these sources. They are representative of the type of assistance necessary for the client's particular disability. For example, if a long-handled item is the assistance needed, there are descriptions of several choices of assistive long-handled objects for purchase or use for your client.

Loss of the ability to care for personal body needs and appearance is one of the most difficult adjustments an individual must make following a disability. You, as the caregiver, may find that:

—your client has difficulty accepting the personal care that you perform for him;

—your client, or his family, expect you to perform care, even when he is supposed to assist and increase his own self-care; or

—you and your client are able to improve your relationship and achieve other self-care goals as a result of successfully working together during personal care activities.

Consider the many very personal habits we all have:

No one:
—ever brushes your teeth the way you do,
—ever washes your face to your satisfaction,
—combs your hair exactly the way you want it,
—shaves you as well as you do yourself, or
—applies your cosmetics the way you wish.

Think about your client as you do these things for him.

DRESSING

In our society, we must all wear clothing. We all want to be dressed to some degree like everyone else is dressed. This feeling of wanting to be like others, to belong, starts when we are children and continues into adulthood. A person who has a disability already feels different from others. Other people often react to a person's disability, rather than to the person himself, as if it made him less acceptable as an individual. It is therefore important for persons with disabilities to dress as much like other people as possible.

Styles vary widely among lifestyles and age groups. For example, teenagers tend to prefer jeans and loose shirts, older women may not have considered slacks proper in their youth, and older businessmen may feel they need a suit and tie to be dressed for the day. Choosing what to wear can be fun or frustrating, but the decision belongs to the individual who wears the clothes. The choices of a person who has a disability should be based on his own taste and habits and blended with choices that enable him to be as independent as possible in putting the clothing on and taking it off.

One important way you can assist your client to feel more independent is to encourage him to dress in his own clothing for at least a part of every day. The person's friends and family will react to him more positively if he is dressed. He will feel less "sick" or disabled if he is dressed in his regular clothing.

All clothing must be clean and neat. Wash your client's underwear and socks daily. Remove and wash soiled clothing. Soiled clothes cause skin breakdown and disagreeable odors for your client. If there are difficulties with hygiene or proper amounts and types of clothing, notify your nurse and the family. You cannot keep your client appropriately dressed and clean without the necessary clothing and laundry facilities.

HINTS FOR DRESSING

- Begin dressing with the person's **affected** or weakened side, keeping the arm and shoulder leaning forward.
- Begin undressing with the **unaffected** side.
- Place yourself standing next to the **affected** side.
- Encourage your client to dress out of, or sitting on the side of, the bed as much as possible to keep the idea of independence on his mind—and on yours too.
- Have your client do whatever he can for himself and use assistive devices.

Often a minor adjustment or a clever adaptation can make it possible for a client to be both stylish and independent in dressing himself. The following pages suggest techniques in dressing and clothing adaptations to help your clients toward dressing independence.

Persons who must stay in bed should wear loose-fitting tops with front openings. Baggy pajama tops, shortie nightgowns, and hospital-style gowns are all easy to put on and take off. They are also comfortable for your client to wear in bed without causing skin irritations. If it is cool, bed jackets, sweaters, and flannel pajamas are very useful. The same principles apply to in-the-bed dressing as to other dressing: it should be easy to put on and easy to take off. Use the technique of rolling your client from side to side while assisting him with clothing, if necessary.

As you dress and undress your client, use the same procedures each time. If he needs help remembering, repeat the steps out loud as you do them. Keep him as involved as possible and encourage his participation.

UPPER-BODY DRESSING

All upper-body dressing is easiest if the person is sitting at his bedside in a wheelchair or commode seat. If your client has very weak arms and poor or no shoulder muscles, he may be instructed to wear a sling for support. He would wear the sling as instructed by the nurse or physical therapist, usually when he is out of bed. A sling is placed over the outside of his clothing while he is indoors. The sling can be made longer to extend over the outside of a coat or jacket.

Blouses, Sweaters, and Shirts

The easiest blouses, sweaters, and shirts for the person with a disability are those with raglan sleeves, dropped shoulders, and loose necklines. Look for large buttons on shirts, and blouses without zippers in the back. Items without stretch cuffs can have a button sewn on the unaffected side with elastic thread. When the person slides his hand through the cuff, it will stretch to allow his hand through, but still give a buttoned appearance. He will be able to button the cuff on the affected side with his unaffected hand.

Buttons on the front of a shirt can be buttoned with assistance of a buttonhook (Figure 6-1). The shirt may be stitched half-way up the front, appearing buttoned, but put on over the head as a slip-on shirt. Velcro tape can be placed on the top two or three buttons to finish closure of the shirt. If the client uses a buttonhook assistive device, this can be used instead of Velcro. Use a shirt with a full tail, not a tapered one.

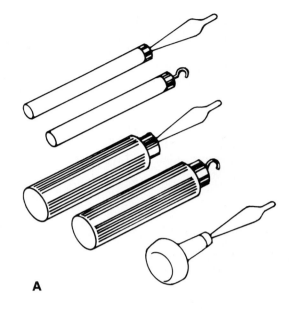

A

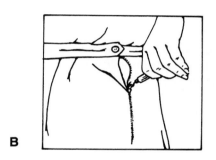

B

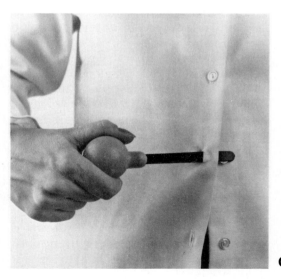

C

Figure 6-1. *Various styles of button hooks enable a client to button and zip his own clothing.*
Courtesy of Lumex, Division of Lumex, Inc.

Begin dressing standing on the person's *affected* side.

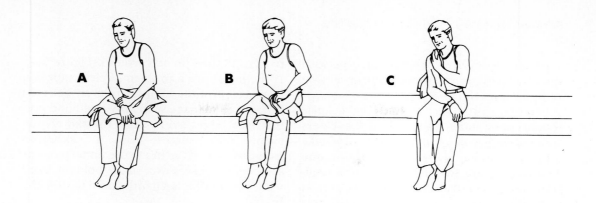

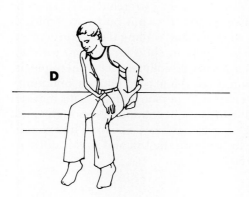

Figure 6-2. *Dressing in a shirt (or button-style dress).*

*A, Check your client's ability to balance before beginning. The client who has one side of the body affected should sit down to put on a shirt or shirt-button styled clothing. Lay the shirt **inside-up** with the collar at his knees.*

*B and C, He uses his **unaffected** hand to lift the **affected** hand into the armhole and to pull up the sleeve over his **affected** shoulder.*

*D, He uses a tossing movement to place the shirt and other sleeve behind him. He can reach behind him with his **unaffected** hand and insert it into the shirt sleeve to finish dressing.*

Put the *affected* arm into the shirt first to dress (Figure 6-2).

Undress the *unaffected* arm first (Figure 6-3).

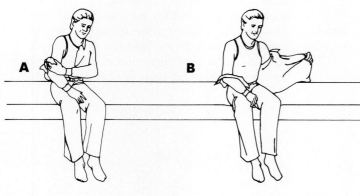

Figure 6-3. *Removing a shirt.*

*A, The client sits safely. He uses his **unaffected** hand to slide the shirt off his **affected** shoulder.*

*B, He holds the front placket of the shirt on the **unaffected** side to pull it away from his body and off his shoulder.*

*C, He can sit on part of the shirt-tail to assist while he pulls his **unaffected** arm out of the other sleeve.*

*D, He uses his **unaffected** hand to slide the sleeve down his **affected** arm and the cuff over that hand.*

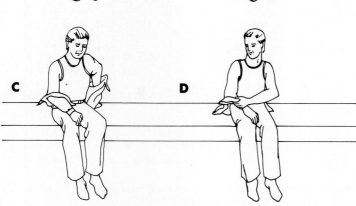

If both sides are affected, such as with spinal cord injury, begin with whichever side your client prefers.

Pullover shirts, sweatshirts, and T-shirts should all be loose-fitting. V-neck sweaters and undershirts are easier to put on and take off because they have more neck room. These shirts are *put on the person with hemiplegia using the affected arm first.* The person with spinal cord injury will use both arms together. A person with multiple sclerosis or arthritis will place his weaker or most limited arm into the shirt-sleeve first. The other arm is inserted into the other sleeve before pulling the shirt down over the head. Many times a shirt will go on easier if the person brings his head forward and down alongside his hands and then raises his hands and head together pulling on the shirt.

Coats, jackets, and heavy sweaters are treated as if putting on a cardigan or a button-down-the-front shirt. Start dressing the affected arm, but pull the sleeve up onto the person's shoulder before starting to dress the other arm. This is necessary to keep the sleeve from falling down due to the extra weight of the coat.

Brassieres

Bras are a particular problem for women. Often a regular back-fastening bra is easier to manage than a front-closing bra. The bra is put on backwards, being fastened in the front, and then turned around (Figure 6-4). If the hooks are a problem, Velcro tape can be placed over the hooks. However, Velcro is difficult to manage with only one hand and the hook edges may irritate the skin. Some clients have success with a clothespin snapped to hold the bra to the underpants or slacks. This serves as a stable holding hand while the **unaffected** hand is used to close the hooks.

A bra that is very stretchable lycra can be stitched closed. It is put on by stretching it over the head and pulling it down into place. This is an easy method for persons with upper extremity disabilities such as hemiplegia, amputations, spinal cord injuries, and multiple sclerosis. A person with arthritis may not be able to move her shoulders enough to put a bra on over her head. She may, however, be able to step into the bra and pull it up from her feet.

LOWER-BODY DRESSING

When out of bed, your client should wear underclothing that is loose and non-restrictive. Boxer-style shorts are easier to put on than either jockey or bikini styles. Boxer shorts are also kinder to your client's skin because they absorb moisture and allow free movement without rubbing the skin. Underwear must be kept clean and changed as often as necessary, at least once a day.

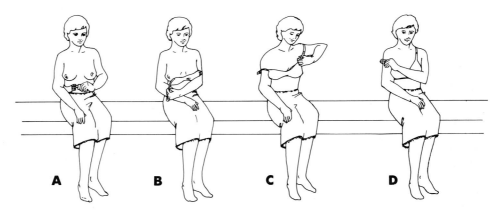

Figure 6-4. *Dressing in a bra.*
   A, *Client must be able to sit and balance safely. She puts the bra on backwards around her waist. Be sure cups are positioned correctly. If she cannot fasten the hooks, velcro may work instead of hooks. Use a safety strap if needed.*
   B, *She turns the bra to the front. She uses her **unaffected** hand to insert the **affected** arm into the strap.*
   C, *She inserts her **unaffected** arm into the other strap and position bra.*
   D, *She uses her **unaffected** hand to position the strap on the **affected** side and to adjust the bra.*

Men are encouraged to select loose-fitting, washable slacks and women to select elastic top, pull-on washable slacks. These styles are useful for both you and your client because they are easy to put on and off, easy to care for, and have a waistband to hold onto during transfers. Many people wear jogging suits because they are stylish, washable, and comfortable. They do not, however, have a waistband to use as a handhold during transfers. If you have no alternative, you may add a belt around the person's waist to use for transfers. This will also work for ladies who choose to wear dresses. Dresses should be washable and open down the front. If your client wears a legbrace, the jogging suit may be too bulky beneath the brace. Other clients find the elastic at the bottom of the leg too tight.

It may be difficult to convince some clients to wear functional clothing and shoes. Jeans are the choice of most young people and may be worn if they are the wide-leg, full-cut styles. The back center seam may cut into the person's skin as it is very stiff and heavy. This is often a problem for the person who has a spinal cord injury, if he is moved or positioned by someone holding onto his jeans. This can cause skin breakdown from rubbing and pressure. Jeans must be kept wrinkle-free. Use a belt if necessary to move or posi-

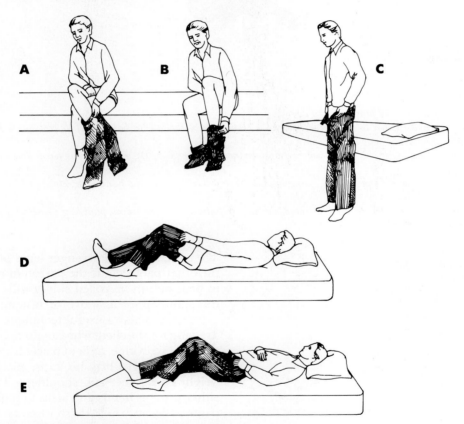

Figure 6-5. *Dressing in pants while standing to balance.*

    A, *Check client's ability to sit or stand and balance safely. Sitting on the bed, he uses his **unaffected** hand to lift his **affected** leg across his **unaffected** knee. He pulls his pants leg completely over his **affected** foot and ankle. If he cannot lift or cross his leg, assist him or elevate his **affected** leg on a box or stool so that he doesn't lean over.*

    B, *He inserts his **unaffected** leg fully through the other pants leg. He uses his **unaffected** hand to pull the pants up on both legs as high as he is able.*

    C, *If he can safely stand, he holds onto the pants and the waist with his **unaffected** hand. He pulls the pants on and adjusts the waist and zipper. He never bends over to pull up his pants.*

    Bridging for dressing:

    D, *If he cannot stand, he lies down on the bed (follow step **B**). He flexes his **unaffected** knee, keeping the foot flat ont he bed.*

    E, *As he pushes down on the bed, his hips will elevate. He can use his **unaffected** hand and arm to pull up his pants and fasten them.*

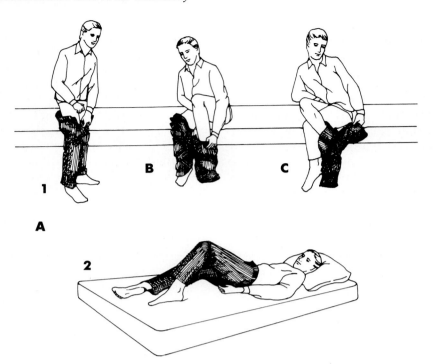

A

Figure 6-6.   *Removing pants.*

A, 1, *Check his ability to stand and balance. Use the side of the bed for balance. If he can stand, he can unfasten his pants and slide them down.*

2, *If he cannot stand, he lies in bed and bridges (as in Figure 6-5,* **D***). He works his pants down onto his legs, below his hips.*

B, *He sits on the edge of the bed, using his* **unaffected** *hand to slide the pants completely off his* **unaffected** *leg and foot.*

C, *He crosses the* **affected** *leg over the other leg. He pulls off the remaining pants leg using his* **unaffected** *hand.*

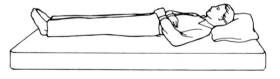

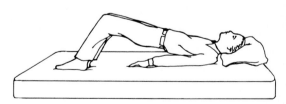

Figure 6-7.   *Bridging is a useful technique for clients who can lift their hips and bear weight on their shoulders.*

tion this person, but not the belt loops, which will break.

Use the same procedure to put on and take off lower-body clothing as you do upper-body clothing (Figures 6-5, 6-6). *The affected or weaker leg is placed into the pants leg first.*

Then the *unaffected,* stronger leg is placed in the other pants leg. If the person must dress in bed, he can be rolled side-to-side to pull the pants up to his waist for fastening.

Bridging is also a useful technique during dressing for the client who can lift his hips off the bed. To bridge, a client places his feet flat on the bed. He lifts his hips, placing his weight on his feet and shoulders. Then he either uses his hands and arms to pull up his pants or assists you to do so when he lifts his hips (Figure 6-7).

The client who is able to stand safely at the bedside and is able to assist in dressing uses the following method. While sitting, the client places the affected leg into the pants leg. Some clients may lift the affected leg over the unaffected leg to do this. The unaffected leg is inserted into the pants leg and the pants are pulled up well over both knees. The client then pulls up the pants as he comes to a standing position. Suspenders may be useful to help pull the pants into position.

If he can stand and balance, but cannot

pull up the pants with either arm, you may assist him by simply pulling up his pants while he stands. If he cannot reach a full standing position, but can lift his hips off the seat, assist him by pulling the pants up as he leans forward and off the seat, especially on his weaker side. *Do not* have your client bend over to pull up his pants from his ankles.

Stockings and Socks

There is a wide variety of footgear available to meet specific needs for clients. For example, the stocking a client wears may be prescribed by his physician. Special stockings are often prescribed to support a client's circulation or to reduce edema in his legs. These stockings are usually made of light-weight, pliable lycra and are used by a client who needs mild support. Heavier, brown-colored stockings, made from a stiffer elastic, are used to provide firmer support. These stockings, which are measured and sized to fit each wearer, are most often worn by clients who have spinal cord injuries. Your nurse supervisor will give you specific instructions about how to put the stockings on your client, when the stockings are to be put on and taken off, and how long they are to be worn.

As a general rule, you should put these stockings on your client each day as soon as he sits at the side of the bed or while he is lying on the bed.

It is easier if you lightly powder the foot, and are sure that the client's feet are dry. The entire foot should be placed in a sock before the sock is pulled up the leg (Figure 6-8). Be careful not to push your fingers through the stocking. This is a good time to check the condition of the foot and toenails. Socks and knee-high nylons should not have elastic tops because they may be too tight around the leg. Similarly, tube socks with long areas of elastic will irritate the skin and cause circulation problems as they become too tight at the top after being worn for long periods. To remove the stocking, simply strip it down from the top, turning it inside out as you go down the leg.

Clients may be able to put on their own socks using fold-at-the heel technique in Figure 6-9.

Some clients have assistive devices with long handles that snap onto the top of socks to enable them to pull their own socks up. Figure 6-10 shows one type of device that can be used for shoes and stockings.

Support stockings are expensive. They must be hand-washed in warm, not hot, soapy water. They are then thoroughly rinsed, and **hung** to dry. The stockings must be washed and hung at least every other day in order to retain their shape and elasticity. (Do not place stockings in the dryer or they will lose their elasticity.) Your client will need several pairs of stockings to rotate, and a spare pair.

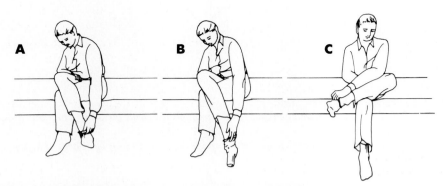

Figure 6-8. *Applying socks. (Check client's ability to balance safely before beginning.)*

A, *The client sits to cross his **affected** leg over his **unaffected** knee. He must be able to reach his **affected** foot without leaning over and losing his balance.*

B, *Using his **unaffected** hand, have the client pull the top of the sock competely over his toes. He works the sock over his foot until his toes are into the toe of the sock. He pulls the top of the sock at the front, then at the back to pull the sock on over his heel and ankle.*

C, *The other sock is applied by using the same technique. The client uses his **unaffected** hand to pull the sock onto the **unaffected** foot. Reverse the procedure to remove socks.*

To remove: Grasp the top of the sock. Pull it down the leg, over the heel, and off the foot.

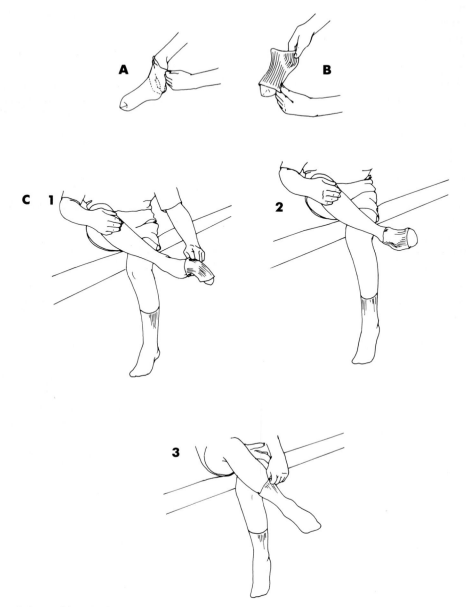

Figure 6-9.   *Fold-at-the-heel technique.*

A and B, Preparing the sock for the client.

A, Hold the sock at the open top with one hand. Reach into the sock with the other hand and grasp the heel area from inside.

B, Pull the top of the sock down over itself so that the inside heel becomes an open area. The top of the sock will extend to beyond the toe.

C, Putting on the sock.

1, Place the open part of the sock over the toes (use the unaffected hand) with the heel area under the foot (on bottom).

2, Pull up the sock onto the toes as far as possible onto foot. The heel of the sock should be at the heel of the foot.

3, Pull the top of the sock over the rest of the foot and heel, and position on the leg. The heel is in proper position. Rib-knot socks are better than long elasticized cuffs (will work for elastic support hose).

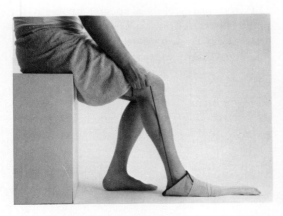

Figure 6-10. *A sock puller with a snap top assists a client to apply his own sock.*
Reprinted by permission of © Bissell Healthcare Corporation/Fred Sammons, Inc.

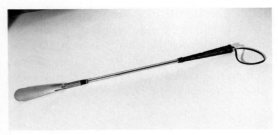

Figure 6-11. *A long-handle flexible shoe horn assists a client to reach his shoes without bending or leaning over.*
Reprinted by permission of © Bissell Healthcare Corporation/Fred Sammons, Inc.

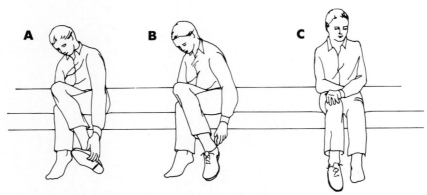

Figure 6-12. **A,** *The client must be able to sit and balance safely. He crosses his **affected** leg over his **unaffected** leg. Using his **unaffected** hand, he puts the shoe onto his foot. Be sure the shoe tongue doesn't buckle under the shoe.*
B, *A long-handle shoe horn may assist him to insert his heel. He places his foot on the floor.*
C, *He slides his foot fully into the shoe, using his **unaffected** hand to push on the **affected** knee. Remove the shoe horn. Repeat for the other shoe.*

On rare occasions a client may have a custom-fitted body stocking that covers his hands, arms, or legs. The body stocking helps to prevent scars following severe burns. Clients who have body stockings need assistance to take them on and off, keep them clean, and eliminate wrinkles. Your nurse supervisor will give you precise instructions and will closely monitor the client who has a body stocking.

Shoes

Shoes are important for your client, whether or not he walks. If he walks, he needs shoes for support. If not, they protect his feet. Flat heels and hard rubber soles are best, and your client's shoes must fit securely for safety during standing and transfers. If you are not sure about his shoes, ask the nurse or physical therapist to check them for you. Keep your client's shoes polished and neat.

If your client wears a leg brace or prosthesis, he should put this on at the side of the bed. Unless he has communication problems, he should be able to assist you with directions about putting the brace or prosthesis on his leg. You will need a shoehorn to get his foot into his shoe with the least amount of trouble. Some clients have long-handled shoehorns that enable them to slip their feet into their shoes (Figure 6-11, Figure 6-12).

Tying shoelaces is a special problem for many clients. Although Velcro and other materials have eliminated some shoe-tying problems, many support shoes require lacing as part of their design. Figure 6-13 shows how a client with right hemiplegia can tie his left shoe using one hand. Reverse the steps for a person with left hemiplegia. Practice the steps yourself before working with your client.

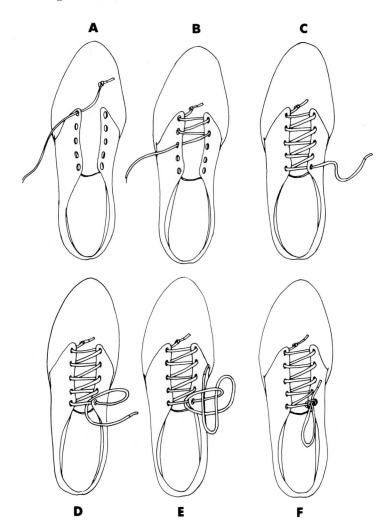

Figure 6-13.   *Technique for lacing and tying a left shoe for a person with right hemiplegia.*

A, *Tie a knot on one end of the shoestring. Begin to lace the open end of the shoestring through the eye at the left side.*

B, *Lace the shoestring across the tongue of the shoe, alternating sides. Be sure to lace in under each eye and over to the opposite side of the shoe.*

C, *The laced shoe should look like this.*

D, *Loop the end of the shoestring under the top row of lacing. Leave the loop open.*

E, *Insert the folded end of the shoestring through the open loop. Pull the folded end toward the ankle and the inside of the leg.*

F, *Tighten the loop. Be sure the shoestring is not too long so client will not trip over the loose end.*

GROOMING

Clients may have disabilities that only affect the daily functioning of certain parts of their bodies. Many persons have upper extremity weaknesses that cause disability for use of both extremities, one extremity, or part of one or both extremities. Others have weaknesses that require them to have support for the trunk of their bodies or have lower extremity weaknesses.

UPPER EXTREMITY WEAKNESS

Persons who have had strokes or have spinal cord injuries, arthritis, multiple sclerosis, muscular dystrophy, and congenital disabilities are examples of clients who may have upper extremity weakness. This section discusses ways to support specific levels of upper extremity weakness so that the client can best help with his own care in grooming. Assistive devices are suggested along with the techniques.

- When the client's shoulder is too weak to lift his hand or arm to his face:
  —Support his elbow from above with a sling.
  —Stabilize his elbow on a lapboard or table.

  —Hold his elbow in your hand to steady and support it.

- When the client's wrist is too weak to support his hand and he cannot use his hand to grasp or hold onto objects:

  —Use a splint prepared by the occupational therapist.
  —"Build up" handles on self-care objects, such as toothbrush, comb, lipstick, hairbrush, or razor.
  —Add longer handles to some of these objects for easier and safer reaching (Figure 6-14).

- When a client has limited range of motion at the shoulder use:

  —light-weight objects.
  —long-handled objects.
  —an electric razor for shaving safety, even though it is heavier and may require your assitance. Keep the razor moving as he shaves, and clean after each use.
  —an electric toothbrush, with built-up handle if needed.
  —assistive devices such as a shampoo brush with a ring that fits over one finger. The brush will enable him to scratch his head or brush his hair.

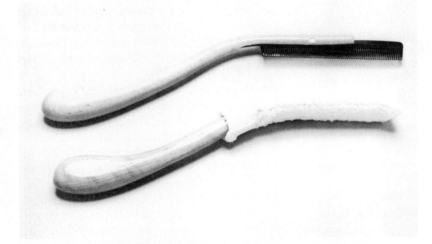

A

Figure 6-14. *Long handles on combs and brushes enable clients to perform their own grooming activities. Courtesy of Lumex, Division of Lumex, Inc.*

Continued.

B

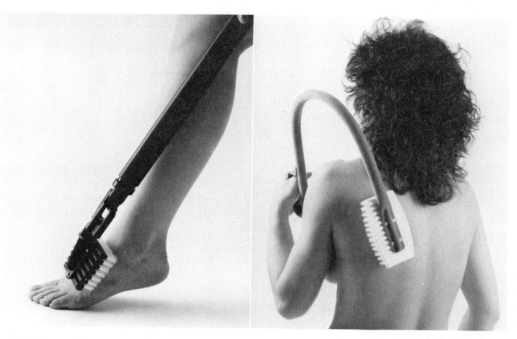

C

Figure 6-14, cont'd.   *Long handles on combs and brushes enable clients to perform their own grooming activities.*
Courtesy of Lumex, Division of Lumex, Inc.

—A mirror placed at a level low enough for him to see himself in the mirror while in his wheelchair or other customary seat. Either a wall- or free-standing mirror may be used.

—assistive devices to help your client open shaving cream cans, toothpaste tubes, or after shave lotion, available from the occupational therapist.

—a suction-cup brush fastened to the side of the sink to brush dentures with one-handed functioning. Apply tooth paste products to the brush after it is attached and before use.

—a washcloth mitt with a Velcro wrist tab to keep it in place while washing and mild liquid soap or soap in a net or dishcloth bag.

—long-handled brushes to reach below his knees and to his back.

Figure 6-15 shows samples of some assistive devices.

● Shampooing is very difficult for the client who has weakened upper extremities and he may require your assistance. Shampoo your client's hair when:

—he is in the shower as part of the routine.

—he is given a bed bath, using a shampoo tray (Figure 6-15 e). A rubber sheet can be folded to form a receptacle. The water will empty into a basin or pail set on the floor.

● Sometimes you may have a client who is able to walk safely, but is unable to use his arms above the level of his waist. He may be able to manage his clothing in the bathroom, but is unable to cleanse himself when needed after toileting. Ask the occupational therapist about the device that will hold paper or cloth so your client can reach and cleanse himself (Figure 6-16).

● In some cases, a client may have low endurance as well as muscle weakness. He may not be able to complete his grooming by himself or he may have to use both hands at some point. He should continue to do what he can and try to increase his endurance; then you can finish the task. If your client has other deficits, sich as visual deficits following a stroke, you may have to remind him to groom both sides of his body.

● When a client cannot grip well with his hands, a *Universal Cuff* may be useful.

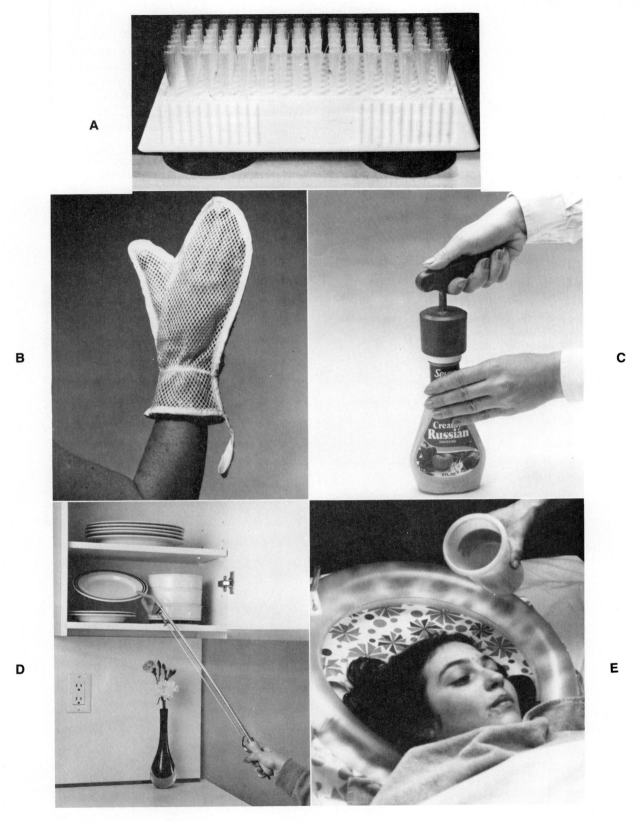

Figure 6-15. **A,** *Suction cups hold this nail brush firmly in place for the client to use.*

   B, *This mesh hand mitt holds a bar of soap for a client who is unable to grasp or hold soap.*

   C, *A client may be able to grasp the handle of a cap turner when he cannot grasp and turn a small cap.*

   D, *Reachers can assist clients to reach objects from wheelchair height.*

   E, *A bed shampoo tray assists clients with grooming.*

   A and B reprinted by permission of © Bissell Healthcare Corporation/Fred Sammons, Inc.; C and E courtesy of Lumex, Division of Lumex, Inc.

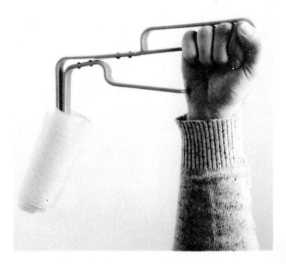

This assistive device fits around his hand. He can insert a self-care item securely into the pocket of the Cuff and use the item without having to grasp it. Insert a comb, lipstick, hairbrush, or a safety razor in the pocket once he has mastered the technique.

Figure 6-16. *A toilet paper holder assists client to cleanse himself after toileting.*
Reprinted by permission of © Bissell Healthcare Corporation/Fred Sammons, Inc.

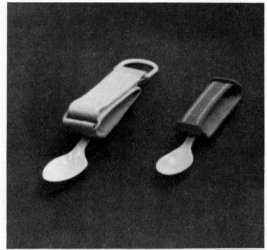

A

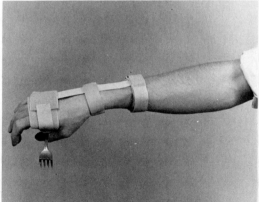

B

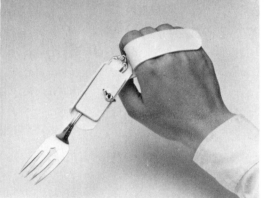

C

Figure 6-17. **A,** *A universal cuff can grip many self-care items.*
B, *Universal cuffs may be combined with wrist splints for support and stability.*
C, *This universal cuff uses a C-clip and a different style pocket.*
Reprinted by permission of © Bissell Healthcare Corporation/Fred Sammons, Inc.

*E*ATING

Clients who require assistance to feed themselves may become frustrated, even losing their appetites. It is difficult for many clients to accept having someone else help them with eating. It may cause them to feel helpless or as if they were sick so that they had to be fed. If a client finds it difficult to eat neatly, keep him tidy so that food does not dribble down his chin and cause him to become upset with his attempts to eat or feed himself.

On the other hand, our eating habits are very personal—choosing which bite to take, in what order, and what amount. A client who requires assistance may also eat slowly; he may tire easily. If he can partially assist himself, you may have to finish feeding him if he becomes fatigued. Monitor your own feelings about assisting your client with his food so that your frustrations do not affect your client's ability to feed himself, be nourished, and enjoy a comfortable atmosphere.

Assistive devices and equipment are becoming widely available, not only in medical supply catalogues and home care specialty supply catalogues, but also in numerous gift and mail order catalogues. Check with your therapist and nurse supervisor to see whether equipment or devices are appropriate for your client and whether the items can be made at home if the client's budget is lean. There is a temptation, on the part of families, clients, and caregivers alike, to want to order more items than necessary in attempts to make the client's eating easier and help him become more independent.

Clients who have weaknesses in their upper extremities have access to an increasingly wide variety of adaptive equipment to assist them with feeding themselves. Assistive devices and equipment mentioned earlier for grooming—elbow slings, wrist splints, the Universal Cuff, and holders—are all used for eating as well. One of the more common adaptations is a "built-up handle." The utensil or aid with a built-up handle may be purchased or made at home.

The home model is made by slipping a

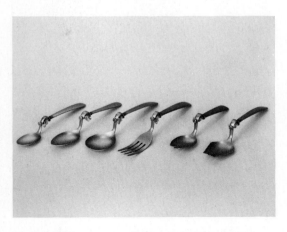

Figure 6-18. *These eating utensils have adjustable swivel handles designed to keep food on top of the utensil without spilling.*
Reprinted by permission of © Bissell Healthcare Corporation/Fred Sammons, Inc.

foam hair curler over the handle of a fork. The idea behind building up the handle is to create enough bulk or surface area for the client to hold onto if he cannot close his hand around a smaller handle. It also enables him to control the movements of the utensil by using larger muscle movements rather than fine motor-control movements.

A similar spoon is called a swivel spoon (Figure 6-18). No matter which way the client's hand turns, the bowl of the spoon swivels to remain upright, preventing spills. A client must be able to grasp the handle and bring the spoon to the dish and back to his mouth, but the design of the spoon enables him to do so without spilling the contents.

Clients who use built-up utensils often benefit from a dish or plate equipped with a stop. A client may be able to get food into a spoon if he has something to push against with the spoon to trap the food into the spoon. Children's feeding dishes may have a stop feature; look for those with decorations that are not childish for adult clients. Figure 6-19 shows a metal plate guard that clips onto the edge of a standard plate as a stop; it is removed for washing (Figure 6-19). Some

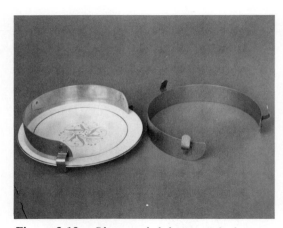

Figure 6-19. *Plateguards help "trap" food onto a utensil and keep food on the plate.*
Reprinted by permission of © Bissell Healthcare Corporation/Fred Sammons, Inc.

clients use utensils that are combinations of a knife and fork or a fork and spoon to assist them.

Cutting food is another area that is difficult for some clients who are able to perform other self-feeding tasks. The motion of sawing back and forth with a knife in one hand and a fork in the other may be difficult or impossible for some clients, often for different reasons.

For example, the person who has one hand amputated or has a weak hand following a stroke may be unable to press down hard enough to cut. Similarly, the person who has multiple sclerosis or arthritis may have this difficulty. A person with quadriplegia will not be able to press down or hold the food in place, requiring other ways to cut.

One method that may work uses a shallow flat dish to hold the food. The client grasps a

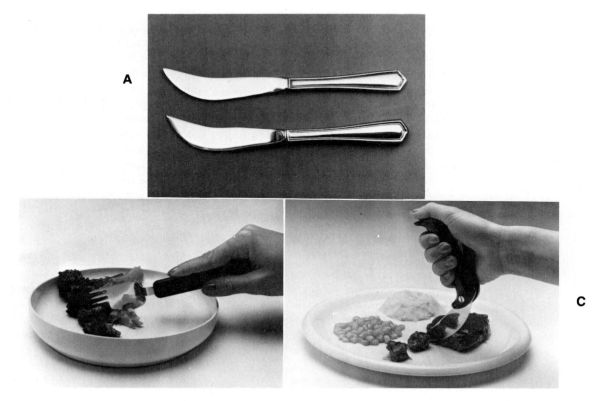

Figure 6-20.   A *and* **B,** *Utensils with rounded edges can be rocked back and forth to cut food.*
C, *This rounded knife is collapsible.*
Reprinted by permission of © Bissell Healthcare Corporation/Fred Sammons, Inc.

sharp steak knife or collapsible knife that is equipped with a rounded blade (Figure 6-20). The knife is manipulated in a rocking motion over the food. With practice, many clients become successful using this type of knife. A rounded fork can also assist with cutting food.

It will also assist your client if the food itself is stabilized. Large items such as baked potatoes can be skewered into place so that a client can eat around the potato. Divided plates with high divisions are useful for trapping food into sections. Long, flexible straws eliminate the need for a client to pick up a cup or glass to drink; even a cup holder can assist a client who cannot hold a glass or cup in his hands (Figure 6-21).

One thing that affects self-feeding but is often overlooked is the surface of the table. The surface must be close enough for the client to reach easily and at a comfortable height for bringing utensils to and from his mouth. The surface must be non-slip so that plates, cups, or other objects do not move away from the client, especially if he has to exert pressure away from himself to trap food. Simple assistive measures include:

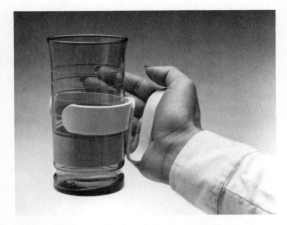

Figure 6-21. *A C-clip glass or cup holder may enable a client to drink independently.*
Reprinted by permission of © Bissell Healthcare Corporation/Fred Sammons, Inc.

—non-slip pads,
—double-stick tape on the bottom of a plate or cup,
—a wet washcloth under the plate,
—weighted bottom plates,
—a glass holder with a straw holder, and
—long-handled utensils.

SUPPORTS FOR CLIENTS WITH TRUNK WEAKNESSES

Clients may have weakness or lost strength in their abdominal and back muscles that causes weakness in the trunk. They will have difficulty with:

—maintaining balance while sitting,
—sitting in proper alignment,
—sitting for any length of time because of low endurance, and
—breathing, because they have little support from diaphragm and lower chest muscles.

Do not apply a trunk support unless your nurse supervisor has approved the use of the device and given you instructions about how to place the support on your client. Clients may have supports in their homes that are incorrect for their current condition. Supports used for clients who have trunk weaknesses are:

- *Binders*—A binder is a wide elasticized support that is wrapped around the abdomen and fastened in place with Velcro strips. A binder is used to support a client's lower abdominal muscles. Wash binders in mild soapy water, rinse, and hang to dry.
- *Corsets*—A corset is a rigid trunk support that is individually fitted to the person. It is fortified with bone stays and has adjustable hook-and-eye fasteners. Wash corsets in mild soapy water, rinse, and hang to dry.
- *Back braces*—Back braces are the most rigid support devices in this group. A back brace has metal upright supports that fasten with leather straps. It is individually fitted and extends from the individual's shoulders or underarms through the full length of his trunk. Cli-

ents who require back braces may wear them 24 hours a day, but almost always while they are out of bed. This brace is not washable.

- *Molded braces*—On occasion, a client may wear a molded plastic brace covering his trunk area. These braces are not removed except by the physician.
- *Safety strap*—Safety straps are similar to moveable seat belts. They are made from canvas or similar materials, can be buckled or fastened at various heights as needed, and can be washed. They are not to be used as restraints. A safety strap can be a useful device, but does not allow you to leave your client sitting alone. Use a safety strap if your nurse supervisor agrees when:

—your client continually slips down or falls over when sitting and his poor trunk strength is the only thing that keeps him from getting up,

—needed to hold onto your client during a transfer or while getting in and out of the tub, and when

—your client has poor sitting balance when in the tub.

He will need a safety strap around his chest and secured around the back of the tub seat. This client may become safe in the tub, but he cannot wash his lower body with the strap in place.

SUPPORTS FOR CLIENTS WITH LOWER EXTREMITY WEAKNESSES

Lower extremity weakness will not cause problems for a client's bathing unless he insists upon standing or stepping into a shower or tub. Instead assist him with a sitting transfer to a seat in the tub. It is NEVER safe to allow your client to step into a tub or shower. Do not let the client stand to bathe if he has lower body weakness. (Review tub seats and other equipment for bathing in Chapter 5.)

SEATING

Seating is often overlooked as an important part of daily living for the person with a disability. Whenever anyone sits for a long period of time, body heat and pressure build at the bony prominence areas of the buttocks. A client who has reduced circulation or

mobility, a sense of feeling pressure, or related disabilities is at high risk for developing reddened skin areas. A reddened area can develop on the skin of the buttocks within a matter of hours, especially after repeated sitting.

The most common types of cushions, coverings, and paddings are discussed in the following sections. Bed coverings are included with the seating options because many of the same materials are used for both bedding and seating.

1. *Foam*—Foam is available under many brand names. The variations in foam are: thickness, density, hardness or softness, amount of waterproof covering (most foam is not waterproof and must be covered), durability, size of foam block, and cost.

---

*Things to Consider When Seating
a Client*

—length of time he expects to sit
—his disability and ability to move and
shift weight
—his body weight and size
—his general health status and nutritional level
—his risk factors, such as poor circulation or paralysis
—his fit on the seating device
—how the seating device fits into his
chair or wheelchair
—his fit into his chair while using the
seating device
—whether he is incontinent
—the covering of the seating device
—the filling or composition of the seating device
—the durability of the seating material
—the cost of the seating and available
funds

---

2. *Gel*—Gel cushions are heavier and
more expensive than foam as well as
being waterproof or water-resistant.
They vary in weight, price, style, and
covering. The gel may be damaged if
the cushion is torn or split from improper handling.
3. *Air*—Air cushions are available with
sealed or unsealed construction. An air
cushion may cause increased pressure
on a client's skin if it is over- or under-
inflated.
4. *Combinations*—Two common combinations of cushion filler are water combined with foam in a sealed pouch, or
gel combined with different densities of
foam.
5. *Molded or contoured*—This type of cushion is molded to fit the individual client
and his wheelchair. A combination of
several materials or of different densities of a material may be used to construct this type of cushion. These are

the most expensive types of cushions
and usually have their own covers.

PADDINGS, COVERINGS, AND BEDDINGS

1. *Plastic sheet coverings or waterproofed mattress covers*—These coverings are the
best protections for mattresses used by
a client who is incontinent. A mattress
pad or bed blanket should be placed
between the client and the plastic covering, especially in warm weather, so that
the plastic does not become irritating or
"sticky." Keep all coverings wrinkle-free
and do not allow them to dry out and
begin to leak. Frequently used coverings for bedding are:
2. *Sheepskins*—Sheepskins are often used
for wheelchairs as well. They may be
real sheepskins, which are commercially cleaned, or Kodel synthetics,
which may be machine washed and
dried. Due to their special properties,
the benefits of sheepskins are numerous. They are soft, allow air circulation, provide cushioning for some clients, and keep the client warm in the
winter and cool in summer (Figure
6-22).
3. *Air*—Air is used in several varieties of
alternating pressure mattresses, all of
which are equipped with electric
pumps to regulate the air flow. Cover
the mattress with a sheet so that your
client does not lie directly on the plastic
covering. In some cases, clients use an
air mattress designed for camping, being careful that it is not over inflated.
4. *Flotation Mattresses*—A flotation mattress can be used with a regular mattress, in place of another mattress, or on
either a hospital or a regular bed. Common types of flotation mattresses include:
a) *Water mattress*—Water mattresses
have become popular for the general public as well as for clients who
require cushioning. They are available in many styles, thicknesses,
sizes, and with heating elements.
Check the water level, the temperature, the amount of support the bed
offers a client, and his positioning

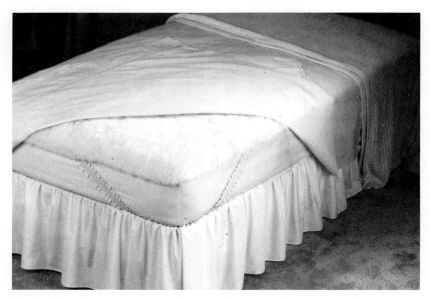

Figure 6-22.   *Sheepskins offer many benefits to clients. They are used in bed, wheelchairs, and car seats. Reprinted by permission of © Bissell Healthcare Corporation/Fred Sammons, Inc.*

while on the bed. Water beds that have firm bumpers around the water mattress are better for moving clients into and out of bed. Some persons do not like the sensation of sleeping on water mattresses; others rest better than ever before. If your client is considering purchasing a waterbed, he must be sure that the floor in his room, especially on a second story, and the structure of his housing will support the weight of the bed.

b) *Gel mattress*—Gel mattresses or combination mattresses containing gel and foam are becoming popular with disabled persons. These mattresses support the body while relieving pressure on the bony prominences, may be used with or without an underlying mattress, are available in sections that are easily moved or cleaned, and are comfortable for the client. There is enough motion in the gel mattress that you must be cautious when moving a client into and out of his bed.

Have your nurse supervisor review any new mattress material with you and practice moving your client into and out of bed the first time.

AMBULATION

Many of your clients will need assistance with ambulation or walking. You must have specific instructions from the physical therapist and the nurse supervisor before assisting your client with ambulation. *Never* take your client up or down stairs without supervisory direction to do so, even if you assist him to ambulate about his home. A client who needs assistance with ambulation may be:

—relearning to walk after an illness or injury;
—learning to walk with paralysis or paresis;
—learning to walk using a prosthesis, crutches, or braces;
—learning to walk using new rhythms or patterns such as for cardiac rehabilitation, to strengthen muscles, or to overcome pain; or

---

Basic Rules When Ambulating with a Client

- Have detailed instructions and practice sessions before working with your client to ambulate.
- Know your client's strength and endurance.
- Do not attempt activities beyond your ability or instructions from the therapist or nurse.
- Understand the purpose of your client's ambulation—is it exercise, working toward independent walking, learning equipment, or other?
- Know how to use any equipment and find out if your client knows how to use the equipment.
- Have equipment checked by the physical therapist or nurse supervisor before using it the first time; recheck it your-

self before each use; do not use faulty equipment.
- Check the walking area for safety hazards and obstacles, before starting to ambulate with your client.
- Be certain that your client is able to rise to a standing position and to sit again after ambulating.
- Guide and support your client as he walks, but do not push, steer, or rush him.
- Assist him to walk with as normal a gait as he is able; if he has an unusual or abnormal gait, poor walking posture, or changes in his gait, ask the physical therapist to check your client's ambulation with you.

—walking with limited endurance, stamina, or balance.

Some clients will always require the supervision of a physical therapist for ambulation activities. These clients are not walking in order to get from place to place, but rather for their own satisfaction and to keep their muscles strong.

AMBULATION WITH A CANE OR ONE CRUTCH

A client who uses a cane, a wide-base cane, or single crutch to assist him with walking will hold the cane or crutch in his hand opposite the affected leg (Figure 6-23). He will ambulate by:

- moving the cane forward and placing the tip on the floor, just ahead of the unaffected or stronger leg and slightly out to the side of his foot,
- taking one step forward with the affected leg, bringing his foot even with the cane,
- placing his body weight on the affected leg and cane,

—stepping forward with his unaffected or stronger leg, stepping just ahead of his affected foot, and
—repeating steps to walk.

You assist by:

- standing at his side that is away from the cane (or crutch if only one is used); if he uses a walker, stand behind him while he is moving.
- using a transfer belt, safety belt, or strap around his waist, if necessary, to steady and support him.
- holding the strap or belt with your hand that is closest to the client, placing your other hand at his shoulder to assist him if he loses his balance.

AMBULATION WITH TWO CANES OR A WALKER

When your client uses two canes or a walker, he will use basically the same motions. When he uses two canes, you assist by standing behind him, moving forward as he moves. Hold onto a safety strap or belt to assist him in case he loses his balance. Do not push him for-

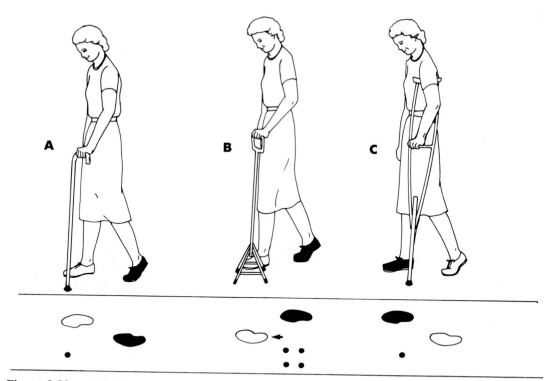

Figure 6-23. *Ambulating with one cane or crutch. Shaded footprints and cane or crutch tips indicate where the foot that bears weight is placed in each step. (This client has his right foot affected).*

A, *The client moves the cane forward, placing the tip on the floor just ahead of his **unaffected,** or stronger leg, and slightly out to the side of his foot. Then he takes one step forward with his **affected** leg. This brings his foot even with the cane or crutch.*

B, *He shifts weight to the **affected** leg and cane or crutch. Then he steps forward with his **unaffected** leg, stepping just ahead of his **affected** foot and **C,** He continues by shifting weight to the **unaffected** leg and repeating the process.*

ward. Assist the client who uses a walker in the same manner.

A client who uses crutches to walk will have been taught a specific step and gait pattern by the physical therapist. Some clients are taught to "swing through," placing both crutches down in one step, then swinging their bodies ahead of the crutches as the next step. This is not a stable gait; it requires strength and balance.

Most clients walk with crutches using walking patterns similar to that for using two canes. Other clients may have been taught to use two- or three-point gait patterns. You must be sure to understand what your role is in assisting these clients. Safety precautions are extremely important to prevent falls. Check the condition of the crutch tips. Be sure the client is not injuring himself under his arms with either crutch. Use a safety or transfer belt. Request directions and supervised practice from your nurse supervisor

and physical therapist (Figures 6-24, 6-25, 6-26).

AMBULATING UP AND DOWN CURBS AND STAIRS

The physical therapist or nurse supervisor may instruct you and your client about ambulation activities that involve going up and down stairs (or curbs when out of doors). The same safety precautions and explicit directions and supervised practice are necessary for these activities.

You may assist your client with stairs after you have been directed and supervised by your nurse supervisor or the physical therapist (Figure 6-27).

—*Do not* walk your client up or down stairs unless it has at least one steady handrail

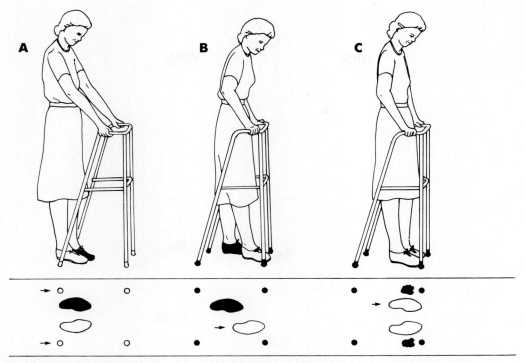

Figure 6-24. *A walker assists many clients to ambulate. (This client has his right foot affected.)*

A, *The client uses both hands to lift the walker and set it ahead of him.*

B, *He steps ahead with his **affected** foot and leg.*

C, *He steps forward with his **unaffected** foot and stands. His hands support his weight on the walker. He repeats this process.*

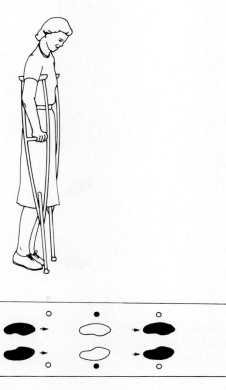

Figure 6-25. *The "swing-through" gait requires a client to have strong arms, weight bearing, and good balance.*

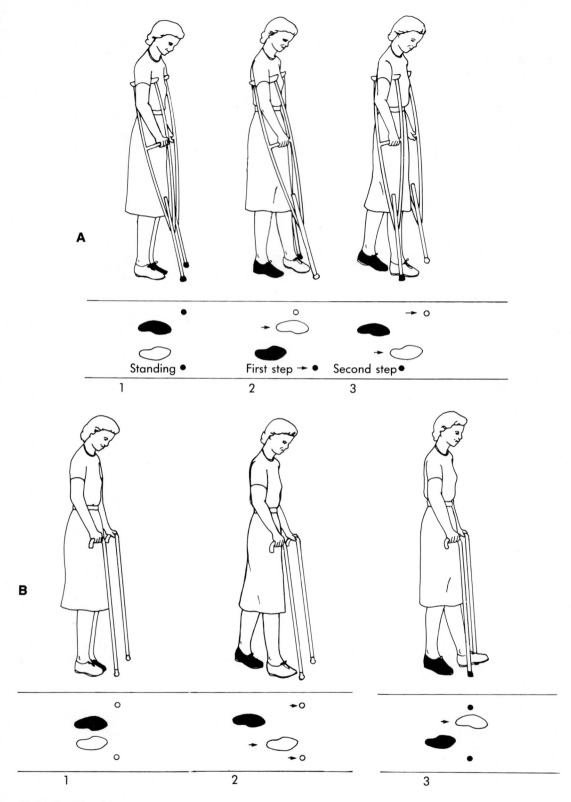

Figure 6-26. *Shaded foot and cane or crutch tip are weightbearing foot for each step.*
A, *A **two-point gait** can enable many clients to become more active in ambulation.*
B, *A **three-point gait** pattern is similar to walking with two canes.*

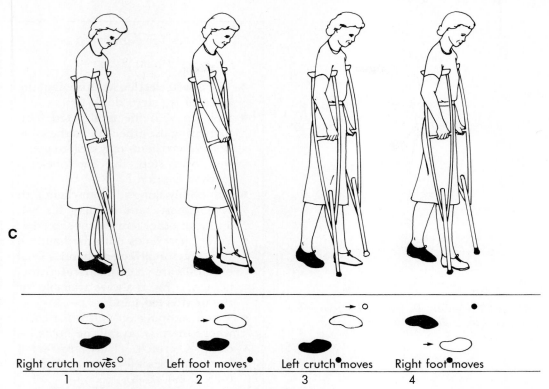

Right crutch moves°	Left foot moves•	Left crutch°moves	Right foot•moves
1	2	3	4

Figure 6-26, cont'd. **C,** *Crutch walking, using a four-point gait, is a slow but safe ambulation technique taught to clients.*

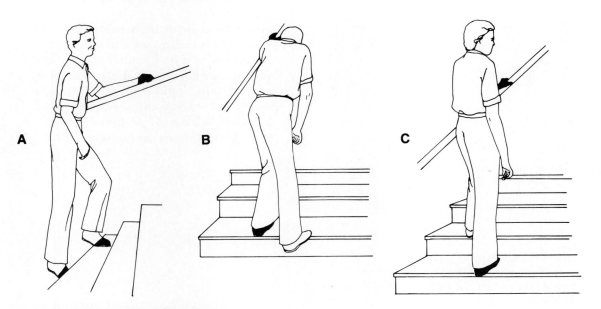

Figure 6-27. *Going up or down stairs.*

A, Step up with the **unaffected** leg. Stay safe. Use the handrails. Use a safety belt if necessary.

B, Bring the **affected** leg up to the same step. Lean slightly forward and onto rail for support and balance.

C, Repeat.   *Continued.*

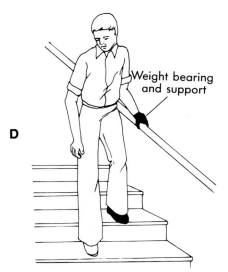

Figure 6-27, cont'd. **D,** *Going downstairs, move the **affected** leg to the lower step; their step down with the **unaffected** leg.*

Rules for Going Up or Down Stairs

- The **unaffected** leg steps up first; the **affected** leg steps down first.
- Step up with the **unaffected** foot, then bring the other foot to the same step. Some clients may wish to go up step over step, but the one-step method is safer.
- Stay evenly alongside your client with your closest hand holding his belt and your other hand at his shoulder.
- Your client holds onto the handrail with his **unaffected** hand. Dual handrails are an excellent safety tool because a rail is always available for the **unaffected** hand.
- When stepping on and off a curb, where there is no rail, he holds his cane or crutch in his **unaffected** hand and uses it for balance (Figures 6-28, 6-29).

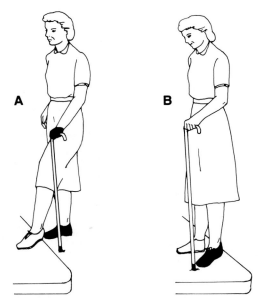

Figure 6-28. *Stepping up onto a curb.*
A, *Step onto the curb with the **unaffected** foot. Keep the cane on the flat pavement. Hold the cane in the **unaffected** hand.*
B, *Shift the weight to the **unaffected** foot while stepping up. Move the cane onto the curb, in one smooth motion, with the weight shifts. Place the **affected** foot on the curb.*

that has been checked and approved by the physical therapist. Handrails are recommended on both sides of the stairs.

—Ask your client if he is ready to go up stairs. If his endurance and stamina are decreased or if he has difficulty breathing, he may have to pause after climbing several steps. Stand at his side and use a safety belt so you can assist him if he loses his balance. If he becomes dizzy, have him sit down on the stairstep.

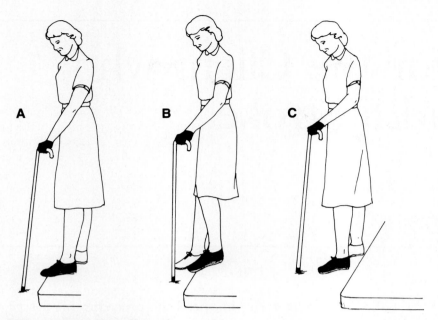

Figure 6-29. *Stepping down off a curb.*

* **A,** *Hold the cane in the* **unaffected** *hand. Place the cane firmly on the flat pavement while standing on the curb. Extend the edge of the* **unaffected** *foot slightly over the edge of the curb.*

* **B,** *Move the* **affected** *leg to the lower surface. Step down with the affected foot. Use the cane to bear weight and balance.*

  C, Step down *with the* **unaffected** *leg and balance.*

CHAPTER 7

Care for the Client who has had a Stroke

OBJECTIVES

When you have studied this chapter and practiced the procedures it describes, you will be able to:

1. Define terms relating to stroke.
2. Recall the causes of a stroke.
3. List the early warning signs of a stroke.
4. Discuss the common sensory, mental, and emotional deficits that may occur following a stroke.
5. Move and position the person who has loss of movement or shoulder pain following a stroke.
6. Provide assistance with activities of daily living for a person who has had a stroke.

OVERVIEW

You may frequently be called upon to care for a client who has had a stroke. More than 500,000 people have strokes each year in the United States. Approximately 350,000 of these people survive their initial stroke. Stroke is the third most common cause of death and the second most common cause of disability, especially among older persons. For example, forty percent of those who survive a stroke have difficulties with speech. Given the rapid increase in numbers of older persons in our society, we can expect the numbers of persons affected by stroke to continue to grow in spite of today's prevention programs.

A major health goal is to keep stroke survivors living as independently as possible so they do not require nursing home care. Persons who have had strokes have a higher quality of life when they can live at home with their families. In caring for a client at home, you will assist the family to care for him and assist him to remain as independent as possible. Caring for the person who has had a stroke in his home can be a very worthwhile and important job.

CAUSES OF STROKE

Understanding the causes of a stroke can help explain what causes some of the difficulties for your client. A **stroke** is an injury that occurs when part of the brain does not receive all the blood it needs to function. (Another term for stroke is **cardiovascular accident, or CVA.**) The brain relies on the blood to carry oxygen to the brain tissues. When the blood supply and its oxygen are cut off from a part of the brain, the brain cells cannot function and may be damaged.

Blood clots are one cause of strokes. Clots that form in the brain's blood vessels may block the flow of blood to the brain. Blood clots may also form in another part of the body and be carried in the blood to the brain. They can lodge in a blood vessel and block the blood supply. Another cause is bleeding (hemorrhage) into the brain from a weakened blood vessel wall.

High blood pressure (hypertension) is often associated with strokes. High blood pressure causes a hardened (sclerosed) blood vessel to rupture. This produces bleeding into the brain. A tumor or swelling that places pressure on the blood vessels in the brain can sometimes cause symptoms like those of a stroke. Even decreased blood flow to the brain from a spasm of a blood vessel can cause temporary or prolonged problems (Figure 7-1).

Most persons who have strokes are older. But younger persons can have strokes from these same causes. The person who has a stroke often has other medical conditions that must be considered in the client's care. For example, many older persons also have diabetes, poor circulation, chronic respiratory diseases, or arthritic conditions. These other conditions make your care for the client more complicated.

A client who has diabetes, for example, used to give himself his own insulin injections before his stroke. He has to do this differently now. You will learn new ways for your client to do things using special assistive devices and adaptive equipment and techniques. Each person who has a stroke has different problems and different disabilities. You need to understand how your client may

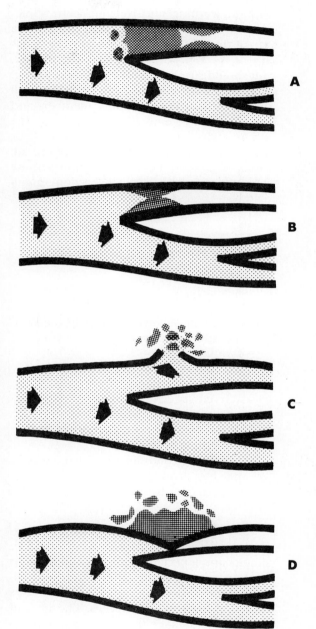

Figure 7-1. **A,** *A blood clot in an artery can block blood flow to the brain. The brain tissues die because they do not receive the oxygen carried in the blood.*

B, *Blood flow through the arteries is slowed when deposits collect inside the artery walls. Not enough blood reaches the brain cells.*

C, *A break, or rupture, in the wall of an artery releases blood into the brain, destroying brain tissues.*

D, *Pressure against the walls of an artery can cut off blood supply to the brain.*

behave after his stroke and how to assist him with his rehabilitation.

The client or family may be concerned about another stroke. Many strokes occur without warning and during sleep. Sometimes there are early warning signs of a stroke that go unnoticed. If your client has any of the signs or complaints listed below, you should suspect that something is wrong. Help him to sit or lie down in a safe place. Call the nurse supervisor, family member, and rescue squad or emergency unit.

The early warning signs of a stroke occur differently for each case. You may see all, some, or none of them. If you observe these symptoms, you should take action immediately.

Early Warning Signs of a Stroke

—dizziness
—headache
—difficulty in seeing
—weakness on one side of the body, including the face
—fainting
—numbness or tingling on one side of the face or a hand
—slurred speech
—unexplained confusion
—sense of anxiety and concern that something is wrong
—worsening condition of a person who has had a previous stroke

---

Your client will not necessarily have another stroke just because he has had one. You should not expect your client's condition to become worse. On the other hand, your client cannot expect to regain lost functions caused by destroyed brain cells. The amount and kind of damage that your client has following a stroke may not be known for some time. By the time you see the client in his home, he most likely will have made some improvements and adjustments. Many people have progressive improvement toward recovery and return of their functions. Your care will not "cure" the stroke. But it can keep the client from having other difficulties and losing functional abilities.

A major stroke can cause severe and permanent disabilities. Little strokes may cause minor disabilities or temporary problems. Brain cells are only damaged in a small area; they are not destroyed. You cannot see the injury from a stroke because it happens inside the brain. You can, however, see some of the effects of a stroke. An injury to the brain that causes paralysis is easy for you and the family to see as a problem. But when a stroke causes injury to the person's memory or judgment, the problems are less obvious and may take a longer time to be discovered. Strokes can cause any number and kinds of problems, and each person is different. You and the family have to be aware of both the problems you can see and the ones you can't.

Since the stroke occurs in the brain, you must understand some things about the brain before you can understand what is going on with your client. The brain is one of the largest organs in the adult body (Figure 7-2). The cerebrum is the largest part of the brain. The cerebrum is divided into two parts, or halves, called hemispheres. There is a right hemisphere and a left hemisphere.

Each hemisphere of the brain sends messages to control movements and sensations for one half of the body. The right hemisphere controls the left side of the body, and the left hemisphere controls the right side of the body. Damage to one hemisphere will cause some degree of paralysis (plegia) or weakness (paresis) to the opposite side of the body (Figure 7-3). This happens because the nerves cross over in the lower brain before they go out to the body. Remember that when the nurse says the client has a *right* hemisphere stroke that the *left* side of the body will be affected, and vice versa. Plegias and paresis are easily noted because of the loss of movement and strength.

The hemispheres control the functions that cannot be readily seen, such as judgment and memory. Each location in the brain is responsible for different functions (Table 7-1).

The nurse supervisor will discuss your client's functional abilities and deficits with you and the family members.

The circumstances following a client's return home following a stroke can be very

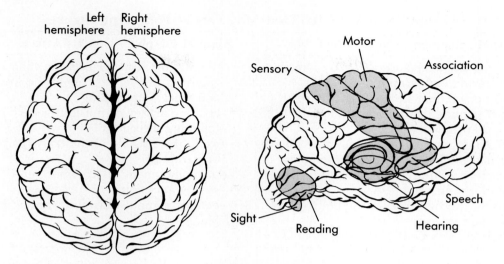

Figure 7-2. *The cerebrum is the largest part of the brain. Specific areas of the cerebrum are responsible for controlling and directing specialized functions of the body. Damage to an area of the brain affects the functions controlled by that area. Thus each client's deficits differ depending on the area of the brain damaged by the stroke and the severity of the damage.*

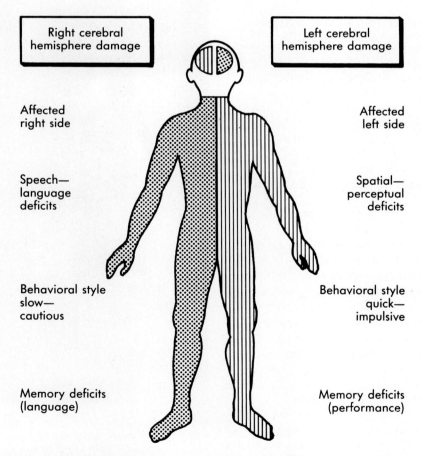

Figure 7-3. *The right side of the body is directed by the left cerebral hemisphere. The left side of the body is directed by the right cerebral hemisphere.*

Table 7-1. Deficits That May Occur Following Stroke

Left Hemisphere Deficits Affect:	Right Hemisphere Deficits Affect:
—using language and doing so correctly	—judging the distance between things
—speaking and writing words	—receiving information about the world and what is happening
—understanding what is said and read	—creating artistic or musical pieces
—performing mathematical calculations and arithmetic	—following directions
—making gestures to communicate ideas	—using the left side of the body (paresis or paralysis)
—performing skilled hand movements such as writing, drawing, cutting food, and sewing.	—using judgment or "common sense"
—using the right side of the body (paresis or paralysis)	—paying attention
—behaving cautiously or being anxious	—behaving impulsively and without inhibitions

difficult for you and the family. You can help by taking these steps:

Assisting Recovery from a Stroke

- Remind the client of things he has accomplished.
- Discourage undesirable, demanding behavior.
- Remain calm if he laughs or cries inappropriately.
- Be patient if he says yes for no.
- Schedule activities on "good" days and for short periods.
- Make sure he does what he can for himself.
- Use motions and demonstrations to help communicate.
- Repeat the names of objects he has difficulty recalling.
- Treat him like an adult.
- Learn the individual differences of your client and his family.
- Inform the nurse supervisor if he becomes depressed.
- Maintain a safe, clean, comfortable environment.

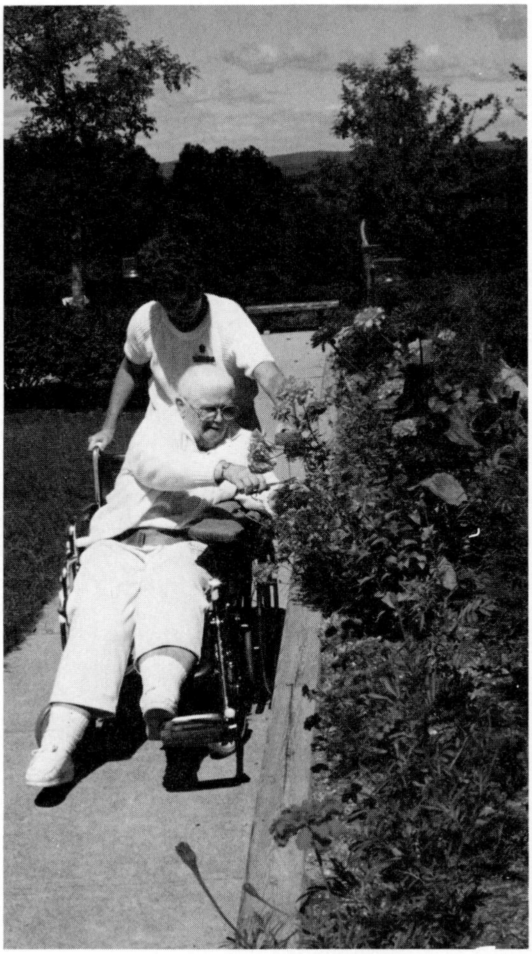

Figure 7-4. *Clients benefit from maintaining their hobbies and interests. Assist your client to be as independent as possible while enjoying his environment and activities.*
Photo courtesy of NJ Rehab Magazine.

Common difficulties and problems for persons who have had a stroke are discussed in the following pages. Related communication problems are covered in Chapter 3.

PHYSICAL DIFFICULTIES FOLLOWING A STROKE

Your client will have some or all of the difficulties listed in the following sections as a result of his stroke. Some may be very severe and others may be so slight that they are barely noticeable. For the safety of your client and yourself, be a good observer and listener so you can learn about your client's strengths and problems. Do not overestimate your client's capabilities or endurance. Report any changes in function or behavior to the nurse supervisor.

DIFFICULTIES RELATED TO MOVEMENT

A person who has had a stroke will have loss of movement due to **muscle weakness, paresis,** or **hemiplegia.** The nurse supervisor will assess your client in a number of areas. She may give you specific instructions and directions based on her assessments. These will change as your client's abilities change.

The nurse supervisor will evaluate your client for:

—normal body movements,
—muscle actions,
—balance and coordination,
—posture and alignment,
—feelings and sensations,
—awareness of position, and
—involuntary movements.

Encourage your client to be aware of his affected side and to use it whenever possible. Do not allow or help your client to perform a movement that is not one you were taught is within his normal range of motion, or one that may be painful to him.

Spasticity can cause problems as well, but the muscles themselves are not the problem. The stroke has caused the brain to send mixed-up or incomplete messages to the muscles. Exercise the muscles, as directed. Use proper positioning and alignment so they do not *atrophy,* weaken, or develop *contractures.*

The client may have difficulties with balance and coordination that affect his physical functioning. Balance and coordination are different when the person is sitting than when he is standing. A client who has hemiplegia or hemiparesis cannot depend upon his body to maintain good balance. It is essential to maintain safety because he has a tendency to fall. However, if your client becomes fearful of falling, he may become so anxious that he will hesitate to do activities that he is capable of doing. You must be aware of his abilities before you begin positioning, transferring, or otherwise moving your client. Good body mechanics, proper equipment, and safety precautions are essential.

Immobility may be caused by weakness or paralysis of a part of the body. A stroke commonly affects only one side of the body. Weakness, or paresis, for the person who has had a stroke is either **right hemiparesis** or **left hemiparesis.** Paralysis occurs on one side of the body, either **right hemiplegia** or **left hemiplegia.** This means that he cannot move one arm, one leg, or one side of his face. He may not be able to feel where that part of the body is positioned, or what it is doing or touching. The arm or leg may feel dull, heavy, and awkward.

His muscles may be **flaccid** (limp and floppy). If the arm or leg has spasticity or too much muscle activity, the person will have the opposite problems. The arm or leg will be stiffened and tightly clenched. The person typically clenches his hand and holds his arm close to his side with the elbow bent upward. Neither you nor the person can easily move the arm or leg or open a tightly clenched fist. At other times, the spastic movements may increase when the person is tired, upset, or fearful.

He may have prescribed exercises for assisting him with reduced mobility. If he can stand or walk, encourage him to get up for several minutes every one or two hours. This is especially important if he spends a great deal of time sitting in a chair. If he is in bed, turn or assist him to turn every hour and a half (more often if directed). The client's care plan may include equipment or supplies

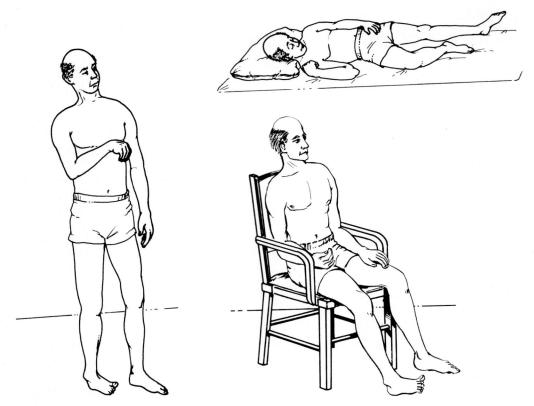

Figure 7-5. *Following a stroke, clients tend to assume an* **undesirable,** *typical "stroke posture." Note that the client's head appears to lean toward his affected side while he faces the other way. DO NOT allow your client to stand, lie down, or sit in these* **incorrect** *positions.*

to help prevent pressure areas. Examples include: eggcrate mattresses, sheepskin pads and booties, elbow pads, wheelchair and chair cushions, or waterbed mattresses.

Each person who has had a stroke has individual combinations of sensory losses. He may have retained some senses, but lost awareness of his body parts. For example, he may feel temperature but not know where his body parts are placed, or vice versa. This combination produces the poor **"stroke posture"** often assumed by clients following a stroke (Figure 7-5). In a stroke posture, the client's head appears to lean toward his weakened side, but his face looks away. His arm, hand, leg and foot are turned inward and downward while coming close to his trunk. He seems to lean toward the weakened side but without any support from that side. Avoid allowing your client to assume this posture. It works against his rehabilitation.

Try to put yourself in the client's place. Sit as if you were a person who had right or left

hemiplegia as described above. Then try to do several activities of daily living, such as making a transfer or eating. Notice that you are looking at the world from a different level many inches below what you see when you are standing. Notice how losing the use of one side of the body affects the ability of the whole body. Discuss your feelings about this trial experience with your nurse supervisor. Think about what it felt like for you when you work with your clients.

When your client does not pay attention to his affected or paralyzed side, remind him gently and point to that side. Encourage him to scan by turning his head and looking at his affected side during activities. The person who has paralysis or paresis must be reminded about the position of body parts since he is not aware of how they are placed. For example, he may tend to let his arm fall off the wheelchair arm on the affected side. He must learn to remember that his body parts are there even when he cannot feel them. Safety measures for the client who has paralysis or paresis include protecting him from such things as:

—hot bathing water
—hot liquids to drink
—heating pads
—ice packs
—cigarette burns
—sharp objects
—pressure on the area
—other items he cannot feel

Remember that helpful equipment can become harmful if not checked and monitored. A catheter may help to empty the bladder, but the tubing can produce a pressure area if it rubs the skin. Heating pads can cause burns. Pillows and pads assist in positioning, but can lead to contractures if improperly placed.

Shoulder Pain

A common problem following stroke is pain in the weakened or paralyzed shoulder. This happens because some muscles are weakened or not working and others are overused or misused, causing pain or strain. The shoulder and arm should not be moved into positions that cause pain. Whenever the client complains of shoulder pain, inform the nurse supervisor. Learn how to properly support your client's paralyzed or affected arm.

The client may have a sling to use as a support for his arm when he is walking or transferring from one place to another (Figure 7-6). Be sure the nurse supervisor approves the way the client wears his sling. An improperly used sling can cause postural and other difficulties for the client.

The most common supports are armboards that fit onto the wheelchair arm, pillows used as supports, or purchased armrest cushions. The client's arm must be placed in the proper alignment as illustrated in Figure 7-7.

Never use the person's affected arm to position or pull him or to help him to transfer, stand, or move. If the person tends to lose his balance while sitting, insert pillows alongside his trunk to keep him from leaning or falling to one side. Prop his arm on other surfaces such as a table. Remind your client to check the position of his arm.

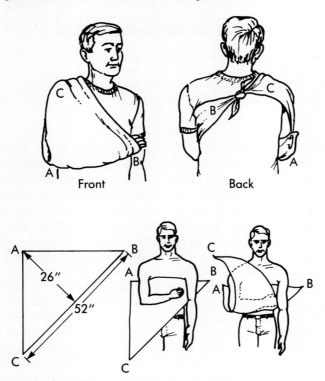

Figure 7-6. *A sling is not recommended for all clients. If your client does wear a sling, it must be properly constructed and positioned.*

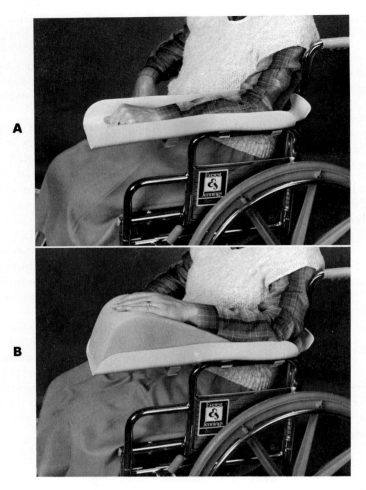

Figure 7-7.   **A,** *Proper support for an affected arm is very important and can prevent further disability for the client. A wheelchair armboard is commonly used equipment.*
   B, *Armboards may be padded and elevated to suit each client's individual needs.*
   Reprinted by permission of © Bissell Healthcare Corporation/Fred Sammons, Inc.

When a person has a problem with his balance or loss of feeling, he will tend to let his arm fall off the wheelchair arm and to slip down in his chair toward the affected side. To prevent this, seat him as far back in the wheelchair as possible. Lock the wheelchair or stabilize the chair. Be sure his feet are flat on the floor. Follow the instructions for moving him back into the wheelchair as described in Chapter 4. Use body mechanics that use leverage as well as your leg muscles when moving or lifting. Do not use your back muscles to lift or move clients.

Even when some clients are properly situated, they continue to slide forward, slip down or out of their wheelchair seats. Check the material that covers the seat as well as the client's clothing so they are not sliding on each other too easily. If the sliding becomes a safety hazard, the nurse supervisor may obtain a physician's order to use a binder, transfer belt, or cloth. The nurse supervisor will show you how to secure the client in his seat and explain when this can be done. Do not use or consider the binder, belt, or cloth as a restraint. Be sure your client's feet are securely and properly placed on the footrests. Never leave your client's position unchanged for longer than two hours.

Encourage your client to take as much responsibility as possible for making his own moves and changes. Practice with him so that he is shifting his weight in his wheelchair every 20 minutes. Assist him if he becomes tired or frustrated, or if his muscles become tightened. Given simple directions or point out directions to him.

Dressing

Dressing is an activity that your client will have to relearn and practice with your guidance and maybe some help.

Rules for Helping a Client who has had a Stroke to Dress

- Let him do as much as he possibly can for himself, even though it is faster and easier for you to do it for him.
- Know what he can and cannot do.
- Be sure that your client is sitting straight.
- Stand on his **affected** side as you work.
- Use the **affected** side to **start** dressing your client.
- Put the **affected** arm or leg into the clothing first.
- Encourage him to look at the **affected** side as he works.
- Give simple instructions or point to give directions if he hesitates.
- Begin **undressing** by **removing the unaffected** arm or leg from the clothing first.

The section on assistive devices in Chapter 6 will give you ideas about techniques in dressing and grooming aids, such as button hookers, long-handled shoehorns, sock pullers (Figure 7-8), and one handed devices.

EATING AND NUTRITIONAL DIFFICULTIES

Your client may have a great deal of difficulty with eating, and as a consequence, may not be well-nourished. There may be a combination of reasons for eating problems. Clients with paresis, paralysis, or visual deficits may have difficulty feeding themselves. Samples of utensils and dishes designed to assist him are presented in Chapter 6. If your client is older, the normal changes of aging can be aggravated by functional losses. This can lead to becoming poorly nourished and losing stamina and endurance. He often will require special diet modifications to deal with other health problems. Additionally, the stroke may affect his ability to readily swallow food.

Dysphagia, or difficulty swallowing, is an eating problem that frequently occurs following a stroke. *Read the information* about clients who have difficulty swallowing, chewing, and seeing while eating, and the emergency actions for choking. Both are detailed in Chapter 2. This is *essential information* for you to know before caring for a client who has had a stroke. Also read about dysarthria in Chapter 3.

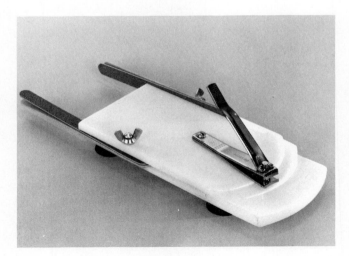

Figure 7-8. *Many assistive devices are available to enable clients to participate in self care activities. A client who is able to use one hand can cut his own nails with this assistive nail clipper.*

Reprinted by permission of © Bissell Healthcare Corporation/Fred Sammons, Inc.

BOWEL AND BLADDER DIFFICULTIES

After a stroke, a client may lose control of the voluntary muscles that control bowel or bladder functions. He may have difficulty with controlling his urine, his bowel movements, or with both bladder and bowel functions. Your client may not know when he needs to go to the bathroom. The lack of bowel and bladder control can force a client to stay home, limiting his social life and sense of self-worth. Few clients are willing to go out and be around others when fearful of bladder or bowel **incontinence** or soiling.

Do not add to your client's dilemma by blaming or shaming him if he becomes incontinent. Many clients are so upset and distressed by their incontinence that they do not discuss it with anyone. There are some things that can be done to help. Read the sections about bowel and bladder training in Chapter 2. Work as a team member with the client, family, and nurse supervisor to combat and conquer your client's bowel and bladder difficulties.

CHAPTER *8*

Care for the Client with a Traumatic Brain Injury

OBJECTIVES

When you have studied this chapter and practiced the procedures it describes, you will be able to:

1. Define terms relating to brain injury.
2. Describe the types of head injury.
3. Match body functions with lobes of the brain.
4. List common difficulties following brain injury.
5. Describe the importance of using structure in the client's home environment.
6. Discuss the expected range of stresses for the family and client.
7. Know basic principles for home care of clients with brain injuries.
8. Perform specific actions in care of clients with brain injuries.
9. Prepare for a potentially aggressive or violent situation.

OVERVIEW

Every year more than 700,000 people are hospitalized in the United States with some type of head injury; 100,000 people die and between 50,000 and 90,000 others are disabled in some way by brain injuries. Causes of head injuries are similar to causes of spinal cord injuries. For example, a large number of those who receive head injuries are people under 30 years old who are injured in automobile and motorcycle accidents. Other common causes are falls, being hit in the head by an object such as a rock or baseball, receiving a penetrating wound such as from a bullet, or a medical condition such as a hemorrhaged blood vessel.

Head injuries are described as either open or closed wounds. Some head injuries are only surface injuries to the scalp. Others are deep wounds with fractures to the skull. The degree of brain injury cannot be determined by the amount of visible damage. A closed head injury may cause more long-term damage or brain trauma than an open head injury. What happens to a person with a head injury depends on the part of the head and brain injured, the severity of the injury, and the care he receives.

TYPES OF HEAD INJURIES

SEVERITY OF INJURY

The terms **concussion** or **minor head injury** and severe head injury are used to describe the seriousness of the injury. The person who has a minor head injury may have:

—lost consciousness for less than 20–30 minutes,
—headache,
—visual changes,
—general weakness,
—short-term memory loss,
—dizziness,
—nausea and vomiting,
—irritability, or
—lack of ability to remember events before or after the injury.

Clients may have a rapid and complete recovery following a concussion. Others develop prolonged problems that last for years or for life, affecting different functions and abilities.

A **severe head injury** or **traumatic brain injury (TBI)** usually involves a **contusion,** or bruising of the brain. There is a loss of a level of consciousness that may last for days to weeks or longer. In severe cases it can lead to death. If the person is in a state of profound unconsciousness or **coma,** more problems can be expected. In all head injuries there is potential for hemorrhage, edema of the brain, and nerve damage.

A classic example is what happens to the brain in a car accident when the person's head hits the windshield. The brain hits the front of the skull on the first impact. Then the brain bounces to hit the back of the skull for a second injury on the rebound. At the same time there may or may not be neck and spinal injuries, fractures, and open wounds. These people have intensive hospital care that may include mechanical ventilators, heavy medication, and surgery to reduce pressure, swelling, and bleeding in the skull.

Your nurse supervisor may describe your client's brain injury by using a number or level such as Level 6. This number is a score that is used to describe the client's mental status and functional abilities after the in-jury. The level or number score will indicate a great deal about what your client can do and how he might behave. The nurse supervisor will explain what your client's level or number means about his abilities and actions.

LOCATION OF INJURY

The location of the injury and part of the brain injured will affect your client's actions and abilities. Read more about the parts of the brain for specific body functions in Chapter 3. The cortex is the largest part of the brain and is divided into two halves or hemispheres. There are 4 lobes in the cortex. Each lobe has control over specific functions. When a lobe is injured, the specific functions controlled by that lobe are affected. The following illustration, Figure 8-1, will help you understand the relationship between the location of the head injury and your client's disabilities.

Match the following brain lobes and body functions with those in the illustration. The frontal lobe of the cortex is important for planning and carrying out behavior and for motor functions of movement. The temporal lobes are used for speech, hearing, and memory. The occipital lobes at the back of the brain are used for vision functions. The parietal lobes affect the sense of touch and loca-

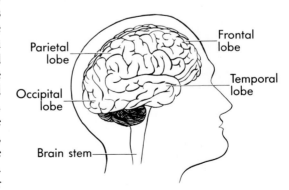

Figure 8-1. *Each lobe of the cerebral cortex of the brain controls specific functions. Specific functions are interrupted when a particular lobe is injured. (See also Figure 7-2.)*

Common Difficulties Following Traumatic Brain Injury

—memory loss—this may be loss of memory about things that occurred before the injury or difficulty remembering things from day to day

—inability to follow directions, except one step at a time

—distractability and short attention span

—irritability which can become aggressive behavior

—lack of "common sense" about social situations, right and wrong, or appropriate behavior

—disorderliness, messiness

—boredom and depression

—lack of recreation and friends

—inability to manage independent dressing, hygiene, or grooming

—inappropriate sexual behavior or advances

—vulgar language

—bowel and bladder incontinence

—paralysis or paresis as with hemiplegia

—spasticity, tremors, and rigidity

—easily fatigued

—difficulties communicating, especially verbal communication and aphasias (discussed in Chapter 3)

—dietary or nutritional changes such as loss of appetite or constant desire to eat

—family problems due to stresses of injury

—difficulty getting continued education or job due to aftereffects of injury

---

tion in space. The parietal lobes also bring together all information from the senses.

Each client will have different difficulties and his particular abilities may change over time.

HOME CARE

When the client is ready to return home to live, he will need a carefully **structured plan** to enable him to live agreeably in a home setting that includes his family and other people. The nurse supervisor will work closely with the rehabilitation center or traumatic brain injury center to develop a care plan that contains step-by-step instructions suitable for the home setting. The care plan will be a schedule of predictable events and activities for each day. Things should be done in the same ways and at the same times each day. This schedule will reinforce the activities for the client. He will be practicing and repeating tasks each day. At the same time he will be relearning the tasks and activities.

Recovery from traumatic brain injury (TBI) occurs in stages or levels. The amount of time for each stage of recovery varies for clients. Not all clients will have complete recovery. Some clients will have complete recovery over time. Other clients who seem to be progressing well may become very depressed and regress to childlike behavior.

This happens when a client gets well enough to realize what has happened to him. As he realizes the situation, he becomes depressed even though he appears to be progressing. He may be grieving for the loss of his "old self." This can be a very difficult time for the client and the family. You can help by being supportive but firm and reinforcing your client's positive behaviors. Discuss the client's behavior changes with the nurse supervisor so she can include specific actions to help him in the care plan.

Both the client and his family may belong to **support groups.** Support groups are composed of individuals and families who are dealing with the challenges of a family member with a traumatic brain injury. Although he is able to return home, there are many challenges for the client, family, friends, and caregivers. For example, the client may have problems that cause disturbances with his mental functioning, behavior or emotions, and physical abilities. Everyone in the family and support group needs to understand the changes that have taken place.

STRESSES OF CHANGE

Bringing the brain-injured client home is usually a difficult adjustment for the family. They look at a person they knew before the injury but the person they see does not have the same personality. If the wife or husband is injured, the marriage partner may feel married to a stranger. Children may not understand the behavior of an injured parent. The family may be fearful or overwhelmed by the responsibilities of care.

Most family members will experience grief and loss. Your nurse supervisor can talk with you about specific responses appropriate to each family's particular way of working through their grief and loss. When a child is injured, the family may have a great deal of guilt about the injury. Their reactions may last a long time and may become a chronic sadness or sorrow. They may continue to grieve for "the child that might have been" if the injury had not occurred. The child himself may mourn his own loss, feeling angry and frustrated about his condition. Families and clients may take a long time to adjust and put their lives back together. It is normal for a family and client to experience grieving, anxieties, and concerns about the future.

These emotional problems place tremendous stresses on the daily family life in addition to those caused by the demands of physical care and financial worries. The nurse supervisor will work with the family to identify support groups and organizations that can provide reassurance and encouragement. You may be an active part of that process.

WORKING WITH PERSONS WHO HAVE HAD BRAIN INJURY

The environment must be arranged so the client can use the world about him to help him function. For example, if he has become very forgetful because of a memory loss, things that he needs should always be kept in the same places. He may learn to write notes as reminders to do things. When the environment becomes predictable and structured for him, he can begin to relearn ways of doing things. He must relearn things because he cannot remember how to do them. Relearning takes time and repeated practice; each success must be reinforced.

The client's world must be organized so there are patterns of organization in whatever he does. In this way he can relearn how to do things for himself and relearn what is acceptable in our society. His family, friends, and caregivers must work together to keep daily tasks and activities very structured. He needs set routines and timetables.

For example, when directed by the nurse supervisor, use lists, calendars, and similar reminders to help the client keep in touch with reality (Figure 8-2). They may lessen the confusion he feels about the world around him. Clocks help some clients, but are confusing to others. A reward system may be helpful. Be sure to reward the positive behaviors by carefully following the guidelines set by the nurse supervisor. The family and friends may assist by describing the client and his interests before the injury. If this does not upset them, it is a simple way of learning what the client likes to do and what may appeal to him. Study these basic principles for the care of persons with brain injuries.

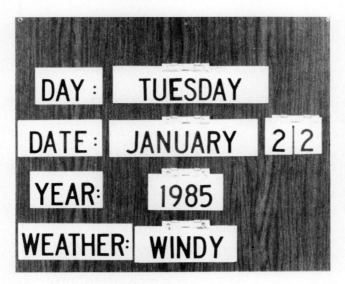

Figure 8-2. *Calendars and information remind clients about what is happening in the world around them so they are less confused.*
Reprinted by permission of © Bissell Healthcare Corporation/Fred Sammons, Inc.

Care for Clients who have had a Traumatic Brain Injury (TBI)

- Assure a safe environment.
- Follow step-by-step directions for care and activities that are part of the client's structured environment.
- Provide correct information to the client, he may not remember day to day or recall from the past.
- Allow the client time to organize his thoughts.
- Know when he is fatigued.
- Be courteous and considerate:
  —ask if he likes to be touched,
  —remove things that annoy him,
  —call him by name,
  —introduce yourself, if he does not remember you,
  —tell him what you are doing before you do something for him,
  —be pleasant, and
  —reinforce desirable behaviors.
- Use the television or radio for short times, as directed.
- Tune television and radio to programs that do not cause him to have negative reactions or behaviors. Use meaningful and informative shows instead of violent ones.
- Direct his attention away from vulgar language and sexual acts; be firm, but non-threatening.
- Provide physical care according to his disabilities while encouraging independence.
- Discuss concerns with the nurse supervisor before they become problems.

---

*T*HE AGGRESSIVE OR VIOLENT CLIENT

A client will not necessarily be violent because he has had a head injury. He may never become violent or he may commit a violent act once. However, some clients have troubled thoughts about violence and have problems controlling aggression. You must understand what to do before you are in a situation with a person who becomes violent. You and the nurse supervisor should discuss the situation openly. There are specific actions you should be aware of before any violence occurs:

1. *Be prepared by having a plan of action* before violence occurs. The nurse and family will work with you to develop the plan. If there are things that agitate him, remove them. Keep the room quiet, at a comfortable temperature, and keep the lighting low. If certain activities reduce his agitation, provide these at the first sign of upset. Substitute a pleasurable activity to distract him if possible. Alert others if you suspect a violent outbreak.

2. *Do not provoke your client.* A person who has had a head injury may be easily provoked by things that would not anger others. Most violence is caused by the violent person thinking he has lost control over a situation. Or he may feel threatened and even think he is in danger. When he feels in control of his environment, he is less apt to become violent. Make sure you allow him choices and decisions as often as possible. However, if he does not indicate a choice, do not ask him his preferences. Be consistent in what you do; consider his comfort and safety. Once he becomes violent, do not give him choices. Simply tell him what you are going to do. But do not verbally threaten him.

3. *Do not take comments and actions personally,* even when your client directs them at you. You are the one who is there and available, but you are not the cause. He is "acting out" against something else. The things that upset your client are often things he cannot change. This does not mean that you must accept all behaviors and language. However, you can respond more calmly and objectively when you realize that you are not the target of the client's anger. Inform the nurse supervisor and the family whenever a client attempts abusive comments or actions. Discuss the situation and specific actions you should take.

4. *Avoid arguing* with the client.
   —Watch your body language and approach;
   —speak in a soft, unemotional tone of voice;
   —tell your client what you are going to do;
   —keep good eye contact, but do not stare; and
   —try repeating soft words or soothing phrases.
   Do Not:
   —make demanding statements,
   —speak as if giving orders,
   —move suddenly and quickly,
   —stand with your hands on your hips,
   —stand with arms crossed over chest,
   —shake or point your finger, or
   —shout.
   These and similar actions communicate threats to your client.

5. *Be aware of the client's need for his own space.* Do not get close enough so that an agitated client can reach you. If he grabs your wrist, release yourself by quickly bending your elbow and pulling your straightened wrist up. Your wrist will escape through his thumb and fingers. Twisting your wrist or pulling away will not release you.

   Similarly, do not place yourself in potentially awkward positions. For example, do not kneel or bend down in front of your client when assisting him. Do not stand so that you are in the corner of the room without a clear exit.

6. *Do not wear jewelry* or other items that can be used to hurt or control you. Earrings, necklaces, pens on cords around your neck, and scarves can be readily grabbed by clients. They can be used to hold you in his reach. Many clients will try to take hold of your hair. If this happens, do not pull away. The moment you try to pull away, the tension and his grasp will tighten. Do the following instead:

PREVENTING AGGRESSIVE BEHAVIOR

You may not be able to prevent all aggressive or violent behavior. You can, however, work with the nurse supervisor and other health team members to identify things that cause the client to perform negative behaviors. Once you know what they are, you can act to prevent them from occurring. This may prevent some of his outbreaks. The nurse supervisor may direct you to do some of the following activities as part of the care plan.

- Keep a daily log and note the times, activities, or things that cause him to become agitated, aggressive, or violent. Are neatness and cleanliness important to him so that he becomes upset when he spills food or has soiled clothing? The entries in the log may reveal a pattern to his outbursts.
- Find out what is happening with his other activities and treatments. For example, he may visit an outpatient treatment center or have a therapist visit in the home. Find out what he is doing in the visits. Tell the therapists and the nurse supervisor what he is doing in the home. They may include changes in the care plan for activities in the home.
- Ask the nurse supervisor to find out what your client did in the hospital or rehabilitation center before he came home. Learn about the habits that worked well for him just before he came home. For example, he did not like to eat three scheduled meals a day, but wanted to snack all day instead. You may be able to offer him nutritious snacks or several smaller meals at home.
- Work closely with the family and other members of the team. Share things you learn about your client with them. Then everyone can decide to do things in the same way for your client. This reduces the confusion for him. Keep your sense of humor.
- Read about frustration and anger in Chapter 1. Remember that caring for the adult or child who has a brain injury is stressful and challenging for both the client and his caregivers.

> ### *Releasing yourself from a Client who has Grasped your Hair*
>
> - Move slightly toward the pull to reduce the tension.
> - At the same moment that you ease the tension on the grasp, place one of your hands around his wrist and steady his wrist.
> - Use your other hand to push against his palm where it meets with his clenched fingers.
> - Still holding his hand and wrist, lift your hands and quickly slide your hair free. The pressure on his palm combined with the lift and reduced tension will loosen his grasp on your hair. You may be able to pull your hair free by using your hand that is pressing against his palm.
> - Do not free his wrist until you are clear of his grasp.
> - Back away quickly and smoothly as you perform this last step.
> - Practice this maneuver with the nurse supervisor before working with a client.

7. *Avoid a physical conflict.* It is better to leave or escape and get help. If your client does attack you, remain as calm as possible. Realize that even if he is physically stronger than you are, he is still upset and not thinking clearly. If you can think clearly, you will have an advantage over your client's strength. You will do better if you have a plan beforehand. There should also be a plan for getting help if the family is not present. Always report any incidents to the nurse supervisor.

8. *Do not try to get even or punish* a client for his aggressive or violent behavior. Remember that the violence is not directed at you. It is a result of the brain injury.

CHAPTER 9

Care for the Client with a Spinal Cord Injury

*O*BJECTIVES

When you have studied this chapter and practiced the procedures it describes, you will be able to:

1. Define terms relating to spinal cord injury.
2. Outline the differences between level of injury and severity of injury.
3. Describe how spinal cord injury affects functional abilities.
4. Use basic principles for home care of a client with spinal cord injury.
5. Perform special care required by clients with spinal cord injuries.
6. Help prevent complications and further disabilities for clients with spinal cord injuries.
7. Respond properly to an autonomic dsyreflexia crisis.
8. Recognize some of the personal coping patterns and adjustments that clients make following a spinal cord injury.

*O*VERVIEW

Traumatic injuries to the spinal cord occur most often to young men between 17 and 30 years of age. Most of the injuries are caused by automobile accidents. Injuries from diving accidents increase during the summer. Other causes are falls, stabbings or gunshot wounds that penetrate the spinal cord, and sports accidents. A small percentage of spinal problems are caused by tumors or by disease and injuries during military encounters.

Many spinal cord injuries would be prevented by:

—using seatbelts,
—not drinking and driving,
—not riding with someone who has been drinking,
—checking the depth of water *before* diving,
—taking extra care in securing ladders or other climbing equipment, and
—eliminating unsafe sports actions, such as spear tackles in football or wearing inadequate sports gear.

Many persons with spinal cord injuries return to live in the community following long hospital and rehabilitation programs. They have been taught how to manage their care even though they may not be able to personally perform the care. Your client may have, in addition to your services, several attendants or a personal attendant who cares for him. Or you may be the personal attendant.

This chapter instructs you about the special care needs of clients who have spinal cord injuries. You will also learn how to work with your clients as they direct their own care. It is important that you listen to your client about how he wants to have his care done. But you also must perform care as directed by your nurse supervisor. You and your nurse supervisor should discuss any topics about which you and the client do not agree. You should also discuss differences in instructions from the client and from the nurse. The client and the family may also be included in the discussions.

*T*HE SPINAL CORD

The **spinal cord** is the main bundle of the body's nerves (Figure 9-1). The spinal cord nerve bundle fits inside the **vertebrae.** The vertebrae make up the column of backbones that extends from the base of the skull to the tailbone. The vertebrae are hollow in the center so that the spinal cord lies protected inside the bony framework. The nerves travel from the brain and out from the spinal cord to the various parts of the body. They send and receive messages about the body's activities. Although the nerves are bundled within the vertebrae, each nerve begins and ends at a different place in the spinal cord or brain. In the same way, each nerve sends and receives messages for its own specific parts of the body.

LEVEL OF INJURY AND ABILITIES

In this chapter **level of injury** refers to the location of the injury on the spinal cord. The location is described by a letter and number. The letter is the first initial of the section of the spinal cord. The number is the number of the vertebra in that section. There are 4 sections in the spinal column: cervical, thoracic, lumbar, and sacral. Figure 9-2 shows where these sections begin and end and the number of vertebrae within each section. Thus T6 corresponds to the 6th vertebra in the thoracic section of the spinal cord.

The spinal cord nerves enter and leave the spinal cord within these sections. When the

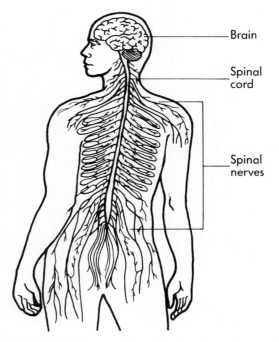

Figure 9-1. *The brain, brainstem, and spinal cord form the central nervous system. The peripheral nervous system includes the nerves that extend throughout the body and the nerve cells (neurons). Nerves transmit and receive messages that connect the brain and spinal cord with the body.*

spinal cord is injured and nerves are damaged, the particular parts of the body that send and receive messages from those nerves cannot function. When you know the level of injury, you can get an idea of what your client will be able to do. For example, when the nerve that signals the legs to move is injured,

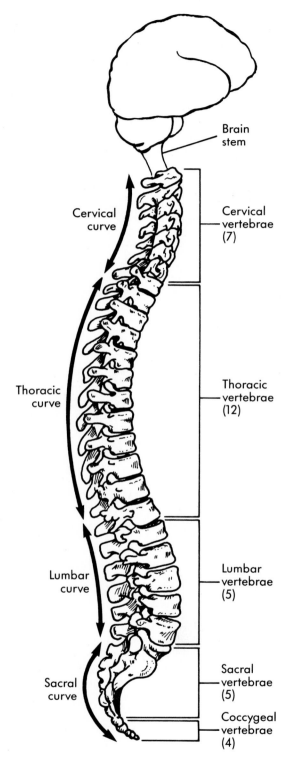

Figure 9-2. *The spinal cord extends from the brain stem through five sections of vertebrae: (1) cervical, (2) thoracic, (3) lumbar, (4) sacral, and (5) the coccyx.*

this interrupts communication between the brain, the nerve, and the legs. The person's legs become paralyzed without the nerve signals. He may be unable to feel sensations of touch or temperature in his legs. Your nurse supervisor will tell you about how your client's nerve injuries affect specific parts of his body.

The actions of all the nerves located below the injury are weakened, interrupted, or stopped. The higher the level of injury, the less muscle function is available to the person. Figure 9-3 shows the expected abilities for various levels of the spinal cord. The nurse knows that the person who has an injury at C2 cannot breathe on his own. He will therefore require mechanical ventilation to assist him to breathe. The nerve that begins in the brain and instructs specific breathing muscles cannot send and receive messages to breathe.

SEVERITY OF INJURY AND ABILITIES

Severity of injury is another factor that determines the extent of a spinal cord injury. This is because the level of spinal cord injury may differ from the level of injury to the bony vertebral column. Lying within the vertebrae, the spinal cord can be compressed, bruised, severed, or partially cut.

Spinal cord injury also affects the actions of two kinds of muscles: voluntary muscles and involuntary muscles. **Voluntary muscles** move when directed by the brain to perform intended actions such as moving an arm and hand to pick up a fork. **Involuntary muscles** also receive messages from the brain and spinal cord. These muscles produce movements such as bladder and bowel activities and sexual functions. Both voluntary and involuntary muscle actions can be affected, depending on the level and severity of the spinal cord injury.

A client may have paraplegia or quadriplegia as a result of his injury. **Paraplegia** means that the injury occurred in the lower part of the back. A client loses use of his legs and torso. He can use his voluntary muscles to move his hands, arms, head and neck, and most muscles for breathing. He can propel his own wheelchair, care for his activities of daily living, and transfer from his wheelchair on his own. Many people with paraplegia are

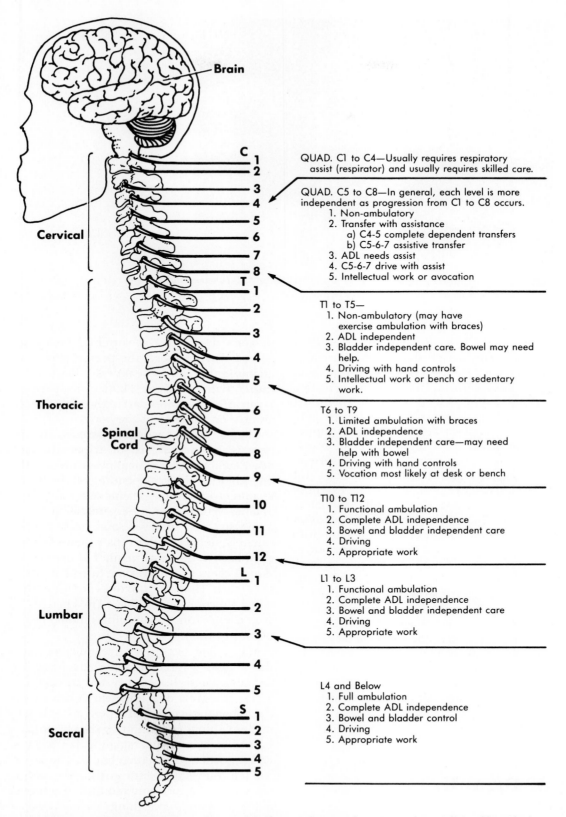

Figure 9-3. *The level of injury on the spinal cord can help to predict what a client will be able to do for himself. The severity of the injury also affects his abilities. Each client must be treated individually; these are general guidelines.*

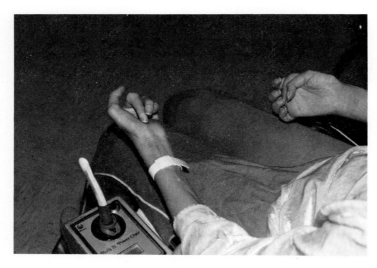

Figure 9-4. *Spinal cord injury results in loss of muscle control, function and strength. Photo courtesy of New Jersey Rehab Magazine.*

able to drive a specially adapted car. He does not have control over some involuntary muscle functions. He must be very careful about good skin care, bowel and bladder activities, and loss of sensation below the level of injury.

Quadriplegia means that the injury damaged the spinal cord near the person's upper back or neck. This higher level of injury causes loss of control for both arms, both legs, and possibly the neck and muscles for breathing (Figure 9-4). The actual extent of his disability must be carefully evaluated. However, many voluntary and involuntary muscle actions are lost. The person with quadriplegia does not have the same potential for independence as the person with paraplegia. However, persons with paraplegia and quadriplegia are able to teach in schools and universities, attend school, manage businesses, and work at other jobs. They must schedule their days to allow time for rehabilitation activities. These activities keep them well, free from complications, and maintain their highest level of functioning. That is a big part of your job with this person.

INDIVIDUAL PATTERNS OF DISABILITY

Each client will have his own pattern of disability. The injury to the spinal cord may occur at a different place from where the person's injury to the vertebral bones occurred. Furthermore, the person may have an injury that causes weakness in body parts, rather than a paralysis. This is called **paresis.** It can affect the lower part of the body or only an arm or one side of the body.

Clients may have **paraparesis, hemiparesis, quadraparesis,** or **triparesis,** and other combinations of weakness with or without other paralysis. Depending on the severity and type of injury, clients may have some abilities return over time. Abilities may return years after injury in some cases. Unfortunately, nerves do not repair themselves or grow back in the same manner as muscles or skin. A client may have some functional abilities return. However, this does not mean that other functions will follow. Any changes in your client's functional abilities should be reported to the nurse supervisor.

Many clients express a great deal of hope that abilities will return, especially the ability to walk. These hopes may not be realistic. There is a great deal of research being conducted on these topics. But persons with permanent spinal cord injuries should not expect to be able to walk again if they are not walking when they return home. The nurse will tell you what realistic goals and expectations are for your client and how to respond to his questions. Some things are not possible for your client. However, you can support other positive things that can be accomplished (Figure 9-5).

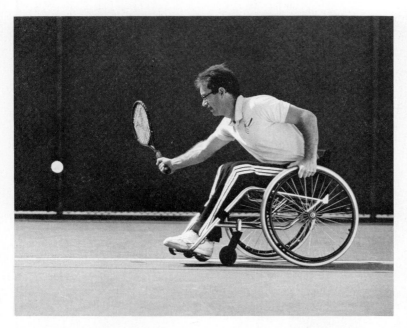

Figure 9-5. *Wheelchair sports activities are gaining popularity throughout the world. Courtesy of Everest & Jennings, Inc.*

*B*ASIC PRINCIPLES FOR CARE

Injury to the spinal cord does not produce mental injuries. Your client may have periods of emotional upset about his condition. This is part of the grieving process, as discussed in Chapter 1. Your client is a normal person who happens to have impairment of certain physical abilities. Once you are aware of what he can and cannot do, your work is to assist him to stay as independent as possible.

Assisting the Client with Spinal Cord Injury

- Understand the use and maintenance of available equipment and assistive devices. Examples include splints, abdominal binders, and TEDS. (Read the chapters on Equipment and Activities of Daily Living.)
- Encourage your client to direct his own care.
- Encourage good health maintenance habits.
- Provide proper nutrition for meals.
- Provide excellent skin care.
- Arrange proper positioning and correct body alignment.

- Follow bowel and bladder programs.
- Assure mobility and range of motion as directed.
- Assist with respiratory programs as directed.
- Observe temperature controls of equipment and in living areas.
- Keep a safe, clean environment.
- Encourage him to stay as independent as possible.
- Treat him as a competent individual.

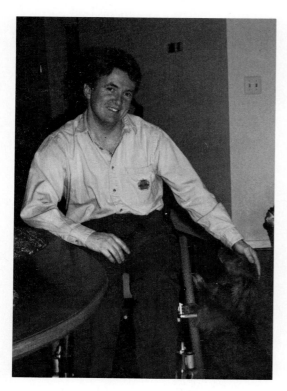

Figure 9-6. *Persons who have a disability are not disabled persons. Photo courtesy of New Jersey Rehab Journal.*

SPECIAL CARE FOR THE PERSON WITH A SPINAL CORD INJURY

THE IMPORTANCE OF CARE

The person with a spinal cord injury has many special care needs. Your care is very important since you are with your client often. The quality of your care will make a difference in his overall health as well as in preventing complications. For example, turning and positioning to prevent skin and circulation problems will also prevent problems caused by immobility. Thus further disability is prevented. A client may be hospitalized if he develops a **pressure sore** or **thrombosis.** He will lose some of his independence and decrease his self-care for activities of daily living. Your client has a great deal of responsibility for directing his own care. But you as the caregiver are responsible for delivering the care. Remember, many problems can be prevented when you deliver excellent care.

Areas of Special Care for Persons with Spinal Cord Injuries

—mobility
—loss of sensation, temperature, and touch
—skin care and hygiene
—bladder program
—bowel program
—respiratory maintenance and assistance
—positioning and alignment
—circulation maintenance
—nutrition and fluid requirements
—emotional adjustments
—family and client relationships
—social and recreation activities
—transportation
—education and job potential

LOSS OF MOVEMENT

The most obvious loss is **paralysis** of movement or the loss of ability to voluntarily move muscles. The type and degree of paralysis varies with the extent and severity of the injury. You need precise instructions from your nurse supervisor about maintaining the range of motion of joints and preventing problems from immobility.

Assistive devices enable clients to perform self-care and maintain independence (Figures 9-7, 9-8). Chapter 3 illustrates TDD (telephone devices for the disabled). They are important for clients in recreational, educational vocational activities.

Excessive immobility can have negative effects on the entire person.

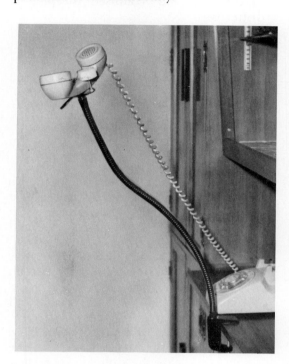

Figure 9-7. *An extended "goose-neck" telephone holder assists the clients who cannot hold the phone to conduct their own conversations privately.*

Reprinted by permission of © Bissell Healthcare Corporation/Fred Sammons, Inc.

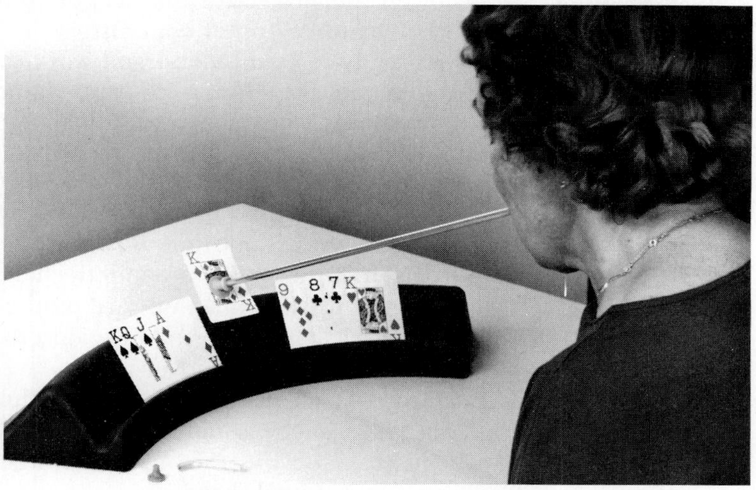

Figure 9-8. *A client who cannot use his hands uses a mouthstick to provide independence for recreational activities. Clients also use mouthsticks to maneuver tools and paintbrushes and to operate computers and typewriters.*

Reprinted by permission of © Bissell Healthcare Corporation/Fred Sammons, Inc.

Negative Effects of Immobility and Excessive Bedrest

—skin breakdown and pressure sores

—muscle contractures, stiffness, and weakening

—joint tenderness and reduced range of motion

—bone weakening, resulting in fractures

—poor digestion

—constipation and impactions or possibly diarrhea

—urinary retention with possible stones or infections

—mental sluggishness and depression

—poor blood circulation with thrombosis formation

—increased, thickened respiratory secretions, reduced respiratory air exchange, and potential pneumonias

—restlessness and confused sleeping patterns

—"sick role—sick person" attitude

ASSISTING WITH RESPIRATORY EXERCISES

Clients who have spinal cord injuries will use various deep breathing exercises to expand and clear the air sacs in their lungs. They are clearing any mucous secretions that may collect in the lungs and maintaining the function of the lung tissues. One exercise is simply deep breathing. Another is turning and moving about every two hours while in bed. The nurse supervisor may instruct you to assist your client to cough. This is done to make the cough stronger, expelling mucus with more force. ***Do not*** *perform this exercise unless directed and supervised by the nurse supervisor.* Practice with your nurse supervisor and for each client *before* performing this exercise with that client. It is very important that you and your client work as a team for this exercise. You may count aloud to signal each step so you will both know when to do your own part of the exercise.

Assistive Cough

Do not perform this exercise if your client has:

—pain,

—injury to his chest or abdomen, or

—any concerns about performing the exercise.

When your client is lying supine:

- Place your hands over the client's xiphoid process (center bone of the rib cage). Move your hands so they are just below the xiphoid process but not on his ribs. You can feel the end of the xiphoid process in the center of the chest between the ribs. The nurse supervisor will direct you to locate the xiphoid on each client (Figure 9-9).

- Ask your client if he is comfortable with the location of your hands.

- Make one hand into a loose fist. Place the fist with the fingers down over the area just below the xiphoid process and not on the ribs. Place the heel of your other hand on top of your fist.

- Get ready to count aloud and work together on the timing of your hand movements with his breathing and coughing.

- Have your client breathe in 2–3 deep breaths. He should breathe in through his nose. At the same time as he breathes in, push the heel of your hand (the hand on top of the fist) in an upward motion. Your fist will move up and in against the area below the xiphoid process.

- Have your client cough as he breathes out. This is one combined motion. As you push, he breathes in and coughs out. Do **not** push hard.

- Repeat 4–5 times. Do this as often as directed. Stop at any time the client becomes uncomfortable or anything changes in his behavior. Report any changes to the nurse supervisor.

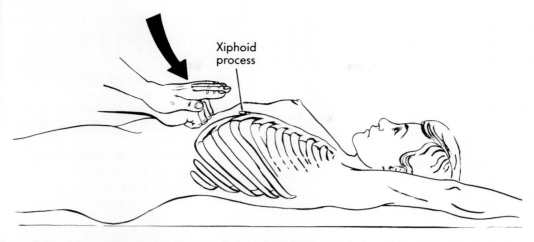

Figure 9-9. *Locate a client's xiphoid process before you assist him to cough. The nurse supervisor will direct you with the correct placement of your hands and practice in performing the procedure.*

Alternate Exercise

If he does not cough, he may exercise his diaphragm and abdomen using the same technique. Except:

- Place your hands as before. The client is supine.
- He breathes in and you push.
- Count to 3 while your client holds in his breath.
- Have him purse his lips while blowing out the breath.
- Repeat 4–5 times.

LOSS OF SENSATION AND POSITION

Another group of losses includes losses of sensation and touch, temperature awareness, and position of a body part. This means the client's body parts affected by the spinal cord injury are very vulnerable because he does not have sensations. He cannot experience how his body feels and he cannot feel what he touches. He is unaware of things that touch him or that he may come up against. This means that he cannot feel temperatures of hot or cold, cannot feel pain, and cannot feel pressure on his skin. Furthermore, he cannot feel where his body parts are or how they are positioned. He must look to find out. You must look also because he will not complain of pain if he is not sitting properly or if he has a scrape or cut. Make it your rule to

look carefully at your client. Be observant and anticipate problems that can arise.

BOWEL AND BLADDER PROGRAMS

Clients who have spinal cord injuries with loss of voluntary control over their bowel and bladder functions can have successful regulatory programs for these functions. Bowel and bladder programs are covered in Chapter 2. Your client may use suppositories, and occasionally medications to stimulate his bowel program. Many clients eat diets that include high fiber foods to promote bowel activity. Fluids and foods that acidify the urine may help to reduce bladder infections. Your nurse supervisor or the dietitian will discuss the dietary care plan with you. Examples are included in the Appendix.

THE SPECIAL IMPORTANCE OF SKIN CARE

When a person has a spinal cord injury the communication is interrupted between the brain, the spinal cord nerves, and the skin below the level of injury. The person has no feelings of sensation, pain, pressure, or touch. The skin has many other functions to perform in the body, but when the feelings are not communicated, the skin's job becomes more difficult to carry out. You and your client must think about what the skin does for the body and how to prevent skin breakdowns.

The person with a spinal cord injury has special concerns about his skin. The primary concern is to prevent **pressure sores** from developing. A pressure sore is an area where the skin has broken down, causing redness. There may be breaks in the skin, ranging from cracks to large open ulcers or wounds. Pressure sores remind you that any kind of pressure on the skin for an extended length of time can cause sores. Many clients cannot sense the pressure to tell you about it themselves.

Two other types of pressure that cause sores are skin shearing and skin friction. These occur when the skin rubs or slides across any surface or object. Think about the red areas that appear on your own skin after sleeping with your legs crossed or about "sheetburns" on your elbows after a day or so in bed. Think about the layers of the skin to picture how skin cells are damaged. When the client moves in one direction he slides the outer skin layer in the same direction. The deeper layers of skin containing the blood vessels and other tissues do not slide with him. They go the other direction. As the person shears his skin, the skin layers are literally torn one way against the other. This damages the cells, causing many of them to die. (Skin is discussed in Chapter 2).

Preventable Skin Problems

The following situations can cause skin problems for the person with a spinal cord injury. Think about them and look for similar situations that could affect your client. Prevent them from happening.

If you were in any of these situations, you would either complain about discomfort or take some action to remove the source of your discomfort. The person with spinal cord injury is not made aware of the problem by his body defense mechanisms. He must learn to check his condition and think about possible problems before they happen. For example, many disabled persons use timers to remind them to shift their weight and use mirrors to be able to see parts of the body they cannot otherwise monitor. You and your client may

> *Causes of Skin Problems for Clients with Spinal Cord Injury*
> —Rough or rumpled material on seat or bed linens.
> —Seat or bed too close or touching a heat source, a radiator, heating pad, or the sun.
> —Sitting in the back of a van with the van heat or air conditioning vented only to the front of the van.
> —Burns from hot water, cigarettes, matches, coffee, or soup.
> —Contact with cold metal, chemicals, or frostbite on hands or feet, such as bare or stockinged feet on the floor of a car.
> —Scrapes, injuries, cuts, or insect bites.
> —Arms or legs at "odd" or incorrect positions.
> —Spills of hot foods on skin or clothes.
> —Wet or soiled clothing or cushions.
> —Pinched arm, leg, or skin between surfaces.

think of other preventable problems and how to watch for them before they become troublesome (Figure 9-10). Be sure to talk to your nurse supervisor before implementing any new techniques.

SPASTICITY

Spasticity is the term used to describe involuntary and uncontrollable muscle movements. Spasticity often occurs for persons with spinal cord injuries. It may also follow stroke, Parkinson's disease, and other conditions. Spasticity is a response to an increase in muscle tone; there may be tremors and rigidity. Spasticity can affect the arms, legs, or areas of the trunk. The amount and location of spasticity varies with individuals.

Spasticity can be triggered by such things as changing positions; the stimulation of heat, cold, or pain; and by tight-fitting clothing, shoes, or assistive devices. Some persons have spasticity in response to treatments or procedures. Your client may have medications to control or reduce spasticity. Although spasticity can cause problems in positioning and mobility, some clients have

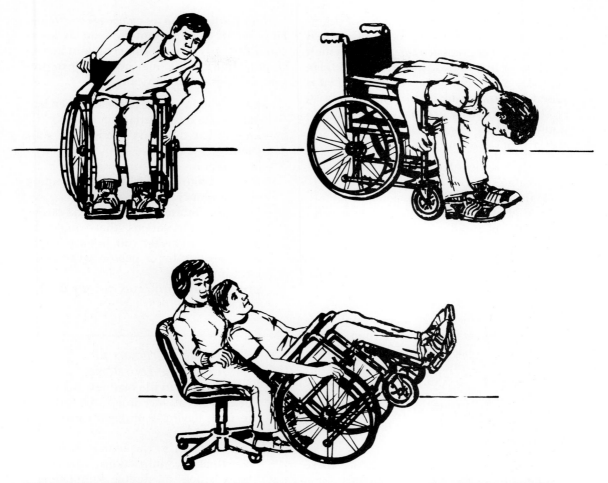

Figure 9-10. *Clients must shift their weight regularly to prevent pressure areas from developing. Weight shifts are simple techniques that help prevent complications.*

learned to use spastic movements to accomplish other movements. A general rule is to move the muscles slowly when working with a client who has spasticity. Discuss any spasticity with the client and the nurse until you are all comfortable with the proper way to work with these muscle movements.

Spasticity can improve and then become progressively more severe. Inform the nurse supervisor if the client's spasticity:

—causes him to develop skin problems,
—interferes with his performing activities that he could previously accomplish, or
—becomes upsetting to him.

There are medications, exercises, and treatments that the physician can prescribe to reduce some of the spasticity.

POSTURAL HYPOTENSION

Postural hypotension is a decrease in blood pressure that occurs when a client who is lying down changes position to sit up or stand up. The part of the nervous system that regulates the blood pressure during these changes in movement is not fully operational due to the spinal cord injury. These clients also have low blood pressure readings and reduced urinary output while sitting. Thus they are particularly susceptible to drops in their blood pressures.

Most clients who have spinal cord injuries wear support stockings, TED stockings, or binders around their abdomens to help prevent postural hypotension. They also move slowly in progressive increments when changing positions, especially from lying down to sitting up or transferring. For example, a client may have the head of his bed raised 15–20 degrees at a time until it is high enough for him to transfer from his bed. He may stop a few minutes each time the bed is raised to allow his blood pressure to adjust.

The signs and symptoms of postural hypotension are:

—sweating;
—pale, colorless face;
—weakness;
—fainting, may lose consciousness;
—blood pressure lower than baseline; and
—weak but rapid pulse.

How to assist your client:

- Call for assistance. Notify your nurse supervisor. If the client does not respond in 1–3 minutes, call the rescue squad or emergency medical unit.
- If your client is in his wheelchair, tilt the wheelchair backwards. Tilt the chair until he is horizontal. Keep the chair in this position for 4–5 minutes. *Slowly* set the chair upright.
- If your client is in bed, help him lie so he is nearly flat in bed. Elevate his legs 10–15 degrees.

The nurse supervisor will practice these movements with you **before** you care for a client with a spinal cord injury. You should have experience tilting an occupied wheelchair backwards before you do so with a client in it. Also check the bed to decide how the legs would be elevated if necessary. The person with quadriplegia does not usually have his head lowered. Be very clear about how to implement the instructions from the nurse supervisor.

AUTONOMIC DYSREFLEXIA

Autonomic dysreflexia (autonomic hyperflexia) is a high blood pressure crisis caused by some irritating stimulation that occurs below the level of injury. Autonomic dysreflexia is a potentially life-threatening crisis for the person with spinal cord injury because the person's blood pressure can become high enough to cause death. This crisis can happen to persons who have quadriplegia or a high level of paraplegia (T6 and above).

Many clients never have autonomic dysreflexia. However, it is important for you to know about the early signs of this crisis and how to respond quickly. You may not be able to prevent this crisis, but you can:

—know whether your client has ever had autonomic dysreflexia.
—know what can start a crisis for your client.
—be observant.
—act quickly to prevent it from becoming an emergency.
—know that autonomic dysreflexia can be caused by irritations that would be minor irritations for you, but are potentially serious for a person with spinal cord injury.
—prevent many problems with good rehabilitation care.

Possible Triggers for Autonomic Dysreflexia

1. An irritation to the bladder, such as being too full, needing to be catheterized, having a plugged catheter, or spasms.
2. An irritation to the bowel, such as constipation, impactions, passing large stools or digital stimulation during bowel program, or enemas.
3. An irritation to the body from pressure or pain, such as tight clothing, belts, or equipment; prolonged pressure on an area, including an ingrown toenail; a pressure sore; burns; or hitting the body.
4. Discomfort from normal body activities, such as menstrual cramps or stimulation of the genitals as in sexual activity.
5. Something that is an irritation to your client as an individual.

Signs of Autonomic Dysreflexia

Your client may tell you (he may or may not know) or complain about some of these signs:

—feeling anxious or nervous;
—blurred vision;

—trouble breathing or stuffy nose;
—chills, "goosebumps," or clammy skin;
—pounding headache; or
—sweating (above the level of injury).

You can observe and check for these signs:

—red, flushed face with profuse sweating. His blood pressure may be high and increasing and his pulse rate may be slowed. The nurse supervisor will know the client's baseline readings for blood pressure and pulse.
—no fever, but chills.
—skin blotching from being flushed, then paled.
—cool, clammy, sweaty skin below the level of injury.
—seizures.

What To Do

You should know what to do immediately if this crisis ever happens. The best things to know are the signs that autonomic dysreflexia may be happening so that you can act immediately.

1. Place the person in a sitting position.
    a) *Never* lay the person down. Sitting will help to keep his blood pressure lower.
    b) Elevate the head of the bed, raise the back of a reclining wheelchair, or prop him up with pillows.
    c) Raising up the person's head, shoulders, and trunk will help to lower his blood pressure.
2. Call for help and notify the nurse as soon as possible, but there may not be time to wait for assistance to arrive.
3. Check for any of these irritants and correct them: *If the client does not feel immediate relief when a possible cause of the problem is removed, continue to look for possible causes and remove them until he has relief or until help arrives.*
    a) Check indwelling catheter for kinks and straighten it out. If it is plugged or clogged, call the nurse supervisor, rescue squad, or emergency unit. The emergency room staff will remove the catheter and replace it.
    b) Check for tight clothing, belts,

shoes, elastic stockings, binders, or equipment. Loosen or remove it.
    c) Look to see if the leg bag is too full. If so, empty it. Reconnect the bag and the catheter tubing. Urine should flow into the bag. If not, he may have a full bladder. Read number 4 below.
    d) Check the rectum for large stools or an impaction. If stool is not passed, notify the rescue squad so that the stool can be removed.
    e) Keep the client's head elevated and continue to reassure him as you take action.
4. If the client uses intermittent catheterization and he cannot do this himself, call the family member who can perform the catheterization. If no one is available, call the rescue squad and the nurse. The person must be catheterized to relieve the irritation to the bladder causing the high blood pressure.
5. **Do Not** leave your client. If a family member or friend is near, contact them. Call the nurse or the office to tell them what is happening, but do not leave the client. Reassure your client that you are taking action and that you will not leave him.
6. If the client gets worse or passes out, call the rescue squad and tell them that the person must go to the emergency room immediately. Stay with the client so that you can tell the rescue squad and the emergency room staff what is happening. Your client may pass out and not be able to tell others what is wrong.

This emergency may never happen, but you must know what to do if it ever does. Prevention is the best method.

THROMBOPHLEBITIS

Thrombophlebitis can result from prolonged immobility and decreased blood circulation. It is best to prevent the conditions that may lead to thrombophlebitis. Preventive measures are:

—active or passive range-of-motion exercises to keep an active blood flow,
—regular exercise and mobility,

—wearing TED stockings if ordered,

—reporting signs and symptoms to the nurse supervisor, and,

—if able, point and flex the client's feet throughout the day.

Your client should not:

—become immobile, or

—wear girdles or tight knee-high stockings.

Signs and Symptoms:

—Early signs are muscle aches in the calves (your client may not be able to feel these),

—increased warmth in the lower leg (the skin will be warm to the touch),

—the lower leg or calf will increase in size, and

—there may be a reddened area on the skin.

Your client may be unaware of the changes in his lower legs due to his decreased sensations. The nurse supervisor may instruct you in specific ways to check your client's lower legs on a regular basis. You may do this when assisting him with personal care.

PERSONAL ADJUSTMENTS TO SPINAL CORD INJURY

ADJUSTING TO LIFE STAGES

Persons who have disabilities following a spinal cord injury vary individually in the ways in which they adjust to the changes the injury produces in their lives. There are, however, some predictable patterns of adjustment and reactions that may be experienced by your client. Your client will also develop his own methods of coping with his situation. Some ways of adjustment and coping can help a person work through crisis times in his life. Other ways are not productive; they may even retard or prevent positive adjustment and coping.

One important consideration in the way a person deals with a crisis such as spinal cord injury is his stage of life and his stage of personal development. In other words, we must consider how old and how mature he is, what else has occurred in his life, how successfully he has dealt with past situations and crises, what his personal strengths are, and what family, religious, or other resources he has to assist him.

Many clients with spinal cord injuries are in their late adolescent or young adult years. They will have the same personality traits, goals, and experience levels of able-bodied persons in the same stage of life. Additionally, many persons who have spinal cord injuries are living longer. They must be respected in terms of their individual life stages and changes as older adults as well as in terms of the lifestyle changes and coping necessary because of their spinal cord injuries.

THE GRIEVING PROCESS

Grieving may be particularly marked for a client who has spinal cord injuries; he may have lost many functional abilities if his injury is severe. Too often, he will forfeit friends, career, marriage, and important resources as a result of his disabilities. Although these losses are not inevitable, it takes time to restructure his life. He may experience the different stages in the grieving process for many years following his injury.

Recent studies report that the person with a severely disabling spinal injury may grieve for three or more years after he returns home. Other changes and factors in his lifestyle, his support from his family and friends, his basic personality, and his resources influence how he copes with this process. All clients who have spinal cord injuries will go through the grieving process, each one in his own way and time.

This does not mean that your client will not nor cannot have a productive and happy life. The grieving process is a necessary coping and adaptation reaction so that he can set new directions for his life as it is now. Furthermore, other research studies show that clients do not view their quality of life as good or poor based solely on their disabilities. *Read about the grieving process* in Chapter 1.

Review your role and activities in each case with the nurse supervisor on a regular basis. This is important if you are in the home of your client for a long period of time. Your client will change by working through the various stages to adjust and cope with his injury and by growing and developing through his life stages. Work closely with the nurse supervisor about how you can respond to your client so that you will be a positive influence in your client's changing life.

CHAPTER 10

Care for the Client with an Amputation

OBJECTIVES

When you have studied this chapter and practiced the procedures it describes, you will be able to:

1. Define terms relating to amputations and prosthetics.
2. Assist with correct procedures for ace bandage-wrapping of a residual limb, if directed and supervised.
3. Report signs of potential circulation problems.
4. Discuss special considerations for the client who has an amputation, such as phantom limb sensations, falling safely, and preventive care measures.
5. Practice correct positioning for the person with a lower limb amputation.
6. Assist your client with donning and doffing his prosthesis.
7. Provide care and basic maintenance of a prosthesis and related supplies.
8. Combine amputation care with care for other disabilities for the client with multiple conditions.

OVERVIEW

This chapter discusses the special care needs of the person who has had an amputed body part. An **amputation** is the partial or complete removal of a body part, usually an arm or leg. The limb remaining after the amputation is called a **residual limb;** it is *not* a "stump." Some types of amputations are not as common as they once were due to medical advances such as antibiotics and microsurgery. However, people of all ages still may require amputations. Men between 60 and 70 years old have the most amputations. They are usually needed because of complications from peripheral vascular or circulatory diseases and diabetes mellitus. Others are the result of injuries, tumors, or birth defects. Amputations of the legs below the knee are the most common. Occasionally legs are amputated above the knee or at the hip joint.

The person who has had an amputation has to make a number of adjustments in his activities of daily living. Persons who have amputations may have a **prosthetic device.** This could be an artificial leg, arm, hand, or foot. Prosthetic devices may be temporary or permanent, motorized, cosmetically designed, and equipped with joints and movable parts. Each prosthesis is made and fitted for the individual who will wear and use it. Each one is selected for an appearance that matches the person's body shape and skin color. The client works with a **prosthetist** to fit the prosthesis so that it functions as well as possible as a replacement for the amputated body part (Figure 10-1).

There are some differences in care and problems between persons with amputations of the upper and lower parts of the body. The person with an amputation from the upper body, such as an arm or hand, will have several physical care requirements that differ from those of the person with a lower body part amputation. However, there are many assistive devices for improving self-care developed specifically for upper or lower body amputations.

Assistive devices are used by clients when cooking, dressing, grooming, conducting business activities, and participating in sports. Chapter 6 provides photographs and detailed information about assistive devices. Persons with disabilities often are very creative about ideas and tools to assist them in conducting activities independently. You and your client may find new ways to adapt everyday items and clothing.

Some persons have limited activities following an amputation. Others are able to continue active lifestyles (Figure 10-2). Some persons who have had leg amputations still go skiing. Others with amputations of both arms wear prostheses so they can fish and hunt. Outdoor camps are becoming popular for children and young adults who wish to learn how to adapt their disability for sports, camping, hiking, and similar recreational activities.

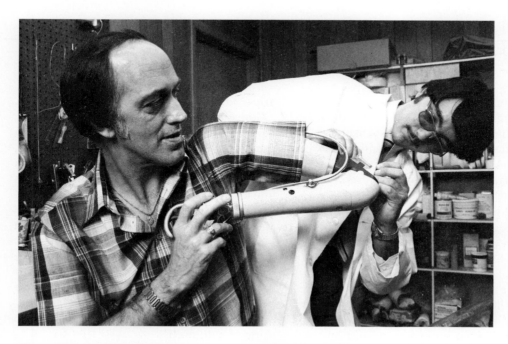

Figure 10-1. *Optimal functioning of a prosthesis depends on obtaining the correct prosthetic device and the proper fit.*
    Photos courtesy of Motion Control, division of 10 MED. Inc., Salt Lake City, Utah.

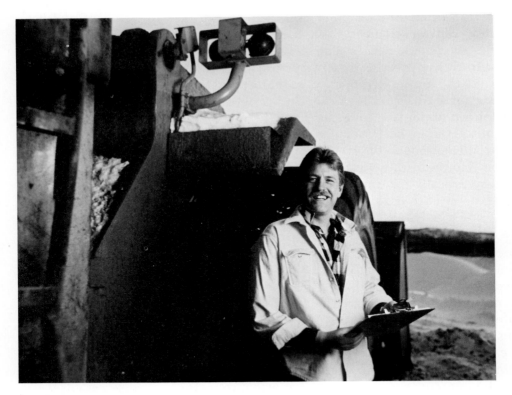

Figure 10-2.   *Prosthetic devices enable persons to continue active lifestyles. Notice the cosmetic appearance of the arm and hand prosthesis in this photograph.*
Photos courtesy of Motion Control, division of 10 MED. Inc., Salt Lake City, Utah.

Successful management of an amputation

Assistive devices are important for the person with an amputation. There are also other factors that also determine how successfully the person with an amputation manages his lifestyle. As you read through the following list of factors, think about how each one affects your client.

The older person who has an amputation may struggle with a chronic medical problem that adds to his physical and mental stresses. Diseases like diabetes or peripheral vascular and circulatory problems can lead to painful gangrene followed by amputation. The amputation may cure the immediate problem with gangrene and so the person feels *physically* better. That same person may feel *psychologically* unhappy because he has lost a part of his body. He may mourn the loss of what he could do before the amputation or grieve about the change in his appearance.

The client mourning the loss of his body part needs attention and support in addition to care of the amputation itself. For example, a client may feel so "incomplete" after an amputation that he cannot or will not dress himself with the same care as before the surgery. He will not maintain personal hygiene and grooming. He may say that he is not a "whole person" or that he is no longer useful. Taking care of himself may no longer be important. Be patient and a good listener if your client has these reactions. Tell the nurse supervisor and the family if he acts depressed, mentions suicide, or neglects to do things for himself.

You client may change his attitudes toward family and friends. He may become overly conscious of how others view him. All per-

---

Factors Affecting Successful Management of an Amputation

- The acceptance of his amputation by himself and family, friends, and co-workers.
- The quality of hospital care and teaching, including care in a specialized rehabilitation facility.
- The quality, appearance, and useful functioning of his prothesis.
- The available resources, services, and support groups.
- The degree of pain, infection, or problems with healing.
- His age, general health, strength, and endurance.
- The type, location, and severity of the amputation.
- His attitude and motivation to overcome everyday problems.
- His participation in social and leisure activities.
- The reason the amputation was necessary and future health needs.

---

sons who have contact with a person who has had an amputation must **react to the person, not to the amputation.** In our society there are many negative references to persons with amputations. Tell your client about positive examples. These include athletes who have prostheses and other well-known personalities who use prostheses and have managed their lives successfully. The nurse supervisor and the physical or occupational therapist will plan activities that your client can complete to feel in control and successful (Figure 10-3).

Your client may have periods of grieving for the loss of his body part. The person may have some grieving for loss of abilities as he works to regain as much function as possible. He must deal with his individual grieving about the loss of a body part. Be supportive but do not allow your client to neglect his self-care or other activities that lead to independence. All of us are important and useful for more reasons than the arrangement of our body parts. We are more than our parts, together or apart.

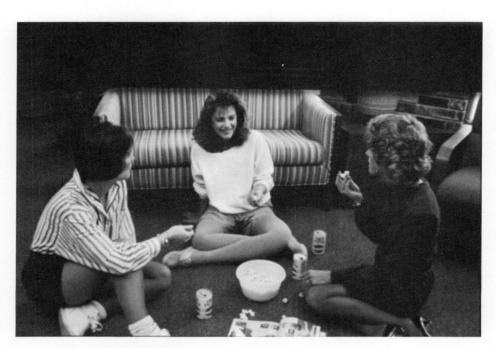

Figure 10-3. *Clients can lead normal, active lives using a prosthesis. In this photograph the client is sitting cross-legged while wearing a lower limb prosthesis.*
Photo courtesy of Otto Bock Orthopedic Industry Inc., U.S.A.

ACE BANDAGE WRAPPINGS

The hospital nurses, aides, and therapists have given your client care and directions which you must understand and continue to follow in the home. Your nurse supervisor will instruct you about specific care for the person's amputation site. Your client may have instructions to wrap his residual limb with an ace bandage. This is done to improve circulation, reduce swelling, and help to correctly shape his limb.

You do not wrap a client's residual limb. The nurse supervisor will direct and supervise this procedure. Directions for wrapping the residual arm or leg with an ace bandage are explained and illustrated below for reference. If your client has difficulties with the wrapping or does not seem to be performing the procedure correctly, notify the nurse supervisor.

You will NOT perform this procedure. However, you need to know if the client or family is wrapping correctly or incorrectly.

Correct ace bandage wrapping procedures are very important. The ace bandage wrappings are applied in a criss-cross figure 8 pattern. *Pressure is applied away from the body on*

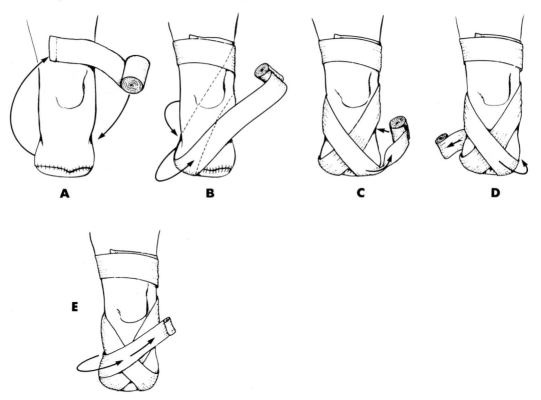

Figure 10-4. *Ace bandage wrapping is performed under the direction of the nurse supervisor. These illustrate a lower limb below-knee wrap for your reference.*

A, *The residual limb is wrapped with an Ace bandage. The first wrap anchors the bandage without applying any pressure.*

B, *The bandage is looped behind the limb to cover the lateral lower corner of the residual limb. The skin is pulled forward with the wrap.*

C, *Continue the wrap up and around behind the leg. This wrap is below the first anchoring wrap, but slightly overlapping the lower edge of the wrapped bandage. Begin to add tension (one half to two thirds of bandage stretch) to the wrap. If the client feels throbbing, loosen the tension.*

D, *Wrap the opposite inner corner so the entire residual limb is covered with ace bandage wrapping. Continue with one half to two thirds stretch tension to the wrap, unless the client feels throbbing.*

E, *Continue wrapping in a figure-eight style. Each wrap only slightly overlaps the preceding layer. There must be no wrinkles or sags in the wrap. Pressure is distributed from the proximal portion of the wrap to the distal portion.*

the amputated end of the limb. Too much pressure can cause throbbing, cut off blood supply, and create a poor shape to the residual limb. Ace wraps should be firmly wrapped *without wrinkles* and *fastened with tape.* Do not use metal clips or safety pins. These may fall off the wraps into a bed or chair and cut or scrape the client when he lies or sits on them. Ace bandages should be hand-washed daily. They are laid flat or hung to dry. This helps them to maintain the elasticity that makes them effective.

The ace wrappings should extend far enough on the residual limb to include all tissue that will be enclosed in the prosthesis. The wrapping for an above-the-knee amputation (AK amputation) should extend to the person's groin. A below-the-knee amputation (BK amputation) should extend above the knee (Figure 10-4). This usually requires two bandages. These may be sewn together to make one longer ace bandage. Notify your nurse supervisor or the physical therapist if you have questions about the appearance of an ace bandage wrap. Also report any signs or symptoms of possible circulation problems.

"STUMP" SHRINKERS

"Stump" shrinkers are special sock-like wraps used to prevent or decrease edema after an amputation and to reshape a residual limb so a prosthesis can be fitted as soon as possible (Figure 10-5). The stump shrinker slips over the residual limb. Many clients and physicians prefer them to ace bandage wraps. Stump shrinkers come in a variety of lengths, materials, and styles. Most stump shrinkers are made of an elasticized material. The below-the-knee shrinker will extend above the knee joint so that it will not slip off the residual limb. The above-the-knee shrinker will extend high on the thigh. The client will wear a non-elastic belt with straps fitted to the shrinker to keep it in place.

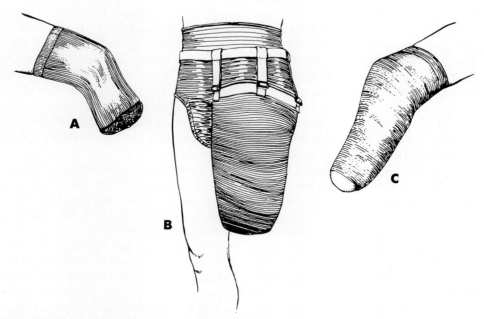

Figure 10-5. *Many clients wear commercial "stump shrinkers" to reduce edema following a limb amputation. These are fitted elastic supports.*
   A, *Ventilated below-the-knee style.*
   B, *Styled for above-the-knee amputation, this version includes a belt, straps, and contoured, crotch.*
   C, *A stump shrinker styled for below-the-knee amputations has a padded distal end.*
Courtesy Truform Orthotics and Prosthetics, Cincinnati, OH.

Stump shrinkers are worn day and night as directed. You must check the skin and circulation just as for the ace bandage wrappings. Notify the nurse supervisor if the stump shrinker seems to fit differently or to have changed in size. Your client's leg may have changed in size. If it is enlarged, it could be due to edema or to a developing problem such as a thrombosis. To care for stump shrinkers, wash them by hand in mild soapy water, rinse, and lay flat to dry. Clients will need a second shrinker to wear when one is drying.

Signs and Symptoms of Possible Circulation Problems

—Skin color changes, either paler or darker skin;
—shiny skin that is tight or puffy;
—distended veins;
—complaints of itching or throbbing;
—skin temperature changes to warm or cold;
—changes in limb shape, or one limb larger than the other;
—complaints of pain or discomfort, including tingling; and
—skin redness, breakdown, bruises, or cuts.

COPING FOLLOWING AMPUTATION

THE PROPER WAY TO FALL

Your client needs to become as independent as possible, but in a safe manner. Increased mobility and a prosthesis usually mean new experiences after an amputation. Clients with walking prostheses can expect to have to learn how to cope with some difficulties. They must be taught how to fall down without hurting themselves—and how to get up again.

Your client has been taught by the physical therapist how to fall to lessen the chance of injury. He is taught to fall toward his able side if he finds himself falling. During a fall he can expect to have a reflex action that is difficult to avoid. The reflex causes him to automatically reach out with the amputated leg. This would place the weight of the fall onto the amputed limb. The trauma may cause the end of the residual limb to break open along the old suture line. Severe bruising or fractures are possible. The client may complain of severe pain and may become anxious and frightened.

If your client does fall, do not move him until you have directions from the nurse, physician, or rescue team. Call the rescue team if your client is in shock or bleeding.

Ask for instructions for emergency measures until help arrives. Remove the prosthesis if necessary to thoroughly check both his residual limb and the prosthesis for damage.

Once a person has had a serious fall, it may be difficult for him to be as venturesome and independent as before. If your client falls without injury, let him get himself up, using the way he was taught. Most clients are taught to get up by putting their weight to the able side. This lets them get on the able knee. Using the arms for support, one hand is placed on the able leg as the leg is extended. The prosthetic leg is pulled up as he gains an erect posture.

You will have to be sure that you and the family do not become unduly concerned about your client's increased mobility. Mobility is the key to independence and a better lifestyle. A safe environment, proper shoes and equipment, and attention to preventing falls are the best ways to avoid problems. The person should learn to set realistic expectations for what he can or cannot do without losing functional abilities. For example, when dealing with wet, icy walking surfaces, strong winds, or uneven footing, the person wearing a prosthesis may use a cane and walk slower.

Similarly, it takes more energy than usual to walk with a prosthesis. Your client needs to learn his level of fatigue and abilities. He needs to plan to avoid overexertion that leads to accidents. Each client advances at his own rate within the limits of his abilities. A person who formerly walked only around his home or strolled several blocks to the office should not be expected to take up skiing with a prosthesis.

Clients wearing prostheses eventually progress to a walker or crutches. Be sure the house has been inspected for safety. Be sure the family and other caregivers in the home cooperate with *keeping* the house safe. Work with the client, your nurse supervisor, and the physical therapist to learn exactly what your client has been taught to do when using the walker or crutches. You will be told:

how far he can walk,
for how long,
where he can go, including stairs and out of doors, and
the exact techniques he has been taught.

Ideally, the physical therapist and the nurse will work with the person while you are in the home. This lets you see the procedure for yourself.

CHANGING DOMINANT SIDES

Some clients have lost an arm or leg on the **dominant** or usual side. These clients have more difficulties with other activities. For example, right-handed clients will have to learn to use their left hands to do things. They will also have to learn how to handle the prostheses. The nurse supervisor or therapist will give the client special exercises or activities that will help him if he has to change his dominant hand or leg. Loss of a dominant arm or leg may also affect balance. The therapist may have given him exercises to improve his sitting and standing balance and exercises to strengthen his muscles.

PHANTOM PAIN

"Phantom limb sensations" or "phantom limb pain" are other situations you may encounter while caring for a person who has had an amputation. The person may feel that the amputated limb is still there. Sometimes he may feel pain. This situation usually leaves within 4–6 months after the surgery. However, some persons experience "phantom" sensations and pain for years. If your client complains of this situation, notify the nurse supervisor. She will plan exercises or other activities to assist your client.

Phantom sensations and pain are very real to the client. You should not ignore the concerns or think that your client has emotional problems. The person's brain remembers the part before the amputation and is telling the person that the arm or leg is still there. It may be telling him that pain is still there also. The person feels what the brain is telling the body to feel. Your client may have difficulty with phantom sensations. If so, the following may be part of his care plan:

You may be instructed to assist him to:

- Take a short walk wearing the prosthesis.
- Place pressure on the end of the prosthesis by either
  —donning the prosthesis and pushing the foot against the footboard of the bed or
  —looping a towel, belt, or binder over the end of the amputated limb. Then the client pulls on the ends to apply pressure to the amputated limb.
- Place both limbs in the same position, close his eyes, then breathe deeply, as he relaxes both extremities.

CARE WITH LOWER LIMB AMPUTATIONS

Amputations of the lower extremities may involve the foot or may be as large as the entire leg up to the trunk. Most lower extremity amputations are below the knee so that the bend of the knee is still available. These are called **BK** for *below knee* amputations. The other usual amputation site is just above the knee into the thigh region. These are called **AK** or *above knee* amputations.

Many clients who have leg amputations do not wear prostheses and need a wheelchair. A wheelchair may also be used for an older person who has been ill for a time and has low endurance or little strength. Wheelchair procedures are discussed in Chapter 5.

Whenever your client is in a chair, his amputated limb *must be kept as straight as possible and elevated.* **Do not** allow your client to sit with his amputated limb bent at the knee. Keep the knee of the amputed limb straight when he is seated. This will give him a straight posture when he stands with his prosthesis. Some people have both legs amputated. Therefore, both legs must be raised and supported as straight as possible.

To do this, elevate and lock the wheelchair leg rest on the same side as the amputation. Place a small foam cushion or a folded bathtowel (inserted inside a pillowcase) on the leg rest. Be sure there are no wrinkles or lumps. This soft pad will prevent pressure areas from developing on the back of your client's leg. This simple technique at the appropriate time will help your client avoid a problem and be more successful later.

You may have to transfer a person with a below-the-knee amputation from the wheelchair to another chair or commode. You must keep the knee as straight as possible. This means that you must have some support for the residual limb. You can use another chair to support the residual limb or a stool or cardboard box with pillows on top.

With an amputation *above the knee*, the residual limb will be short enough to rest on the chair seat. However, some persons have very long upper legs which extend over seats of wheelchairs or kitchen chairs (Figure 10-6). The seats of their chairs may have to be extended with a piece of smoothed wood or heavy cardboard. The extension must be strong enough to support the weight of the leg. Cover the board or cardboard with a piece of foam or folded towels and a smooth pillowcase. Watch for pressure areas. If the person's leg is very flabby, watch for pressure on the outer side of the leg.

Encourage your client to do the following if ordered by the nurse supervisor or therapist:

—turn prone during bathing, bed changes, or backrubs;
—lie prone for several times during the day; and

> ***Never*** *Allow Your Client with a Lower Limb Amputation to:*
>
> —place a pillow under his hip or knee when in bed,
> —lie in bed with his knees bent,
> —put a pillow under his back when he is lying on his back in bed,
> —put a pillow between his thighs,
> —lift or crank up the lower end of the bed under his knees,
> —let the residual limb roll in or turn in toward the other leg,
> —let his legs fall outwards while lying on his back,
> —hang his residual limb over the edge of the bed or chair,
> —sit with his residual limb bent, or
> —stand with crutches or a walker and rest his residual limb on the handle or crossbar.

—use an overhead trapeze to strengthen his arms and to lift and turn in the bed.

SPECIAL CARE TECHNIQUES

Never lift or crank the lower part of the bed under the knees or use pillows to elevate the person's knees while he is in bed. This statement may sound opposite to the rule of keeping the legs elevated while in the wheelchair. When you raise the knees while the person is in bed, it forces his hips to bend. This can cause a contracture that will keep him from being able to stand with the prosthesis flat on the floor. If the person has an above-the-knee amputation, he may sit with the residual limb pointing up in the air.

Your client may want the bed elevated because it may feel more comfortable to him. If there is a need to elevate the leg, the bottom of the bed can be elevated on blocks of wood. These can be purchased from a surgical supply house or made by the family or volunteers. Two-by-four or four-by-four pieces of lumber that firmly support the bed are used. They do not slide and are not dangerous to others walking about the bed and the room. Your nurse supervisor will initiate this action if necessary.

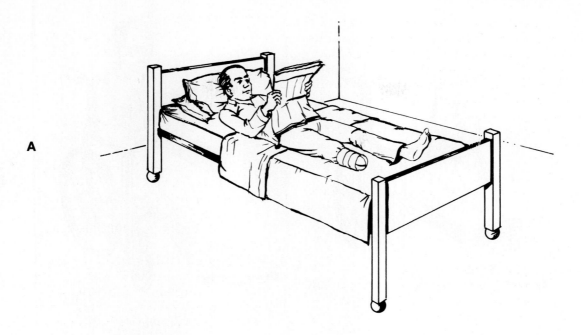

A

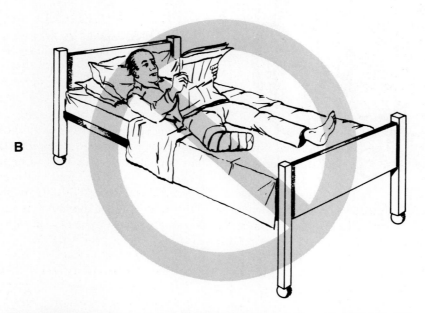

B

Figure 10-6. **A,** *DO position a client to lie in bed with his residual limb straight.* **B,** *DO NOT allow a client to roll his legs inward.* *Continued.*

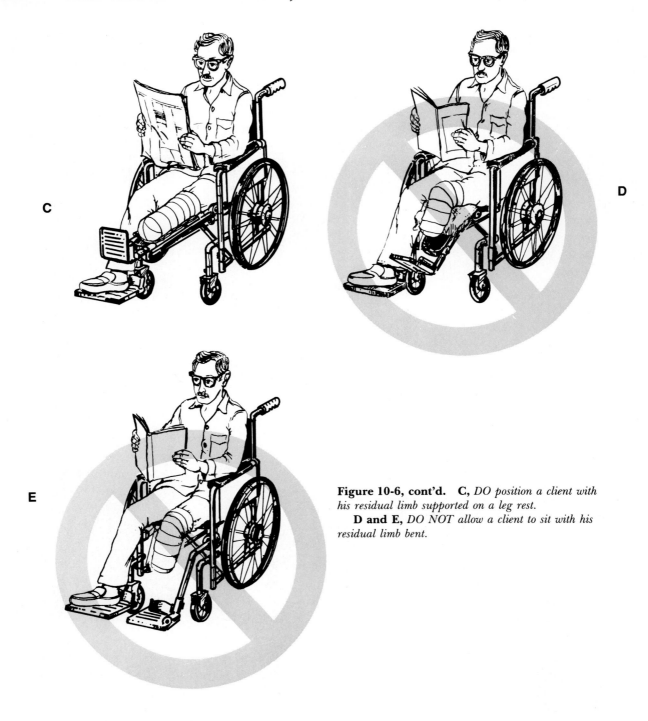

Figure 10-6, cont'd.   C, *DO position a client with his residual limb supported on a leg rest.*
   D and E, *DO NOT allow a client to sit with his residual limb bent.*

Some older persons with poor posture, arthritis, or osteoporosis did not stand up straight before a leg amputation. These clients need to keep their posture as straight as possible. However, they may never be able to walk using a prosthesis. They may have prostheses for cosmetic purposes, but not for walking. It may be important for this client to be seen by himself and others as a whole person with two legs, even if he cannot stand or walk on them. Encourage these clients to perform standing transfers only if you and they are taught by a physical therapist. Practice with the therapist there to direct you before attempting to transfer the client alone.

DONNING AND DOFFING

Donning and doffing are the terms used to describe the process of putting on and taking off a prosthesis. To don, or put on, a prosthesis is one of the first tasks learned during rehabilitation. The person usually wears a special sock over the dressing of the amputated area. (The seam of the sock is arranged so that it does not touch the suture line at the amputation site.) Your client should be very sure not to have wrinkles in this sock. Seams and wrinkles could cause skin irritations and blisters. The size of the amputated leg decreases over time. The physical therapist will supply additional socks to maintain the correct fit.

Some prostheses have velcro straps or other fasteners to keep them in place once they are donned. Your client may have to stand to adjust his prosthetic leg. Other maneuvers may be necessary to get him set into the prosthesis. The physical or occupational therapist will show you how to assist your client if your help is required.

The series of photographs show a client who can independently don an above-the-knee prosthesis and its cosmetic cover. Prostheses and covers will vary. Clients will require different amounts of assistance. Fig. 10-7.

Doffing is also taught at the rehabilitation center or hospital. Each client is taught techniques to suit his special needs. Follow instructions from the center or the therapist about handling and storing the prosthesis when it is not in use. Always make sure your client is in a position with good balance and in a safe environment for donning or doffing his prosthesis. Your client may feel more secure if his prosthesis is stored near his bed or chair. Consider how much more in control he will feel if his prosthesis is within reach.

Some clients have more than one prosthesis (Figure 10-8). Be sure to get clear instructions from the nurse supervisor or the therapist for safe care that will keep your client as independent as possible. He may have an upper body prosthesis that ends with either a hook or a solid hand. Check for specific instructions for use and care. Avoid using any products that contain grease or solvents. Do not immerse the prosthesis in water or remove the coverings.

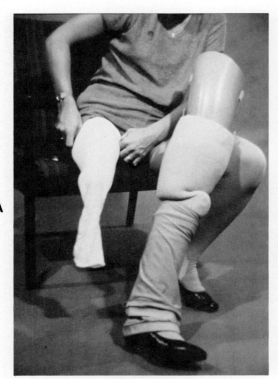

A

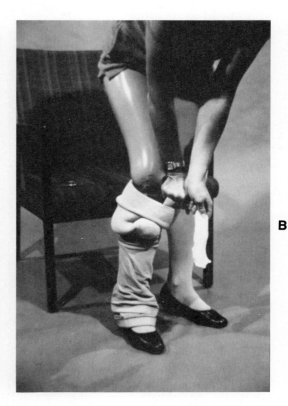

B

Figure 10-7. *The steps in donning an above-the-knee prosthesis with a cosmetic cover. Photo courtesy of Otto Bock Orthopedic Industry Inc., U.S.A.* *Continued.*

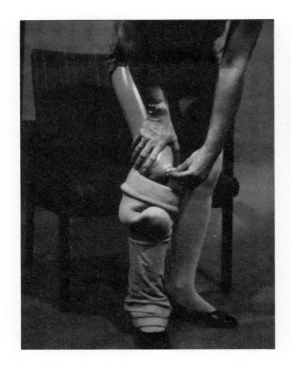

C

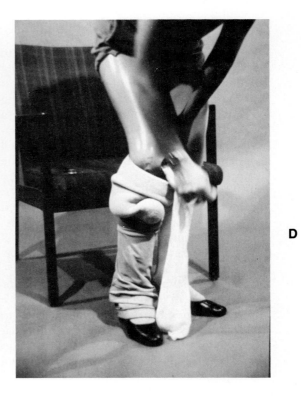

D

E

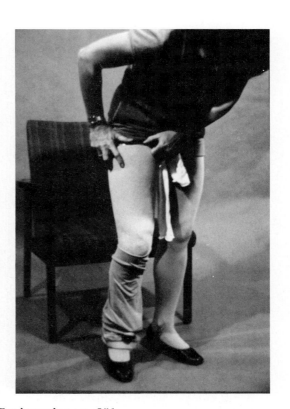

F

Figure 10-7, cont'd.   For legend see p. 251.

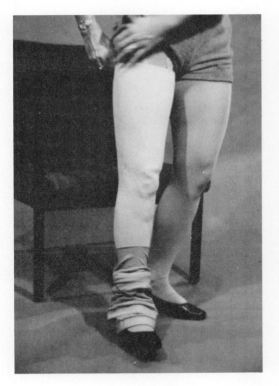

G

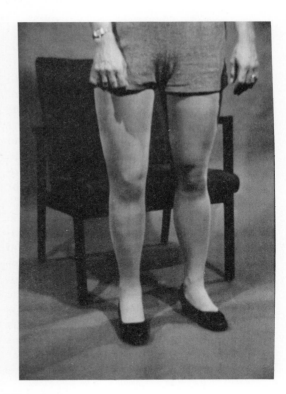

H

Figure 10-7, cont'd. For legend see p. 251.

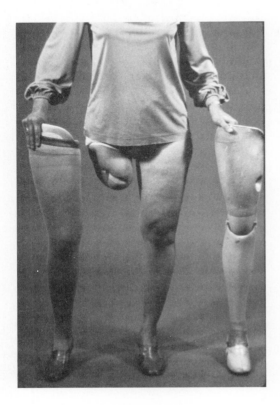

Figure 10-8. *Some clients have more than one style of prosthesis.*
Photo courtesy of Otto Bock Orthopedic Industry Inc., U.S.A.

CARE OF THE RESIDUAL LIMB

Hygiene is as important for the person with an amputation as it is for everyone else. Unless there are orders to the contrary, clients should bathe daily. Specific instructions for hygiene of the amputated area will depend on its severity and stage of healing. In fact, hygiene is especially important if the amputation was performed because of diabetes or poor circulation.

The amputation may not stop the disease that necessitated the amputation, such as diabetes, for example. Your client may develop problems with the other leg or arm if preventive care is not taken seriously. Once the skin of the residual limb is completely healed, the area can be washed with mild soap. Then it is rinsed with clear water, and dried carefully and thoroughly. Review hygiene instructions with the nurse supervisor.

CARE OF THE PROSTHESIS

Make it a rule to check the skin on the residual limb each time the prosthesis is donned or doffed. Your client should be encouraged to check his own skin. However, you must be sure he follows through on this important task. Even minor skin redness or chafing can keep him off his prosthesis for several days or longer. Many clients use a hand-held mirror to check the back of the residual limb.

Part of the client's hygiene is cleaning the prosthesis. Keep the prosthesis clean and dry. A hard outer covering can be cleaned by wiping it daily, using a cloth dampened with rubbing alcohol. The prosthesis is **never** submerged in water. Exceptions are a few specialized prostheses made for swimming (Figure 10-9).

A soft outer covering is cleaned less often and only as needed. A dry cloth slightly dampened with rubbing alcohol or a special water repellent spray can be used. The prosthesis is air-dried. Stubborn spots can be wiped with a damp, not wet, cloth. This soft cover is more easily damaged by contact with sharp objects. Be sure to examine it while

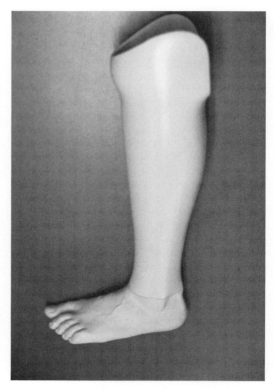

Figure 10-9.   *A hard cover below-the-knee prosthesis is kept clean and dry, but not submerged in water.*
Photo courtesy of Otto Bock Orthopedic Industry Inc., U.S.A.

cleaning. Wipe the socket and feet of the prosthesis in the same manner. Cleaning should be done at least monthly and whenever needed. Your nurse supervisor or therapist will give you any special instructions for cleaning the prosthesis.

Any moving parts, joints, and the socket should be clean and dry. Boots should be worn over prosthetic feet when out-of-doors in rain or snow. Remove the shoe and sock to dry the foot if it gets wet, dirty, or collects sand. If dirt or sand are inside the ankle joint, the prosthetist should clean and check the joint. *Do not attempt to wash or adjust the joint.*

Leather pieces can be cleaned with a leather soap or saddle soap. Leather or nylon parts may retain an odor or become soiled and stained. If so, a prosthetist can replace the parts. The prosthetist can also replace straps, locks, laces, and joint parts. You

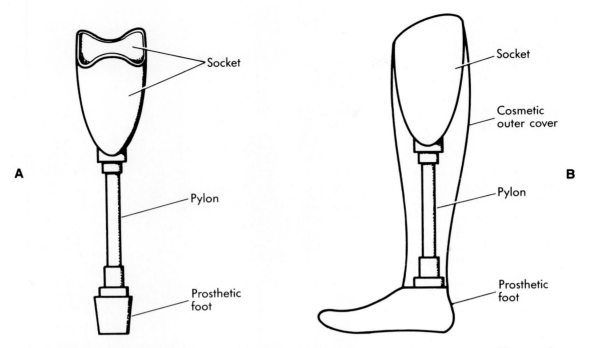

A

B

Figure 10-10. **A,** *Front view of the inner structures of a prosthesis without the cosmetic cover illustrates the construction of the limb.*
 B, *A lateral view shows a prosthesis with the cosmetic cover in place.*
 (Courtesy J. Hodgins, BS, CPO.)

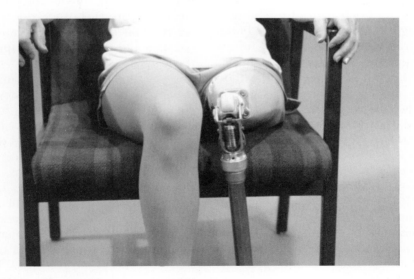

Figure 10-11. *This client is wearing a lower limb prosthesis without the cosmetic cover.*
Photo courtesy of Otto Bock Orthopedic Industry Inc., U.S.A.

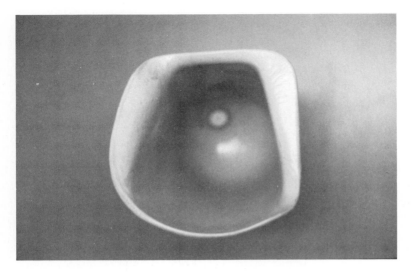

Figure 10-12. *The inside of a hard prosthetic socket must be fitted to the client's residual limb. This will avoid pressure areas, for proper functioning and for comfort.*
Photo courtesy of Otto Bock Orthopedic Industry Inc., U.S.A.

should check these parts to be sure they are working and not worn or soiled. Never attempt to fix or adjust the prosthesis yourself. Always check with the client, family, and nurse for special instructions for prosthetic care.

Additionally, good hygiene includes the liner or soft insert of the prosthesis. The liner should be cleaned like the prosthesis, but using a *well-wrung-out* cloth. The liner requires nightly cleaning to remain odor-free and to reduce infections. A good time to clean the liner is when your client goes to bed at night. This will allow the liner to thoroughly dry and air out overnight.

One of the most important things for you to do each day is to check all moveable parts of the prosthesis. You are looking for any loose parts or excessive movement in the joints. Loose parts can cause your client to have a fall or to develop skin or postural problems. If the equipment makes squeaks or other sounds, the prosthetist should check the prosthesis. He will oil moveable parts and check the alignment. Figures 10-10, 10-11, and 10-12 show features and parts for prostheses.

PROSTHETIC SOCKS

Care of prosthetic socks is an important daily hygiene task. Prosthetic socks must be changed daily or as often as necessary to prevent perspiration build-up. Perspiration collects on the socks and causes skin breakdown to begin. The person with a relatively new prosthesis tends to require more changes of prosthetic socks due to swelling of the residual limb. The socks come in different sizes and thicknesses. A supply of prosthetic socks (several sizes and thicknesses) must be available for your client as *he may change the socks 2–4 times in a day.*

Wool socks can be washed, but they are dried slowly away from direct heat. Nylon socks are machine washed and dried. Good quality socks will not have seams. If your client uses socks with seams, the seams should run from side to side. They should not run front to back across the suture line. Your client may even wear several prosthetic socks at the same time. He may use extra socks to create various levels of thickness inside the socket of the prosthesis. This may be necessary because of some shrinking of the amputated leg over time. Persons with upper limb amputations traditionally use a thick sock. Some clients elect not to use socks. The nurse, client, and prosthetist will decide if this is workable.

PELVIC BELTS

Clients who have above-the-knee amputations often wear a prosthesis attached to a pelvic belt (Figure 10-13). Do not remove the leather straps that connect the prosthesis to the belt unless the physical therapist directs you to do so. The straps are marked to indicate where they are to meet with the buckles. Likewise, any padding for the pelvic belt must be kept in position. There is a joint that bends for sitting. If it becomes difficult for your client to sit while wearing the prosthesis, add a drop of 3-in-1 oil to the joint. Wipe the joint and the leather straps with a slightly damp cloth to keep them clean.

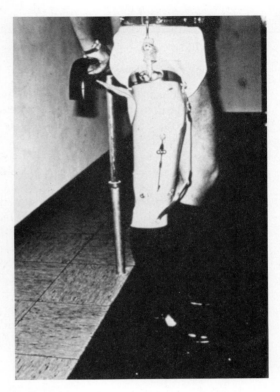

Figure 10-13. *A pelvic belt assists a client with an above-the-knee amputation to keep his prosthesis in place.*
Photo courtesy of Otto Bock Orthopedic Industry Inc., U.S.A.

CLOTHING AND SHOES

Most people can wear their own clothing after an amputation. Some alterations may be necessary if they have lost weight. Other alterations are made to make it easier to use the bathroom or for ease in dressing. For example, men who wear suspenders can more easily pull up their slacks or pants when dressing or toileting. Suspenders not only pull up the pants, but keep them in place while the zipper and button are closed. Loosely fitted clothes such as jogging sweatsuits are comfortable, warm, and easy to put on over a bandaged part. However, they may be difficult to pull on with one hand while trying to balance in the bathroom and have no fly front for the men.

Shoes are very important for safe transfers or ambulation. This is important regardless of the level of amputation or the condition of the other leg. Many clients like to slip on loafers rather than shoes with ties for ease in dressing. Loafers must be firmly constructed and in good condition. Slip-on scuffs, shoes with heels (even small 2–3 inch heels), or shoes that do not fit (even though they may have fit prior to the amputation) are not safe for your client. Poorly fitted shoes can cause a fall.

*H*ARNESSES

A person with an upper limb amputation that involves the arm may also have a harness for the prosthesis (Figure 10-14). The harness does not need the nightly care required by prosthetic socks. It is laundered at least every other week using warm water and mild detergent. Be sure the harness has permanent markings to show where it is reattached to the prosthesis and fasteners. It has to be put back together again after laundering. If your client has a hand prosthesis, do not clean or disassemble it unless directed. Do not remove the glove from a hand prosthesis without exact directions from the nurse supervisor or the occupational therapist. Figure 10-15 shows a myoelectric elbow and hand system suitable for some clients.

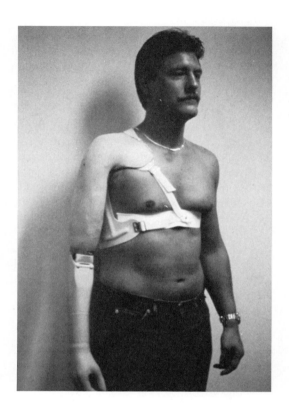

Figure 10-14.   *Clients who have upper limb amputations may wear a chest/shoulder harness to stabilize the prosthesis for smoother fit and functioning.*
   Photo courtesy of Otto Bock Orthopedic Industry Inc., U.S.A.

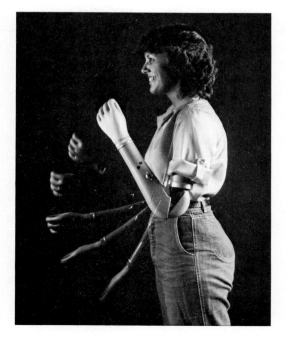

Figure 10-15.   *The "Utah arm" is a myoelectric elbow and hand system developed to enable clients with above and below elbow amputations to function independently, and with high levels of skill, in their daily activities and work. The Utah myoelectric arm features proportional control.*
   Photos courtesy of Motion Control, division of 10 MED. Inc., Salt Lake City, Utah.

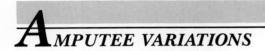

SPECIAL CONSIDERATIONS FOLLOWING AMPUTATIONS

Remember that many persons with amputations are at risk for other problems leading to amputations. You have an important role in preventing further problems. Some ways to do this are to:

—be sure of excellent skin care including footcare;
—follow your client's diet plan;
—maintain exercises and mobility;
—avoid pressure, bruises, and cuts;
—keep prosthetic socks clean;
—check for a safe environment; and
—watch your client's attitude.

AMPUTEE VARIATIONS

Because of improvements in surgery and medical care, many clients with more than one disability are able to survive and return home. For example, the amputation may be one disability while a paralysis on one side of the body may be another. Multiple disabilities are discussed briefly in this section.

AMPUTATION AND HEMIPLEGIA/ HEMIPARESIS

In home care, you may expect to care for an older client who has had an amputation because of diabetes and who then has a hemiplegia following a stroke. If the client has been active and wearing a prosthesis for several years, he is often independent in most of his care. However, when this person has **hemiplegia** or **hemiparesis** following a stroke, he will have further difficulties.

The stroke may affect the side opposite the amputation. If so, he may have difficulty with self-care and balance. If the stroke affects the same side as the amputation, he will have a great deal of difficulty using his prosthesis. For many persons, the prosthesis will have to be refitted and adjusted. The limb may become smaller due to weakness and loss of muscle tone. The person who has an *above-the-knee prosthesis* may now need a lock on the knee so that he can balance and bear weight.

When you care for a client with a prosthesis who has recently had a stroke, you must first focus on him as a client with a stroke. The care for the amputation will follow after the stroke care is established. For example, a person may have a *right* leg amputation, but be paralyzed on the *left* side of his body from a stroke. This person may have to sit to transfer from one place to another. Likewise, dressing, grooming, and hygiene will be conducted as for a person with *left*-sided weakness, the stroke-related weakness.

AMPUTATION AND FRACTURED HIP

The person with an amputation who falls and fractures a hip usually fractures the hip on the amputated side. The pain and discomfort of the hip fracture often deters him from using his prosthesis. Pain may cause the client to resist exercises that maintain his **range of motion.** He may insist on positioning that is not in his best long-term interest. Follow the Do's and Don't's listed earlier in this chapter. Your nurse supervisor and therapist will assist you with proper positioning for this client so that he can regain his abilities to transfer, dress, and bathe.

Additionally, read about assistive devices in Chapter 6 for ideas about special assistive devices. For example, long-handled brushes can assist the person to wash his back and legs while he sits on a tub bench. Special "reachers" will assist him to pull on socks and pants if he has difficulty bending. The client, nurse supervisor, therapist, and the client's family may discover other helpful devices. Many of them can be ordered from catalogs or purchased in prosthetic shops.

CHAPTER 11

Care of Clients who have Chronic Conditions

*O*BJECTIVES:

When you have studied this chapter you will be able to:

1. Define the terms relating to chronic conditions.
2. Discuss the different types of chronic conditions.
3. Identify basic principles of care for common arthritic and other chronic conditions.
4. Know specific actions and precautions for care of the client with an arthritic or other common chronic condition.
5. Perform basic actions that promote comfort and pain control.
6. Assist the client with self-care, maintaining mobility and exercises, as directed.
7. Support the client's interests and help promote positive mental attitudes.

*O*VERVIEW

This chapter describes the care of persons who have chronic conditions. Its sections focus on selected common chronic conditions, arthritic conditions, progressive neuromuscular conditions, and chronic conditions that become terminal, during which clients require increasing amounts of assistance.

A condition is **chronic** when it lasts a long time (three months or longer). Many chronic conditions are not curable, despite today's medical advances. They often lead to disabilities or impairments, and also aggravate other health problems. Chronic conditions frequently occur together, with one condition contributing to the problems of another. For example, persons who have cardiac conditions often develop respiratory difficulties. Persons who have diabetes may develop circulatory problems that can lead to amputations. Clients who have chronic conditions need excellent **care** to prevent additional disabilities and complications and to maintain their health.

This chapter explains how to assist clients who require restorative and rehabilitative care while they are living at home. They may have disabilities or impairments from chronic conditions.

Part I discusses long-term care for persons with selected chronic conditions and diseases, including:

—cardiac conditions,
—respiratory diseases,
—chronic pain,
—Alzheimer's disease, and
—diabetes mellitus.

Part II discusses long-term care for clients who have arthritic conditions and diseases, including:

—arthritis,
—rheumatoid arthritis,
—osteoarthritis,

—gout, and
—lupus erythematosus.

Part III discusses care for clients who have progressive neuromuscular diseases, including:

—Parkinson's disease and
—multiple sclerosis.

Part IV discusses care for clients who have terminal illnesses, including:

—Hospice as a concept for terminal care,
—ALS, and
—AIDS.

PART *I*
Selected Chronic Conditions

*C*ARE OF THE CLIENT WHO HAS A CARDIAC CONDITION

This section discusses care of clients who have *chronic cardiac conditions*. Heart disease continues to be the number one cause of death in our society. Many people require follow-up care after they survive heart attacks or other heart failures and receive cardiac rehabilitation. Other persons have chronic heart conditions and need assistance with activities of their daily living.

This chapter focuses on how you can assist your client to return to an as active and independent life as possible. Many clients who have chronic cardiac conditions can manage to live at home if they have some help and supervision of their cardiac program. Other clients require only temporary assistance un-

til they are better able to care for themselves or regain their strength. Clients often have other chronic conditions or disabilities in addition to a cardiac condition, especially diabetes mellitus and respiratory conditions.

FUNCTIONS OF THE HEALTHY CIRCULATORY SYSTEM

The heart is the major organ in the circulatory system. The heart is located in the chest between the lungs and behind the sternum and rib cage (Figure 11-1). It is a muscle with four separate sections or chambers. There

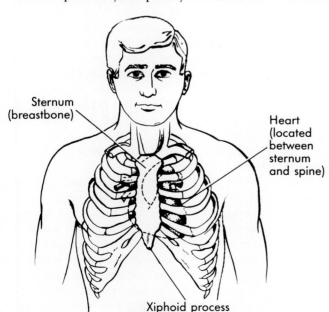

Sternum (breastbone)

Heart (located between sternum and spine)

Xiphoid process (tip of the sternum)

Figure 11-1. *The heart is located in the chest cavity between the lungs. It is behind the xiphoid process of the sternum and the ribcage.*

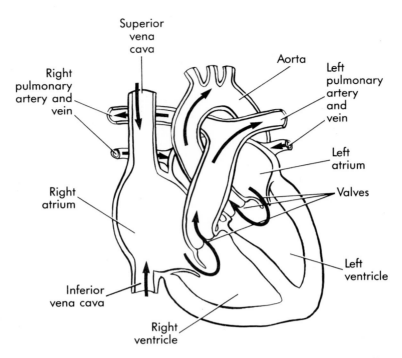

Figure 11-2.   *The heart is separated into four chambers that have valves to control the filling and emptying of the chambers. Major blood vessels carry blood into and out of the heart and throughout the body.*

are two upper chambers, the right atrium and the left atrium (or auricle), and two lower chambers, the right ventricle and the left ventricle. The major blood vessels of the body carry the blood flow into and out of the heart. These are the aorta, the superior vena cava, inferior vena cava, and the pulmonary artery (Figure 11-2).

One-way valves and walls (septae) separate the heart chambers from one another and from the major blood vessels. This is important for controlling the direction and amount of blood flowing through the heart and for preventing overflow or backup of blood. The heart can fill and empty each chamber separately and direct the blood into the proper blood vessel.

Two kinds of blood circulation are useful to understand: the circulation to the lungs and the circulation between the body and the heart. Both systems rely on arteries and veins. **Arteries** are blood vessels that contain **oxygenated blood.** They **leave** the heart to carry oxygen to the tissues of the body. **Veins** are blood vessels containing blood **without oxygen,** but with carbon dioxide. Venous blood has given up its oxygen to the body and is being carried **back to** the heart. The circu-

lation between the body and the heart (Figure 11-3) relies mainly on sending out oxygen-carrying blood and receiving blood that requires more oxygen from the tissues.

The heart moves blood from one chamber to another, opening and closing valves and sending blood to the lungs in a precise cycle. The sounds and activities of the heart movements and valve activities produce the heartbeat. We can count the number of beats, note how regularly the beats occur, note whether they are similar in strength, and describe the type of beat when we take a pulse. The changes in pressure that occur during the filling and emptying of the heart chambers during the heart circulation cycle make the systole and diastole sounds heard when taking a blood pressure.

The heart and lung circulation sends the venous blood to the lungs where the carbon dioxide is removed and the blood is resupplied with oxygen. The blood returns to the heart for distribution to the body. The exchange of the oxygen is discussed with the respiratory system in the next section of this chapter. (The pulmonary vein carries oxygenated blood, but is a vein because it goes back to the heart; the pulmonary artery car-

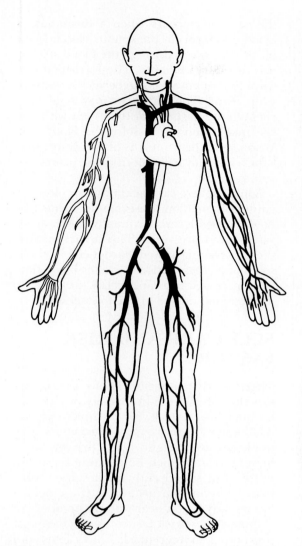

Figure 11-3. *The circulation between the body and the heart carries oxygenated blood to the body tissues and brings oxygenated blood back to the heart.*

ries unoxygenated blood, but is an artery because it leaves the heart.)

CARDIAC AND CARDIAC-RELATED CONDITIONS

Your client may have one of the cardiac or cardic-related conditions on the following list. The physician and nurse supervisor will instruct you about specific measures for each client. The section that follows these descriptions provides general information to help you assist your clients.

Hypertension or high blood pressure is the increased pressure of the blood against the arterial blood vessel walls as the blood passes through the arteries. The blood pressure must regularly rise to greater than 160 systolic and greater than 90 diastolic to be considered hypertension. However, many clients with lower blood pressure readings may be on precautions or at risk for developing hypertension. (Read about autonomic dysreflexia and spinal cord injury in Chapter 9.) Notify your nurse supervisor if your client has these signs or symptoms indicating that his blood pressure may be elevated:

—an increase in his blood pressure reading;
—dizziness, weakness, or fainting;
—headache;
—flushed face;
—heavy or difficult breathing;
—disorientation or confusion;
—nosebleeds; or
—clammy, sweating skin.

Congestive heart disease occurs when some of the blood that flows into the heart from the veins becomes congested in the heart instead of returning through the arteries to the body. Notify your nurse supervisor if your client has any of these signs or symptoms of congestive heart disease:

—chest pain;
—difficulty with breathing;
—audible breathing noises from his chest;
—swelling in his hands, feet, legs, or parts of his face;
—weakness, dizziness, restlessness; or
—is disoriented or confused.

Arteriosclerosis (hardening of the arteries)

Atherosclerotic Cardiovascular Heart Disease (ASHD or clogged arteries)

Post Myocardial Infarction (Post-MI). This term refers to clients who need care after the heart attack.

Rheumatic Fever. A client may have various chronic conditions as a result of having had rheumatic fever. These are secondary to the acute rheumatic fever and often affect the heart. Frequently clients will require rest and prevention of infections.

Angina Pectoris. A client who has angina complains of heart or chest pain. The pain arises from a reduced blood supply to the heart. Angina pain affects particular parts of

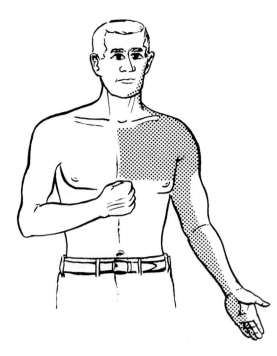

Figure 11-4. *Pain associated with angina pectoris follows a pattern across the person's chest and down this arm as illustrated by the shaded areas.*

the body and may be relieved by rest and medication. Figure 11-4 illustrates the usual path of angina pain in the body.

Peripheral Vascular Diseases. There are several types of diseases related to poor circulation, especially the circulation of the legs and feet. These conditions are related to heart diseases and may cause complications for clients who have diabetes mellitus.

Venous Conditions are often associated with reduced elasticity of the venous walls in older clients, especially if they have cardiac conditions with reduced venous return to the heart. They may also be one of the negative results of immobility and reduced exercise of the lower extremities. Standing for long times, especially in one place, may aggravate venous conditions. A client's therapy may include wearing elastic support hose and elevating his legs while sitting.

—**Varicose Veins.** Enlarged, distended, and swollen veins that most often occur in a client's legs are called varicose. The veins become enlarged when venous blood is not sufficiently returned to the heart. The blood collects in the veins, causing outpouching of the venous walls.

—**Thrombophlebitis** is an inflammation in the vein that occurs when a **thrombus** or blood clot forms in the venous blood. If the blood clot travels through the blood stream, it is called an **embolus.** The formation of a thrombus or embolus can be very serious for your client. The physician may send your client to the hospital for treatment with special medications to dissolve the blood clot. When your client returns home, your nurse supervisor may have specific instructions for you to follow.

Some of these cardiac conditions often occur in combination. For example, clients who have arteriosclerosis frequently also have elevated blood pressures. This occurs because the client has narrowed, hardened blood vessels that increase resistance to the blood flow. This increased resistance raises the pressure of the blood on the arterial vessel walls.

SELF-CARE AND RISK FACTORS

There are certain factors known as **risk factors** that predict the probability of a person having a heart attack. For example, a person is at higher risk of having a heart attack if he smokes, is overweight, is inactive, or eats a high fat or salty diet. Eliminating these risk factors can significantly reduce his probability of having a heart attack. If the person has already had a heart attack, he needs to eliminate these risk factors as one means of preventing another attack. Your clients with cardiac conditions need care to improve their health and to prevent additional problems. Although cardiac diseases differ, the basic care goals for cardiac clients center around reducing risk factors and preventing complications or further disability. Measures to reduce risk may include:

—a controlled diet;
—an exercise program;
—rest and relaxation;
—medications;
—technological assistance or devices;
—a stress reduction plan;
—education of the client, family, and caregivers (you); and
—participation in support or peer groups.

1. *Controlled diet.* A **controlled diet,** usually low in fat, cholesterol, and salt, is essential. Depending on his general nutritional status, he may have a reduced calorie diet to assist him with weight loss. You may work with the client, family, nurse supervisor, and dietitian to develop weekly meal plan guides. The menus will take into account the client's food likes and dislikes. If you do the food shopping for your client, use the weekly advertisements and sales to help stay within the family food budget and meet the dietary restrictions. Carefully follow the diet prescribed by the physician for your client. The diet will be supervised by the nurse supervisor or the dietitian.

The dietary program may require that you prepare foods a certain way, restrict your client's fluid intake, and weigh or measure the amounts of food and liquid he consumes. You may also be asked to weigh the client and to measure the amount of urinary output he produces each day.

Remember that a cardiac client requires rest; eating and digesting a large meal are stressful for the heart. These clients usually prefer to eat light meals 4–5 times a day, rather than 3 large, heavy meals. This spreads the meal activity over the day and reduces the load on the heart.

2. *Exercise Program.* The nurse supervisor will direct you about your client's individual **exercise and progressive activity programs.** You may be given specific exercises to assist your client to perform or he may have his own list of the exercises he is to do. The level of exercise will vary greatly from one client to another. Remind your client to breathe during exercise and to exhale during the more strenuous parts of an activity. For example, exhaling when bending over is easier than inhaling. It makes breathing easier. If your client has any of the symptoms listed below, notify the nurse supervisor or call the rescue squad, emergency medical technicians, or mobile medical team.

Get assistance if your client complains of any of the following:

—chest pains—chest pains with tightness across the chest or between the shoulder blades or sudden pain in the left shoulder that spreads or radiates down the arm;
—difficulty breathing or getting a breath;

—heart palpitations (fast, irregular beats);
—racing pulse or irregular heartbeats;
—dizziness with faint sensations;
—fainting;
—elevated or lowered blood pressure;
—swelling in his hands or feet or "bloating";
—sweating and pallor with cool clammy skin; or
—excessive anxiety or fearfulness.

3. *Rest.* Your client may have set times of the day to **rest** or he may have to take frequent rest breaks, especially after activities such as exercise or meals. He may be more comfortable with several pillows, especially if he is short of breath. As a rule, he should not rest with his feet elevated higher than his head.

If a client has *angina,* he may rest to reduce the pain. Rest does not relieve the pain of a heart attack. The amount of rest your client requires will change as his exercise program is gradually built up or his level of tolerance is increased. Unless instructed otherwise by the nurse supervisor, walk slowly with your client, allowing him to sit for as many activities as possible. Think about conserving his energy.

Keep your client comfortable. Little things may make a difference in his sense of well-being. For example, regulate the temperature so that he is not chilled and place things where he can reach them to help himself.

4. *Medications.* Although you will *not* be giving your client **medications,** you should be aware that he may require your assistance in his own self-administration of medications prescribed by the physician. You may:

—Remind your client of his medication.
—Bring him water or other fluids, if directed, to take the medication.
—Assist with opening a container if he is unable (childproof caps are difficult for many persons to open).
—Contact the nurse supervisor if you or your client have any questions.

Digoxin (also labeled Lanoxin) is a heart medication taken by many clients who have cardiac conditions. This medication stimulates a strong and regular heartbeat. If the client's pulse is too slow, he will delay taking his digoxin. You may need to remind him or assist him in taking his pulse before his medication.

A client who has angina pain may have nitroglycerin tablets to place under his tongue when he has pain. He will have been instructed to take pills two minutes apart. Follow your nurse supervisor's instructions. Generally, if your client has taken 3 tablets and continues to have angina pain, he should be seen by his physician or taken to the emergency room.

If your client has medication to reduce fluid retention ("water pills," or diuretics) he will have to go to the bathroom more often. You may be asked to measure and record his intake and output, and report changes to your nurse supervisor. The nurse supervisor will give you specific instructions regarding potential side effects to look for and report.

Some clients use a partitioned container, a divided box, or a simple egg carton to store their medications. They count out their medications, labeled by name and by each day of the week, into each compartment. The container may be further labeled and divided into the times each day when each medication should be taken. This method assists a client to know whether or not he has taken his medications.

Some medications are now administered through patches worn on the skin behind a person's ear, or on his chest, back, or upper arms. *The medication is absorbed through the skin.* Generally the patches are applied each morning; some are changed every three days. The places on the skin, or sites, are rotated in a pattern so no site is used more than once in a week. Sites for placing patches include the right and left sides of the chest, the right and left shoulder blade (scapulae) areas, and the arms.

You may have to assist your client with the patches.

— Wear gloves. Do not get the patches on your skin. If you do, wash your skin thoroughly with soap and water. The medication enters the body through the skin and may enter your body.
— Rotate sites as directed by the nurse supervisor.
— Remove and discard the old patch.
— Wash the client's skin with soap and water.
— Dry the site thoroughly.

— Assist the client to apply the new patch to the next designated site.
— Record the activity and the site used as directed by the nurse supervisor.

5. *Technology.* An electronic **cardiac pacemaker** is technological equipment that is surgically implanted under a client's skin on his chest wall (Figure 11-5). A client who has an irregular heartbeat or unpredictable heart rate may wear a cardiac pacemaker. The pacemaker sends a controlled electrical stimulation, which specifically initiates heartbeats to a heart node. The most common type of pacemaker works by stimulating the heart node to beat regularly when the client's heart does not beat on its own at a set rate. A less common pacemaker version stimulates the heart to continually beat at a set rate of 60–70 beats per minute.

If your client has a **cardiac pacemaker,** your nurse supervisor will direct you about any specific instructions for your client's care. Some examples are:

— Some pacemakers may be disrupted if worn within 10–12 feet of operating microwave ovens.
— Electrical appliances, including microwave ovens, and power tools may interfere with the pacemaker's operation.
— Report to your nurse supervisor if there are:
  — any of the signs of heart attack,
  — any changes in the color of the skin around the pacemaker site,
  — any pain or swelling in the pacemaker site, or
  — any changes in your client:
    • anxiety or concern about the pacemaker,
    • a pulse rate below the pacemaker rate, or
    • hiccoughs that could result from misplaced electrical stimulations from the pacemaker if it is dislodged or the wires are displaced.

Your client may have an **emergency response unit,** such as a Lifeline Unit, in his home. An emergency response unit is a means by which a person who is alone can contact and summon help in the event of becoming ill, injured, or having another type of emergency. The client carries or wears a transmitter or signaling device, usually on a

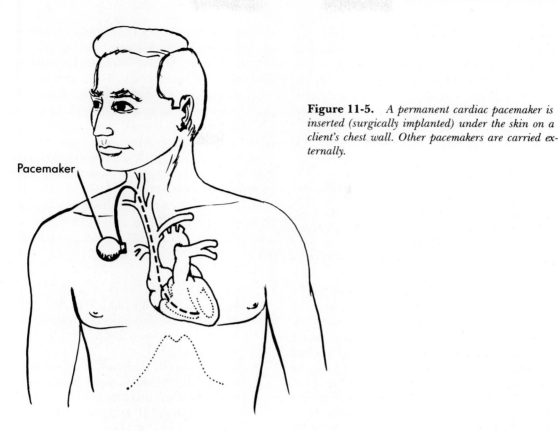

Pacemaker

Figure 11-5. *A permanent cardiac pacemaker is inserted (surgically implanted) under the skin on a client's chest wall. Other pacemakers are carried externally.*

necklace-style cord around his neck. When he presses the device, a signal is sent to a telephone-activated machine in his home. The telephone machine places calls to several persons who have agreed to be responders to his call for assistance.

When a responder answers the call and does not reach the client, he will either come to the client's home or call the emergency medical team or rescue squad that serves the client's area. If none of the responders are available to answer the call or if the signal is sent repeatedly, the telephone device will dial the emergency medical group for the client's area. If your client has a response unit, be sure that he wears or carries his signal device and knows how to use it. You should also know how the unit works, who the responders are, and how to reach them by telephone.

6. *Stress Reduction.* **Personal attitudes** affect how people react to things in their life and what goes on around them. The client who is told that he must **reduce his stress** because of his cardiac condition may have to change his attitudes. For example, the client who has a temper will have to learn ways to handle his anger so that it does not cause him to become stressed and affect his heart. Use slow, smooth movements when you work with him because rushing about may increase his anxiety and stress. He may also have to change his schedule, eliminate alcohol, and reduce his workload.

Some stresses in life cannot be changed or eliminated. Your client will be working to try to change the ways in which he responds to those stresses. The entire family should be involved in working on stress reduction. Few family stresses affect only one family member; there are usually several members involved in the stressful situation. The nurse supervisor may bring a social service worker, a psychologist, or a nurse family therapist (psychotherapist) into the home to work with your client and his family.

7. *Client-centered and Family Education.* Your client and his family will receive a great deal of **teaching and information** about his condition before he comes home from the

hospital or rehabilitation center. You and your client will benefit if you also read and become familiar with the patient education materials. This will help you understand the client's condition and care. Keep your nurse supervisor informed about new or repeated questions your client may ask.

8. *Support Groups.* Your client may ask other questions that are to be answered only by the nurse supervisor. For example, a client who has cardiac problems frequently be-

comes concerned about, and asks questions about, his sexuality. He may also become increasingly depressed or anxious because he fears another heart attack. The nurse supervisor may decide to work with your client and his family in a **support group** setting. A group consists of clients and families who have similar situations and experiences. Membership in a group allows clients and families to have opportunities to help and support one another.

CHRONIC RESPIRATORY PROBLEMS

In order to learn about respiratory problems, it is first necessary to understand how the healthy respiratory system functions. The respiratory system, which is also called the pulmonary system, has four major activities:

1. breathing by inhaling and exhaling air;
2. exchanging oxygen and carbon dioxide, using the respiratory and circulatory systems;
3. moving oxygen to, and carbon dioxide from, the body tissues through the bloodsteam; and
4. coordinating and regulating respiratory activities through the central nervous system.

The functioning respiratory system includes:

- Air routes, or pathways, which begin with passage of air through the nose and nasal passages and continue through the back of the throat and into the trachea. The trachea transports air to and from the area where it forks into a right and a left bronchial tube (Figure 11-6).
- Each main bronchial tube gradually branches into a network of air tubes. These air tubes continue to become smaller and finer tubes called bronchioles. Finally, they become tiny air sacs or alveoli that reach and extend into all parts of the lungs (Figure 11-6).
- The circulatory system of veins and arteries extends into the lungs, where it also branches and extends out into small, fine vessels or pulmonary capil-

laries. The pulmonary capillaries and alveoli mingle (Figure 11-7) so that these tiny air alveoli and blood capillaries can perform the essential functions for oxygen exchange.

- Blood from the body containing carbon dioxide is returned to the heart through the veins. The body has used the oxygen from this blood so it is brought back to the lungs. The carbon dioxide is removed from the venous blood and exhaled out of the lungs. The blood is given new oxygen when the alveoli and capillaries exchange carbon dioxide and oxygen. The newly oxygenated blood is transported back to the heart where it is sent through the arteries throughout the body.
- The right and left lungs function in the same manner, but each lung has its own blood supply, bronchial network, and nerve system. The right lung is separated into three lobes and the left lung has two lobes. The lungs are placed within protective cavities called pleural cavities, which are located on either side of the heart, major blood vessels, esophagus, and the lower trachea. The pleural cavities protect the lungs from rubbing directly against the chest wall and ribs and provide a lubricating fluid around the lungs as they expand and contract during breathing.
- Nerves activate respiration. Respiratory activities are under the control of the central nervous system. Respiratory centers in the brain stimulate the nerves for respiration, coordinate respiratory

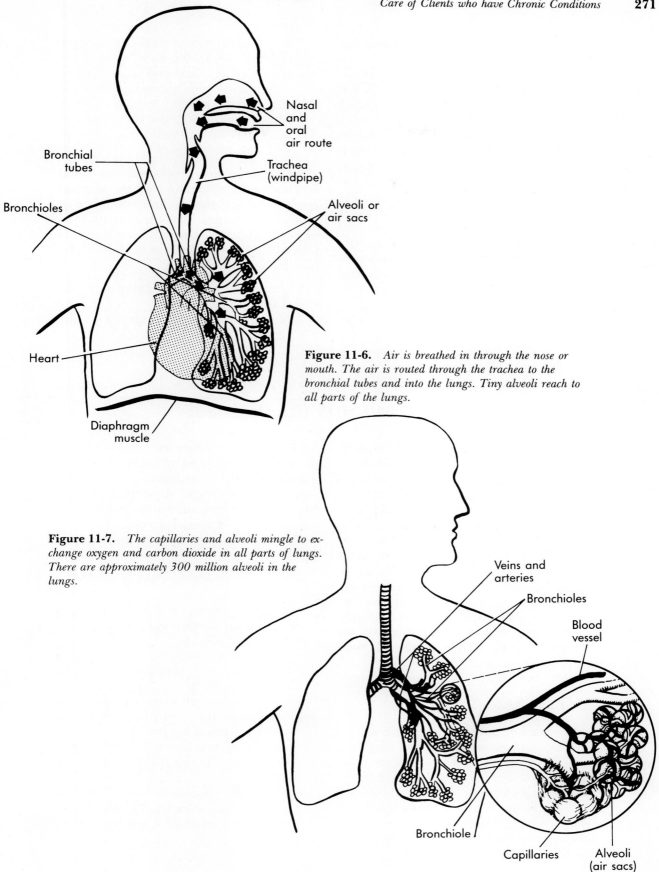

Figure 11-6. *Air is breathed in through the nose or mouth. The air is routed through the trachea to the bronchial tubes and into the lungs. Tiny alveoli reach to all parts of the lungs.*

Figure 11-7. *The capillaries and alveoli mingle to exchange oxygen and carbon dioxide in all parts of lungs. There are approximately 300 million alveoli in the lungs.*

activities, and regulate oxygen exchange with the bloodstream.

- Certain muscles are accessories to respiration. The diaphragm is the most important muscle for respiration. It begins each inspiration when stimulated by its nerve. When it is stimulated it is drawn downward. This changes the pressure in the thoracic cavity (producing a negative pressure), causing outside air to move into the lungs. Once oxygen exchange has occurred, the elastic tissues of the lungs exhale the carbon dioxide-laden air. The pressure changes and the diaphragm rises, helping to force air out of the lungs. The diaphragm muscle is located at the lower border of the thoracic cavity just below the ribs.
- Other muscles may assist with breathing, especially when there are difficulties. The abdominal muscles may assist in raising or lowering the diaphragm, and muscles in the back, around the ribs, the chest, face, and lips may all be used to assist with breathing. When the respiratory system cannot receive proper stimulation, the client may require mechanical ventilation to assist him with breathing.

When there are breakdowns or interferences in the respiratory system, your client may develop chronic lung conditions or pulmonary diseases. These may result from or occur in addition to other health problems. There are two groups of chronic pulmonary diseases:

1) Chronic obstructive pulmonary diseases or COPD, and
2) Chronic restrictive pulmonary diseases.

CHRONIC OBSTRUCTIVE PULMONARY DISEASES

Chronic obstructive pulmonary diseases are the second greatest cause of disabilities in our society. These diseases are mainly caused from smoking or recurring respiratory infections. Workers in certain occupations have developed COPD from breathing toxic substances while on the job. Others have been exposed to polluted air and a few have hereditary forms of these diseases. COPD is aggravated by stress for many people. A client who has an *obstructive* lung disease has resistance to the air *flowing out* of his lungs and difficulty *exhaling*. **Emphysema** is the most common COPD. Other COPDs are **chronic bronchitis** and **asthma**.

EMPHYSEMA

Emphysema affects the tissues and walls of the lungs. The **alveoli** in the lungs are damaged and enlarged, and the tubular bronchioles are clogged by mucus. The lung tissues lose the ability to expand and contract. They begin to "trap air" and cannot efficiently exchange oxygen and carbon dioxide during breathing (Figure 11-8). Clients who have emphysema often have an anterior to posterior enlargement of their chest that gives it a rounded, barrel-like shape. This enlarged "barrel chest" develops as the air-heavy lungs become inflated with trapped air and the chest becomes enlarged.

The client who has emphysema may have signs of:

—difficulty breathing, especially exhaling air;
—fatigue, weakness and low endurance;
—poor appetite and weight loss;
—a "barrel chest";
—"slouched or hunched over" posture as he leans forward attempting to breathe more successfully;
—cough, noisy chest sounds, possibly mucous cough upon rising in the morning;
—physical signs of inadequate oxygen exchange, such as clubbed fingers, dusky skin color, or bluish lips and fingernails; or
—a breathing pattern in which there are short breaths in and extra long breaths out as he tries to push the trapped air out.

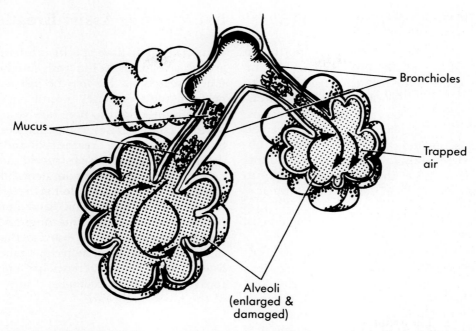

Figure 11-8. *Emphysema causes the alveoli to enlarge and lose elasticity. Air becomes "trapped" in all parts of the lungs. Mucus clogs the bronchiole air routes, and the client cannot fully exhale air.*

Assisting the Client who has Emphysema

- Encourage him to drink plenty of water to help his body thin out the mucus (unless fluid intake is restricted for other reasons).
- Provide a nourishing diet, as instructed. Serve foods that he can manage to eat with his lowered energy level and difficulty breathing. Generally, increased protein and fluids and decreased fat are ordered. Several smaller meals of easily chewed foods may be less tiring for your client to eat.
- Keep his environment clean, free from dust, aerosol sprays, fumes, or other irritants and pollutants.
- Dispose of secretions and used tissues, using universal precautions and infection control procedures.
- Assist him with good oral hygiene.
- Help to prevent respiratory infections as directed by the nurse supervisor or respiratory therapist.

- Assist him with exercises or procedures to help him drain or remove secretions and mucus, under the supervision of your nurse supervisor or respiratory therapist.
- Encourage the use of relaxation exercises if they are ordered.
- Reduce or eliminate things that cause him stress.
- Remind him to use prescription medications, nebulizers, respiratory devices, or other aids for respiration.
- Reduce his exposure to extremely cold air, which may irritate his lungs and start him coughing. Use a muffler or scarf to cover his nose and mouth if he must go out in cold weather.
- Notify the nurse supervisor if his symptoms worsen or he becomes anxious or concerned.

CHRONIC BRONCHITIS

Chronic bronchitis is an inflammation of the bronchial tree of the lungs. Changes in the cell makeup of the bronchial tissues lead to increased secretions of mucus in the bronchial tree. Bacteria grow in the secretions. This leads to infections, damaged or scarred bronchial tissues and, eventually, to obstructed breathing. The excessive amounts of mucus cause the client to cough up sputum, especially in the morning after arising. Follow universal infection control precautions when collecting or handling mucus, sputum, or other respiratory secretions.

The mucus also causes coughing and congestion in the bronchial tree. Drinking water helps thin mucus secretions. An immobile client has a greater risk for excess mucus build-up in his lungs. The thick mucus can collect in one area of a lung. The lung may become inflamed or infected with bacteria or viruses, causing pneumonia.

A client who coughs up blood may have a chronic infection or a chronic lung disease such as bronchiectasis. The long-term condition produces scarring of the lung tissues. Report any sort of bloody sputum or blood-tinged mucus to the nurse supervisor.

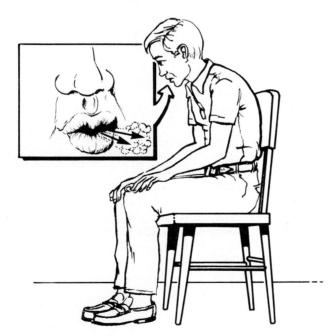

Figure 11-9. *"Pursed lip" breathing assists the client to exhale more effectively. He exhales through his "pursed" lips.*

Exercises to Assist Breathing

Your client may have specific exercises that are designed to assist him with coughing up mucus secretions. He may be instructed to perform these exercises several times each day. It is important to note how your client performs the exercises. If the exercises are to be effective, he must breathe fully and cough deeply. Because of his obstructed and congested respiratory condition, he will have to consciously think about doing this. He will tend to take rapid, "shallow," and inefficient breaths instead of filling his lungs and moving the secretions. Several exercises that assist in deep breathing and help expel mucus are listed below. These exercises are only performed under the direction and supervision of the nurse supervisor.

"Pursed"-Lip Breathing Exercises

1) Ask your client to become as relaxed as possible. If he has been instructed to do certain relaxation techniques, he may use these (Figure 11-9). He should allow his neck, arms, and shoulders to loosen and droop. Ask him to:
2) Lean slightly forward and slowly breathe in.
3) "Purse" his lips as if he were to whistle.
4) Blow air out slowly and evenly to exhale.
5) Relax and repeat until he feels he is getting his breath.
6) Stop and rest if he becomes dizzy.

Try this yourself and you will see why this helps him exhale.

Diaphragm-Strengthening Exercise

The diaphragm is a muscle that assists in breathing. When it is strengthened, it can strengthen your respiration. Do not have your client perform this exercise unless instructed and supervised by the nurse supervisor, physical therapist, or respiratory therapist. They will assure that the exercise is appropriate for the client and that the client's diaphragm is moving properly during the exercise.

Ask your client to:

1) Relax, especially his shoulders, arms, and neck. Ask him to:
   - Sit in a chair with his arms loose at his sides.
   - Tighten his muscles by clenching his hands into fists, shrugging his shoulders, clenching his jaw, and flexing his arm muscles.
   - Continue to breathe in and out while holding the tightened muscles for 2–3 seconds. Relax completely.
   - Repeat the same tightening motions using his feet, legs, and buttocks. Hold the tightening for 2–3 seconds, then relax completely. Try to feel relaxed, loose, and limp.

2) Place both his hands on his abdomen in a resting position, as shown by the supervisor.
3) Breathe in through his nose, keeping his mouth closed.
4) Let his abdomen extend out completely. This should let him feel his abdomen move out under his hands. (Figure 11-10).
5) Breathe out, using pursed-lip breathing techniques.
6) Stop if he feels dizzy.

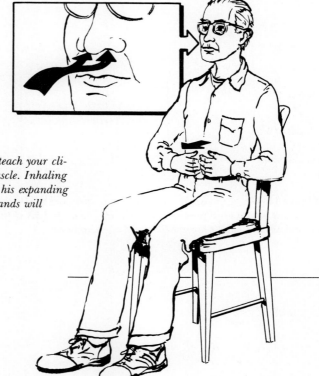

Figure 11-10. *The nurse supervisor may teach your client exercises to strengthen his diaphragm muscle. Inhaling air should cause his hands to move out with his expanding abdomen. As he exhales, his abdomen and hands will move in again.*

Chest-Strengthening Exercise

Do not have your client perform this exercise unless instructed and supervised by the nurse supervisor, physical therapist, or respiratory therapist. They will assure that your client is doing the exercise properly. Stronger chest muscles will assist your client to breathe more efficiently (Figure 11-11).

The nurse supervisor may instruct your client about ways to "cough up" mucus. It is important for your client to clear his lungs of mucus. To do this he will have to cough (Figure 11-12). Swallowing mucus may cause him to be nauseous. The nurse supervisor or respiratory therapist may instruct your client and his family in exercises for postural drainage of mucus or in techniques for an assisted cough.

If he has coughing "spells" that make it difficult for him to stop coughing, inform the nurse supervisor. She can direct you and your client in specific ways to assist him to

Have your client:

1) Stand up to do this exercise for best results.
2) Place his hands on either side of his chest, just at the lower edge. Your supervisor will show you exactly where he is to place his hands.
3) Breathe in through his nose, slowly and smoothly.
4) Allow his lower chest to expand so that he feels his lower chest moving out under his hands.
5) Breathe out, using pursed-lip breathing techniques.
6) Stop if he feels dizzy.

control his coughing and to expel mucus. Try to keep him relaxed during a coughing episode. Have him cover his mouth with a tissue to prevent sprays of droplets or mucus. Use

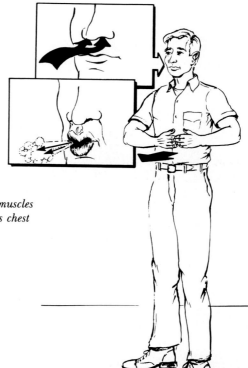

Figure 11-11. *Exercises to strengthen your client's chest muscles will assist him to breathe more efficiently. He should feel his chest expand when inhaling air and relax when exhaling air.*

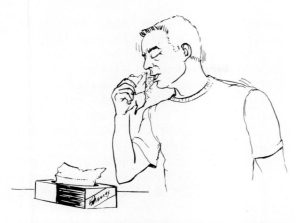

Figure 11-12. *Deep coughing exercises can clear a client's airways of a great deal of mucous. But this takes energy and effort. Assist your client to use procedures as directed by the nurse supervisor.*

proper infection control measures to dispose to wastes.

ASTHMA

Asthma is a disease that causes muscle spasms in the bronchial tubes. These spasms cause the bronchial tubes to collapse or close down, or they may swell the lining of the bronchial tubes. When either of these hap-

pens, air is restricted so it cannot pass through the bronchial tubes or bronchiole air routes (Figure 11-13). Asthma may also occur as an allergic reaction to something the client is sensitive to in the environment.

He should avoid eating foods or handling materials to which he may be allergic. Stress, anxiety, upsetting situations, or excessive exertion may trigger asthmatic reactions. The person having an asthma attack may complain of tightness or closeness in his chest or have difficulty breathing; often there are audible wheezing sounds. A person who is having an asthma reaction can be very frightened. An asthmatic reaction can be life-threatening. Call the rescue squad and your nurse supervisor if your client has difficult breathing during an asthma attack or if your client asks you to call for assistance.

Equipment use

Your client may have equipment such as a suction machine, intermittent positive pressure machine, or other respiratory aids. Check with your nurse supervisor and the respiratory therapist *before you do anything with the equipment*. ***DO NOT*** perform any respiratory procedure for your client unless di-

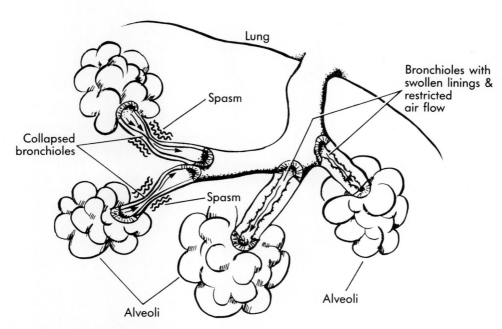

Figure 11-13. *Asthma spasms cause the bronchiole air routes to collapse or close. Or the bronchiole linings may swell as in an allergic reaction, restricting the air flow.*

rected and supervised by the nurse or respiratory therapist.

Humidifiers and Vaporizers

Many clients may have **humidifiers or vaporizers** in their homes. The nurse supervisor or respiratory therapist should evaluate these pieces of equipment before your client uses them. A humidifier or vaporizer puts moisture in the air. Dry air can make the mucus in your lungs thick and hard to cough up. Thickened mucus can contribute to infections and general discomfort. The added moisture from the humidifier or vaporizer can assist in loosening the mucus.

A humidifier or vaporizer is a moist, warm, and dark environment suitable for the growth of bacteria. These items must be cleaned and the water changed according to the directions. Hot-water vaporizers may be safety hazards in the home, especially for children, elderly persons, or persons with disabilities. The water in a hot-water vaporizer is hot enough to cause severe burns.

Air filters or air purifiers may be used for persons who have asthma or allergies. They are also popular in areas where there are people who smoke or where levels of air pollution are high. Some of these purifiers produce ozone, which clients with respiratory conditions should not breathe. The nurse supervisor or respiratory therapist should approve this type of equipment before your client uses it.

Oxygen Therapy

Clients who have lung diseases that reduce pulmonary air exchange may have inade-

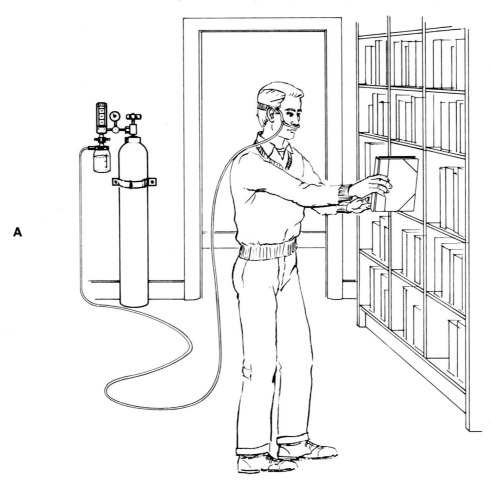

A

Figure 11-14. *Portable oxygen systems are becoming common. These movable systems free clients so they can perform more activities.*

quate amounts of oxygen carried by the blood stream. They may receive oxygen therapy to prevent blood oxygen levels from becoming too low. Oxygen should be regarded as a medication. It is administered under a physician's prescription in prescribed amounts. The amount of oxygen that a client requires may vary each day or week according to the level of oxygen in his blood and the results of other tests.

Oxygen can make it easier for a client to breathe, reduce anxiety, promote relaxation, improve mental alertness, increase his mobility, and enhance his general outlook on life. Too much oxygen can cause a client to feel overly tired, become nervous or anxious, and may cause breathing difficulties and damage the lungs.

A number of different oxygen systems are available for home use. The most common and oldest type of oxygen system is the oxygen tank. Although cumbersome, this type of system is inexpensive, reliable, and easy to use if the client only requires oxygen at night. Small, portable oxygen concentrators are the least expensive systems. Because they concentrate oxygen from the room air, they do not need oxygen tanks. The system requires electricity to operate, but may be adapted to use oxygen cylinders when the client goes outdoors (Figure 11-14 a-b). Liquid oxygen is the most expensive form of oxygen, but a week's supply can be stored in very little space.

Home Oxygen Safety

Oxygen will cause fires to burn at a rapid, destructive rate. Local fire and rescue squads should be notified when oxygen is being used regularly in the home. The family or nurse supervisor can obtain "Oxygen in Use" signs to place on the doors of the home and the client's room. If electricity is required for the oxygen system, utility companies should be aware of the client's high-priority need to have consistent service. Your client should wear a medical alert bracelet or medallion.

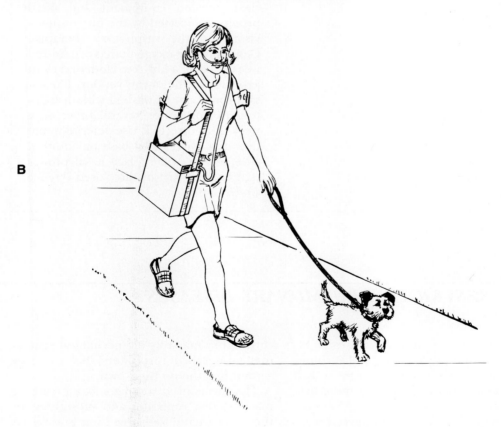

B

Figure 11-14 cont'd.

Home Oxygen Safety

DO NOT:

—allow him or anyone else to smoke in the room where oxygen is administered.

—allow him to go near a stove or other heat source that is turned on. This includes hot water heaters, pilot lights, radiators, electrical appliances such as toaster ovens and irons, and furnaces.

—allow him to go near any open flame or fire.

—use aerosol sprays around oxygen.

—use oil-based creams, hair conditioners, or oily lotions during oxygen therapy.

—use any oil-based product on the oxygen equipment because oil can ignite in the presence of oxygen.

—use grease or solvents around oxygen equipment.

—allow static buildup.

DO:

—follow the directions of your nurse supervisor.

—be sure the nasal prongs are placed comfortably in the client's nose and do not rub or irritate the skin around the prongs.

—check to be sure that there is a steady flow rate of oxygen. Check the tubing for twists and kinks if there is an improper flow of oxygen.

—provide a well-ventilated room for oxygen use.

—store oxygen tanks in an upright position and in a location where they are protected from accidental tipping, being knocked over, or leaking. A fallen oxygen tank may become a safety hazard.

—have a backup system for oxygen systems that rely on electricity for use in case of power failures.

—clean oxygen equipment and nasal prongs as directed by the nurse supervisor and the respiratory therapist. Generally, the oxygen tanks are dusted weekly, using a lint-free cloth or a cloth provided by the supply vendor. The nasal prongs can be washed with dish detergent and water several times each week or as directed. Use detergent that does not have an oil base or additive. The vendor will replace nasal prongs that become stiff or discolored (Figure 11-15 (a-b)).

CHRONIC RESTRICTIVE PULMONARY DISEASES

Chronic restrictive pulmonary diseases cause clients to have difficulty inhaling and exhaling. These pulmonary diseases affect the muscle and nerve activities of breathing more than they affect the lung tissue itself. There are numerous causes, including paralyzed respiratory muscles or damage to the nerves that signal respiratory muscles. For example, your clients who have high levels of spinal cord injury may rely on mechanical ventilators (also called respirators) because they cannot breathe on their own.

The mechanical ventilator is a breathing machine that replicates and substitutes for the client's paralyzed breathing muscles. A client who has a tracheostomy will attach the ventilator to the tracheostomy tube. Various types and kinds of mechanical ventilation are

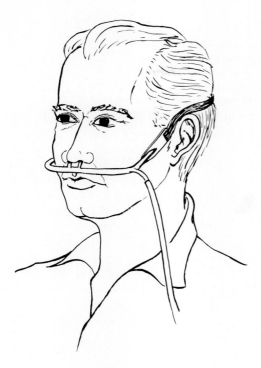

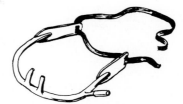

Figure 11-15. *Nasal prongs are positioned in the client's nostrils while he receives oxygen. Be sure they are clean and soft. They should not irritate his skin or rub against the inside of his nostrils.*

used by clients. An authorized vendor or service company will supply and service the respirator. A nurse and respiratory therapist will work with your client.

A **phrenic nerve pacemaker** is designed to support breathing for a client who cannot breathe on his own. Clients are carefully screened by physician specialists before receiving this pacemaker. The phrenic nerve pacemaker has external parts and internal parts. The external parts are a transmitter and antennae. A receiver and electrodes are internal parts that are surgically inserted into the client's chest. The external antennae, which are taped to the client's body, are situated over the implanted electrodes. The electrodes are attached to each of the phrenic nerves, the nerves that initiate respirations.

The respiratory therapist (or the physician or nurse) sets the transmitter controls for the amount, depth, and frequency of respirations for each client. The transmitter sends an electrical signal through the antennae to the receiver and electrodes. This signals the phrenic nerves and causes the diaphragm to contract, beginning each respiration. Only a few persons have phrenic nerve pacemakers.

You will not be responsible for the care of a client who depends on a **mechanical ventilator** or uses a **phrenic nerve pacemaker** unless a registered nurse is with you. However, you should know about these two kinds of technological equipment.

Much of the care for clients with chronic restrictive pulmonary diseases is similar to that for clients with COPD. Be sure to have clear directions from your nurse supervisor about your role in care for these clients.

CHRONIC PAIN

We all know what pain is, but we can neither see nor feel another person's pain. We only understand pain as we ourselves experience it (Figure 11-16). Each person has a different perception of pain and a different tolerance

for it. A client's experience of pain is affected by:

the duration of the pain,
—whether the pain is acute or chronic,
—whether the pain is malignant or nonmalignant,

Figure 11-16. *We understand pain only as we experience it. The transmission and sensation of pain signals in the body and the types of pain may be very complex topics. There is a great deal to be discovered about the causes, experiences, treatment, and relief of pain.*

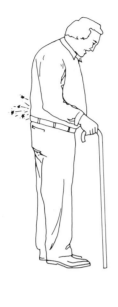
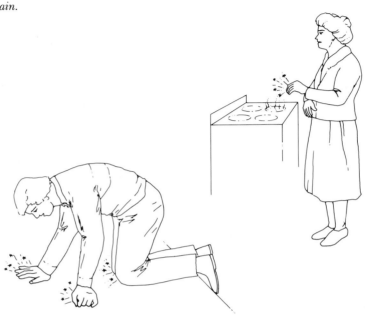

—how tolerant he is of pain,
—his attitudes about pain and the pain experience,
—the methods of pain relief and how effective they are, and
—his functional abilities and mental status.

Acute pain lasts only a short time. The pain eases gradually as the cause is removed, when medication takes effect, or as the body heals. Acute pain may be very intense, but it does subside and may not return.

Chronic pain, like other chronic conditions, lasts 3–6 months or longer. Chronic pain may be mild, severe, or have episodes of becoming severe. Similarly, chronic pain may be constant or recurring; it may be **malignant** (resulting from cancer) or **non-malignant.** Many of your clients will experience some type of chronic pain. You will want to understand whether the goal of your client is *pain relief* or whether his goal is *pain control or management.*

A client who experiences *chronic non-malignant pain* may be treated with techniques designed to help him cope with his pain. For example, a client who has an arthritic condi-

tion will use a combination of exercise, rest, and medications for pain control. Clients who experience pain that does not respond to treatment may visit a pain management clinic. The rehabilitation team at the clinic will examine the client's lifestyle in relation to the pain. If a client has been treated at a pain management clinic he will usually have a specific care plan stating ways for him to deal with his pain.

If your client has chronic non-malignant pain, you may be asked to:

—assist him with exercises;
—assist him with relaxation techniques;
—maintain a calm, soothing environment;
—prepare certain foods or restrict others;
—report specific behaviors and activities;
—play therapeutic cassette tapes; and
—keep a schedule of activities and times of day when he encounters pain. The nurse supervisor may use this information when evaluating the care plan.

A client who experiences *chronic malignant pain* resulting from cancer may receive *hospice* care at home if the disease is terminal. The goal is to keep the client as comfortable as possible, using the lowest amount of medication. This may mean the nurse supervisor may allow the client to take medication as needed, not necessarily on a strict hourly schedule. This client may be receiving large doses of pain-relieving medications administered by the nurse or a family member. (Hospice care is covered in Chapter 12.) If he is recovering from a cancer treatment or from surgery, you will be given instructions for reducing his discomfort. After surgery, he may have specific exercises to assist with restoring the function of the affected area. For example, hand, arm, and shoulder exercises are often ordered by the physician following breast surgery for cancer.

An individual's *tolerance* to his pain is influenced by:

—his personality;
—his cultural background;
—his past experience with pain or painful situations;
—other stresses in his life;
—depression or anxiety;
—fear or apprehension about the painful event;
—the extent of bodily damage and area affected;
—the reason for the pain (is it to gain health or is it part of a disease?);
—the support of family, friends, and professionals;
—the time of day; and
—the type and value of distractions.

Pain outcomes are affected by the use and effectiveness of:

—medications,
—relaxation techniques,
—distraction and imagery (imaging pleasant relaxing thoughts or scenes),
—muscle massage or therapy treatments,
—exercises,
—individual and group therapy,
—alternative or cultural patterns of care,
—assistive devices, such as TENS (see following discussion), and
—how independently the client can function in his activities of daily living and his desired lifestyle.

TENS, an assistive device for pain relief

Your client may use a device called a Transcutaneous Electrical Nerve Stimulator unit or **TENS unit.** A TENS unit is designed to *temporarily* relieve pain. Each TENS unit consists of a small generator with wire leads. At the end of each wire lead is a small electrode. The electrodes, coated with a special conducting gel, are placed on the skin near or over the area to be treated. The unit sends a low level of electricity to the area to interrupt the "pain message" being sent to the brain (See Figure 11-17). The client may have a tingling sensation while using the TENS unit. Each TENS session lasts from a few minutes to 2 hours, depending on the physician's orders. Pain relief lasts longer for some clients than for others; not all clients benefit from TENS. Clients **never** use TENS units without *exact* directions and *supervision* by the nurse or physical therapist.

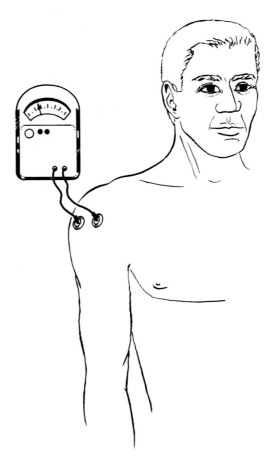

Figure 11-17. *A TENS unit is a small generator with attached electrodes. The electrodes are placed on the painful area. The TENS unit sends an electrical stimulation to the painful area, attempting to reduce or interrupt the "pain message" to the brain.*

*A*LZHEIMER'S DISEASE

Alzheimer's disease is a progressive incurable disease that does *not* occur as part of the normal process and changes of aging. Other disabling mental conditions or **dementias** have some of the same symptoms as early stages of Alzheimer's disease. Dementias are changes in the mental status of elderly person that may result from some type of brain disease or condition. For example, a client who has had a series of small strokes may have lost the function of certain brain cells. Clients with dementias often have:

—loss of memory,
—confusion with persons or places,
—reduced ability with simple mathematic calculations, and

—loss of common awareness, such as inability to keep time.

Some clients may take medications that cause them to appear to have dementias.

Alzheimer's disease produces changes in the chemical makeup of the brain that result in rapid deterioration of the brain cells. The nerve endings in the brain become tangled and loaded with a substance called plaque. Once they are coated with plaque, the brain cells are rapidly destroyed. The disease usually progresses over 7-10 years with increasing disabilities. In some cases, the disease spans 3–15 years.

The cause is unknown, but possible causes include:

—a slow virus that takes several years to emerge.

—heredity; the disease appears more often in persons who have family members with the disease. Children of Alzheimer's clients are 4–5 times more likely to get the disease than are other persons.

—exposure to aluminum, a common but unproven theory.

—a mistaken attack on the brain cells by the person's own immune system. The immune system considers the brain cells to be foreign cells.

Signs or Symptoms

Alzheimer's usually begins to be suspected when the person has a mild memory loss that becomes increasingly severe. Meanwhile, a once calm, quiet individual may become hostile, abusive, and irrational over minor frustrations. Personality changes develop for no apparent reason. The disease progresses somewhat differently for each client because different brain cells are destroyed at different times in each case. Four stages of Alzheimer's disease are used to classify the client's abilities to function physically and mentally.

Stages of Alzheimer's Disease

Stage I

These signs may not be recognized at this stage:

—slowing of memory, reactions, and energy;

—lessened sparkle and spontaneity;

—seeking familiar places, people, and habits;

—easily angered;

—difficulty with new tasks;

—loss of words; and

—slowing of learning.

Stage II

Other persons may become suspicious of a problem:

—increasing slowness of speech and thought, losing "train of thought";

—decreasing ability to make decisions and perform specialized activities, especially mathematical tasks;

—increasing impairment of balance;

—increasing clumsiness, such as dropping things;

—ignoring others' feelings, seemingly unaware of having irritated or embarrassed others; and

—angry outbursts for no apparent reason.

Stage III

The disabilities become obvious problems:

—loses sense of time and place;

—does not always know family or others;

—remembers distant past but not yesterday's events;

—loses daily coping abilities;

—invents words, cannot follow directions unless simple and repeated several times; and

—changes behavior and personality, becoming depressed and lethargic.

Stage IV

The disabilities become severe. The family may not be able to care for the client without assistance and possibly respite care:

—cannot recognize individuals or find his way around;

—poor memory of past and present;

—unable to perform activities of daily living;

—may become incontinent of bowel and bladder;

—may be unable to walk;

—drinks more fluids;

—has no appetite for meals;

—cannot speak and be understood, words are not meaningful; and

—slowed, disinterested reactions, may curl up into a ball (fetal position).

Daily Activities

The client's care plan will generally contain the following directions from your nurse supervisor:

- *A balance of stimulation and calmness*
  —Maintain a calm, soothing environment to lessen his tension and agitation.
  —Include him in daily activities, such as folding laundry, sweeping the floor, or setting the table.
  —Limit distractions while you are talking or giving directions to him. If the radio or television is on, or other conversations are taking place, it is difficult for him to concentrate on what he is doing or you are saying.
  —Play a radio softly, *tuned to the client's favorite station,* if he enjoys this.
  —Encourage him and help him feel useful, instead of feeling a burden.
  —Prevent overly stimulating events.
- *Activities to help him stay oriented to the world*
  —Keep a large calendar, crossing off the days and pointing out the month and year.
  —Place a large, clearly marked, clock in his view.
  —List regular daily activities and the times scheduled for them; refer him to the list.
  —Set a daily routine, using the calendar, clock, and schedule; prepare him for changes, such as an appointment with the physician.
  —Label photographs of family members, pets, and the like and help him refer to them.

Caring for the Client who has Alzheimer's Disease

The primary goals when working with a client who has Alzheimer's disease are to:

- Maintain his quality of life at the highest possible level.
- Assist him to function as independently as possible in a safe environment.
- Be supportive and considerate with the family as the client's health deteriorates.
- Maintain a safe environment.
- Inform your nurse supervisor about changes in his behavior or health and any difficulties for you or the family in coping with the client.

  —Use memory aids to label drawers and cabinets, rooms in the home, and the like; if he can no longer read words, use pictures to identify the contents (See Figure 11-18).
  —Place operating instructions on common household devices such as for use of the telephone.

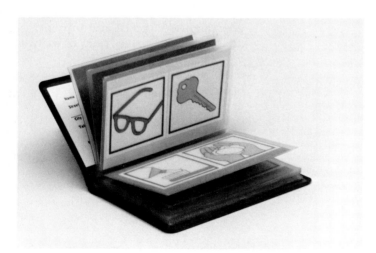

Figure 11-18. *Pictures can become memory aids when a client forgets where things are stored or where they belong.*
Reprinted by permission of © Bissell Healthcare Corporation/Fred Sammons, Inc.

For example, use detailed instructions as follows:

1) Pick up the telephone.
2) Say hello.
3) Ask who is calling.
4) Write down message.
5) Say good-bye.
6) Replace the receiver.
   —Remember that he won't know you either.

Begin each visit by:

1) saying your name,
2) telling him the day of the week, and
3) describing what you are doing. For example, "Mr. Smith, it's 12 o'clock noon on Wednesday. You are going to have lunch now. I am starting your lunch with a bowl of hot tomato soup. It's your favorite soup."
   —List his likes, dislikes, and helpful hints where they can be referred to by you and other caregivers and keep the list updated.
   —Follow the schedule set by the nurse supervisor so he has the same routines every day.

- *Assist him with personal care*
  —Be sure he performs daily hygiene and grooming tasks. Assist him only as necessary.
  —Give specific simple directions, divided into small steps, encouraging him with each step.
  —Limit his choices and reduce his confusion about daily activities. For example, lay clothing items out in the order in which he is to put them on. The nurse supervisor may instruct the family so that client will have only clothes appropriate for the season of year available to him in his dresser. Remove clothing he can no longer wear. The family may use elastic waistbands, Velcro closings, and other simplified dressing aids instead of buttons or zippers to modify the client's clothing whenever possible.
- *Physical activities*
  —If he is able and weather permits, accompany him on several short walks out-of-doors each day. One long walk may tire him, but short walks help break up the day. Walking may help him sleep at night and promote bowel regularity.
  —If he cannot walk out-of-doors, walk indoors.
  —When he can no longer walk, assist him with exercises and range of motion, as directed by the nurse supervisor.
  —Assist him with his personal care in the morning and serve his main meal at noon so that less is expected of him in the evening. Do not put him to bed too early. Many clients' symptoms become worse in the evening, possible because they are tired from coping all day with the confusing world caused by the disease. There may also be more activity and distractions in the evening when family members are home.

Wandering: A Special Concern

Wandering is common to clients who have Alzheimer's Disease and is a cause for concern. Clients can and do wander off. They are unable to identify themselves or where they are, and they may be harmed. Wandering may become a constant behavior for your client, or it may occur intermittently. Just because a client has never wandered does not mean he might not do so. He may wander through his home or try to leave the house, becoming lost.

Some suggestions are:

- Clients who are able to walk should carry an identification card in their pockets at all times.
- Clients who have medic-alert bracelets or necklaces should wear them at all times. If your client does not have a medic-alert tag, ask the nurse supervisor or a family member about it.
- The client's identifications should include:
  The name and address of his home, telephone numbers and family members' work numbers, and the statement, "memory impaired."
- Doors from the home to the outside should have locks that require a 2-step action or a key to be opened.
- Doors may be labeled with signs reminding him not to go outside alone.

Losing and Forgetting

Clients who have Alzheimer's disease often hide things and forget where they are hidden. Sometimes they simply forget where things are kept. This behavior can become frustrating to the client, to you, and to the family. Some suggestions are:
- Store valuables safely.
- Keep extra hearing aid batteries, an extra pair of glasses, and similar items on hand.
- Reduce potential hiding places by locking closets and doors to rooms that are not used or belong to other persons.
- Check for hidden items in common hiding places, such as wastepaper baskets; flower or other baskets; under and between cushions, pillows, mattresses, or carpets; inside shoes and shoeboxes; in drawers, in refrigerators and freezers, or in sewing kits.

Common Annoying Behaviors

Your client can be expected to demonstrate these annoying behaviors. Help others to remember that these behaviors are a part of the disease. He may:

—continually follow you from room to room,
—repeat the same question,
—repeat the same activity or motion,
—refuse a necessary activity such as bathing, or
—be unable to make even simple decisions.

Never contradict or argue with him. These responses make the situation upsetting. Since he will not be able to follow your explanation about the situation, he will only become more confused.

You can:

—Stop him from following you by asking him to help with a simple task, such as folding laundry while sitting in one place. Set a timer and tell him you will return in 10 minutes, then do so.
—Cope with repeated questioning by answering the question one time, then ignoring it. If you try to explain to him that he has just asked the question, he will not remember, but your explanation will keep him focused on the question. Changing the subject may also help direct his attention away from the repeated question.
—Deal with a repeated activity similarly to coping with a repeated question. If the activity is not harmful to him or others, ignore it or try to get him involved in something else.
—Complete a necessary activity by dropping the subject temporarily. Wait a few minutes and then come back to what must be done. Break the activity up into small steps.
—Cope with his lessened ability to make decisions by limiting choices. Ask him simple questions that he can answer with "yes" or "no." You can also use schedules and other time-setting aids.

Maintaining Nutritional Well-Being

As the disease progresses, you may have increased difficulty in getting your client to eat. You can assist the family by sharing techniques that you have used successfully. Some helpful techniques are:

- Plan simple, easy-to-chew meals.
- Serve several small meals, with the main meal at noon, rather than 3 large meals.
- Try serving finger foods.
- Remind him to chew and swallow if he holds food in his mouth.
- Plan a pleasant, calm, undistracted mealtime.
- Pay attention to favorite foods, and special likes and dislikes.
- Plan one-dish meals or one food at a time, rather than too many different choices on one plate; even food can be confusing to him.
- Avoid caffeine drinks if possible and choose decaffeinated coffee and drinks.
- Offer lukewarm, not hot, beverages and soups to prevent him from burning his mouth or becoming burned from hot liquid spills.
- Be sure that he is giving himself or receiving proper oral hygiene care.
- Work with the family, dietitian, and nurse supervisor to plan a well-balanced diet while adapting to your client's reac-

tions to the disease. Make sure that the fluid intake is adequate, but balanced with his solid food diet.

Alzheimer's is a disheartening disease. You and the family will observe the progressive deterioration of your client. He may gradually slip into a state of total dependency and not recognize his family. *It is essential that you and others consciously work and plan so that the client's dignity and quality of life are considered, even when he reaches the final stages of the* *disease.* Family members may vacillate between frustration and grieving during this difficult situation.

Report changes in your client to the nurse supervisor as they occur. You may report any changes in the family behavior as well, so that the nurse can plan to work closely with them during more difficult times. Some families use **respite care** or other alternatives to provide periods of temporary relief from the stresses of caring for a client with Alzheimer's disease.

DIABETES MELLITUS

Diabetes Mellitus is a chronic disease that occurs when the body does not produce enough insulin. **Insulin** is an hormone produced by the pancreas and is necessary for carbohydrate **metabolism** (Figure 11-19). When food is eaten and digested, it enters the blood stream in the form of a sugar called glucose. The blood stream carries the sugar to the body cells, where it is burned for energy. The body needs insulin to get the sugar from the blood stream into the cells. Without insulin, the sugar is trapped in the blood-

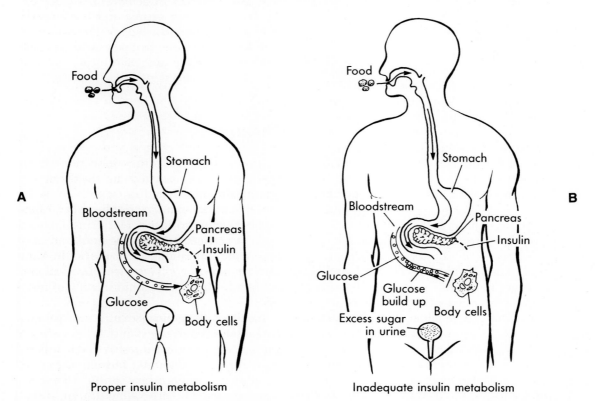

Figure 11-19. **A,** *Proper insulin metabolism occurs when the correct balance of sugar and insulin enter the body cells. The insulin is necessary for the sugar to get into the cell.*
   B, *Inadequate insulin metabolism occurs when insulin does not reach the body cells. Then sugar cannot enter the cells. Instead sugar builds up in the bloodstream. The excess is secreted in the urine.*

stream. The cells do not have enough sugar for energy. Meanwhile, the sugar builds up in the blood. The body attempts to rid the blood of the excess sugar by excreting it through the urine. This is why clients who have diabetes check their urine several times a day to see how much sugar may have accumulated there. The amount of sugar in their urine helps them determine how much insulin they need or whether they need to take more insulin.

When you think about how this process works in the body, it is easier to understand why diabetes causes clients to have the following signs and symptoms.

Signs of Diabetes Mellitus
- increased appetite,
- possible weight loss,
- increased need to urinate,
- increased tiredness or fatigue,
- diminished vision,
- increased amount of time to heal sores, cuts, or bruises, and
- possible itching skin.

Diabetes may begin during childhood or later in life. The cause of diabetes is not known. But if one family member has diabetes, other persons in the family may develop the disease. However, it is not a contagious disease—you cannot "catch it" from your client. Eighty percent of the people who develop diabetes are overweight. Sometimes pregnancy or repeated miscarriages, stressful life crises, or illness lead to a diagnosis of diabetes. It is not clear whether the diabetes is caused by these events, or whether they bring out the symptoms of the disease. Many persons have diabetes and do not know it. Persons who have diabetes should carry a medic alert card or wear a medic necklace.

Most people in our society who have diabetes are middle-aged and older. Many also have other health problems, disabilities, and complications due to diabetes. There are two types of diabetes mellitus. Type I is insulin-dependent or juvenile diabetes. Clients usually develop this diabetes before they are 25 years old. They must have daily insulin injections in order to live. Their bodies do not produce insulin, so it must be added by the injections. They test their blood or urine several times each day to determine how much insulin they need to add.

Type II diabetes or adult-onset diabetes usually develops in clients who are older, over 40 years old. These clients will have strict diet and exercise programs. Many of them are overweight and under-exercised. They may have a physician's prescription for an oral medication to help their bodies produce insulin. Some require insulin injections.

Complications due to diabetes are:

—potential insulin imbalance;
—increased tendency to develop infections;
—circulation problems that may result in the need for amputation;
—impaired vision, glaucoma and cataracts, perhaps blindness; and
—other chronic diseases, especially heart and peripheral vascular disease and kidney disease.

The nurse supervisor will develop a care plan that includes *goals for care* which may include:

- allowing the client to be as responsible for managing his diabetes as possible,
- assisting him to achieve a balance between insulin supply and body needs,
- assisting him to avoid insulin imbalance,
- following preventive care measures, and
- following the care plan to prevent further complications.

Insulin

Insulin is a natural hormone secreted from specialized cells located in the pancreas gland. Insulin in drug form is given to clients to replace the natural insulin when their bodies cannot produce it. Not all insulin must be kept refrigerated. But it should be used before the expiration date on the bottle. Your nurse supervisor will instruct your client and his family about self-administration of insulin.

Insulin is taken by injecting it into the subcutaneous area of the skin that lies between the fat and muscle tissues. A client will require different amounts of insulin each time he takes it. It is necessary for him to test his blood or urine before taking insulin so that he knows how much his body requires at that time. There are a number of urine- or blood-testing products available. Common tests are described later in this section. Whenever pos-

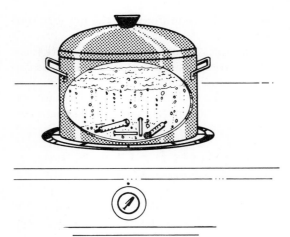

Figure 11-21. *You may be instructed to sterilize equipment in your client's home. Usually equipment is boiled in a covered pan of water for 20 to 25 minutes. Obtain clear instructions from your nurse supervisor about boiling, removing, and handling boiled equipment.*

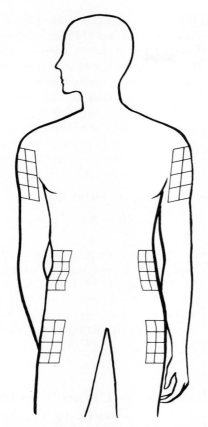

Figure 11-20. *Clients who take insulin injections use a different site on the body for each injection. They protect their skin from damage and infection. Most clients have a pattern or plan for site rotations.*

sible, clients give their own insulin. *You do not give insulin.*

Each time your client administers his own insulin, he will use a different site on his body. He rotates the injection sites in a regular pattern to prevent skin breakdown from continual use of one injection site (Figure 11-20).

A client's particular type of insulin and a diabetic syringe with a needle are prescribed by his physician. These can be purchased at drug stores or supermarket pharmacies. Some clients may still keep reusable needles or syringes in their homes. You may be instructed to assist your client by boiling equipment or supplies in the home (Figure 11-21). Your nurse supervisor will work with the client and his family to assess the client's equipment and personal preferences. Be sure you have a clear understanding of the directions and review aseptic techniques if you are di-

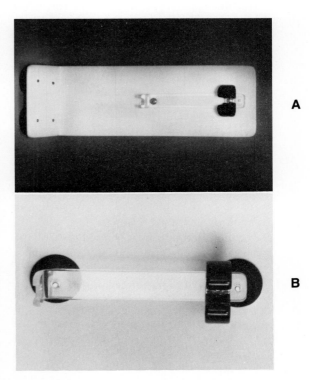

A

B

Figure 11-22. *Insulin holders designed for persons with disabilities may feature insulin bottle holders with,* **A,** *suction cups or* **B,** *self stands. Other styles may have magnified glass panels to enable clients to read the amounts on the bottle and syringe.*

rected to boil equipment in the home to sterilize it.

Examples of insulin and syringe holders designed especially for persons who have disabilities are shown in Figure 11-22 (a-b). These must be boiled and sterilized according to instructions from the nurse supervisor.

Urine Tests for Clients who have Diabetes Mellitus

A client may require different amounts of insulin throughout the day. Testing his urine before eating or before taking insulin indicates to your client how much insulin his body requires at that time. He may use a simple clinitest or clinistix test to check how much glucose (sugar) he is excreting in his urine at a specific time. He tests the amount of acetone, using an acetest or ketostix test. Most clients test their urine three to four times a day—usually upon waking or about 30 minutes before breakfast, before lunch and or dinner, and again at bedtime.

If your client cannot perform the urine test, you may assist him. He may need help with some steps or with all of the testing; allow him to participate, even if you can only show him the test results and have him agree with your scores.

Tests and Procedures

Diabetic Urine Testing

There are a number of urine testing kits available on the market; specific instructions are included with the test materials. The tests use reagent strips or tablets that have a chemical reaction with the urine, showing how much acetone and glucose are in the urine.

The following are general instructions for urine testing:

—Wear disposable gloves; do not touch the urine or the tablet or strip with your fingers. The test materials are poisonous.
—Use a fresh urine specimen from your client; discard the first amount of urine, then obtain a specimen about 30-45 minutes later for the test. Only a small amount of urine is needed.

—Follow the directions carefully. Remember that this is a chemical test that will generate heat; when a test tube is used, the bottom of the tube will become hot.
—Wait the directed amount of time for the chemical reaction of the test to take place.
—Hold the test tube or the strip alongside the color chart to determine the results. Record both the color and the numerical amount that matches the urine test results.
—Rinse materials, throw away disposable items, and clean the area and wash your hands.
—Inform your client of the test results, or report the results to your nurse supervisor, as directed for each client. What you do will depend upon your client's ability to monitor and give his own insulin and the directions from the nurse supervisor.

Obtaining a Urine Specimen from an Indwelling Catheter

(See Figure 11-23 a-c)

1) Wash your hands and wear clean gloves.
2) Empty the leg bag or bed bag.
3) Disconnect the leg or bed bag tubing from the catheter.
4) Allow the urine to drain from the catheter into the specimen cup.
5) Clean the end of the catheter with an alcohol wipe.
6) Clean the end of the leg bag or bed bag tubing with another alcohol wipe.
7) Reconnect the leg bag or bed bag tubing to the catheter tubing.
8) Dispose of the gloves and wash your hands.

Diabetic Blood Testing

Many clients will use self-monitoring kits to directly test their blood instead of their urine for the level of sugar. The client sticks his fingertip to obtain a drop of blood and uses the kit to check the results. This method gives a current reading of the blood glucose

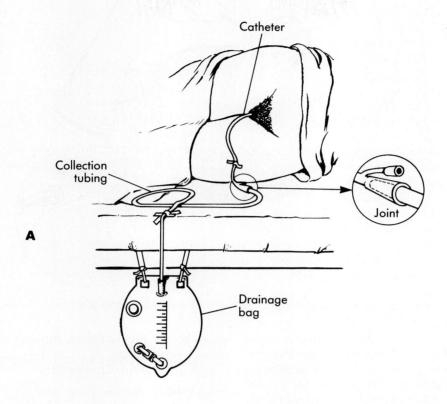

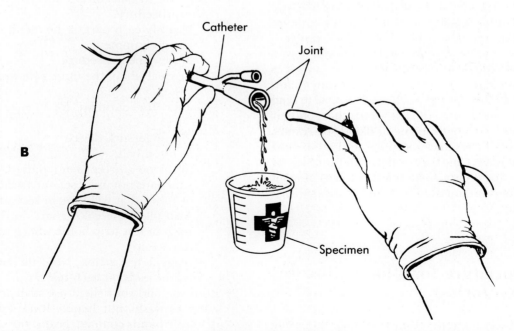

Figure 11-23. A, *To obtain a urine specimen from a client who is wearing an indwelling catheter, first disconnect the catheter from the collection tubing.*

   B, *Drain the urine from the catheter into the specimen container. DO NOT use urine from the collection tubing or drainage bag.*   *Continues.*

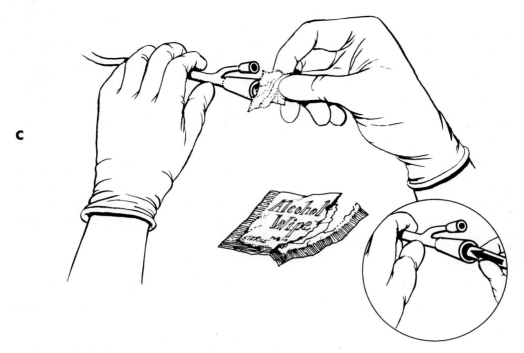

Figure 11-23, cont'd. **C,** *Wipe the ends of the catheter and tubing with alcohol and reconnect them.*

(sugar) level because the measure is direct from the blood. Clients who have unstable diabetes, have frequent imbalance situations, are pregnant, or who use insulin several times a day may benefit from a current reading. The physician will decide if your client is to test his blood glucose level in this manner.

The nurse supervisor will teach the procedure to your client and instruct you how to assist him. Your client should do as much as possible for himself. Even if he cannot manage all the equipment, he may be able to read the results. Many clients keep a chart of their insulin injections, urine or blood test results, times of tests and injections, and other relevant data. Charts provide a reference log or diary of their activities and patterns of insulin needs. You may be asked to assist with a chart.

Procedure for Blood Glucose Monitoring

These are general instructions for using blood glucose monitoring equipment. The procedure and timed steps may vary slightly for the different product brands. It is essential to accurately follow the instructions pre-

pared by the product manufacturer of your client's equipment.

The general instructions are:

1) Prepare for the procedure:
   —Read the instructions for the product and procedure.
      Identify each part of the monitoring equipment.
      Review the procedure.
      Be clear about the timing for each step.
   —Gather the supplies for the procedure:
      —the fingerstick device,
      —a cotton ball,
      —the blood glucose meter, if used. If a meter is not used, set out a watch or timer that will time in seconds. Also place the color chart on the reagent test strip bottle where you can see it.
      —reagent test strips. Note the two yellow pads on each test strip.
2) Both you and your client use soap and water to wash your hands. Rinse and dry your hands completely and put on gloves.
   —Press the button to start the meter. The meter number displayed should be the same as the number on the

reagent strip bottle. If they are not the same, press the program button until they are the same.
—Remove a reagent strip from the bottle. Check the expiration date. Recap the bottle and place it in a safe location and out of the reach of children.

3) Assist your client to use the special fingerstick device to penetrate the skin at the outer edge of his finger. Using the special fingerstick device may make it easier to obtain blood when a client is reluctant to stick himself.
—Obtain a large drop of blood. Avoid dabbing small amounts of blood onto the strip or "milking" his finger to produce blood.

4) Start the meter. When the meter signals, immediately apply the collected drop of blood to the end of the reagent strip. Cover the two yellow test pads completely with blood.

5) Hold the cotton ball ready to wipe the reagent strip. All glucose monitors signal when to wipe the strip. Different manufacturer's monitors have different signals such as displaying a number or beeping an alarm. At the signal, wipe the reagent strip with the cotton ball. Repeat, using a clean part of the cotton ball.

6) Quickly place the strip inside the meter. Insert the strip according to the manufacturer's instructions. The test pads should face the test window. Be sure the window has been cleaned. The glucose score will appear on the meter display.

7) Record the results. Gather equipment and clean the area, discard the gloves, and both you and your client wash your hands. Report any changes to the nurse supervisor.

If your client does not have blood glucose monitoring equipment, you may assist him to use reagent strips for blood glucose tests.

1) Wash both your hands and your client's hands. Put on gloves.
2) Gather the reagent strip, fingerstick device, and watch or timer.
3) Assist your client to gather a large drop of blood for the sample that will completely cover the yellow pads on the reagent strip.

4) Immediately start timing for 30 seconds.
5) Wipe the strip with the cotton ball when exactly 30 seconds have passed. Repeat, using a clean area of the cotton ball.
6) Time an additional 90 seconds (one and one-half minutes).
7) Compare the color of the reagent strip test pads with the color chart on the reagent strip bottle.
8) Record the results. Clean the area, discard the gloves, and both you and your client wash your hands. Report any changes as directed by the nurse supervisor.

Insulin Imbalance

There are two types of insulin imbalances in the body:

1) *too little* insulin or *hyperglycemia,* and
2) *too much* insulin or *hypoglycemia.*

Notify the nurse supervisor, rescue squad, or emergency unit if your client has these signs:

1) Hyperglycemia:

This condition may occur when there is *too little insulin* or *high blood sugar.* The body begins to burn fat for energy because there is not enough insulin to use the sugar in the blood for energy. This causes increased ketones or acetones that can be measured in the urine. This is the acetone test in the urine test as an early indicator of potential acidosis or diabetic coma. The client who feels a great deal of stress or who is sick with other conditions may have high blood sugar (too little insulin). You may expect the client who is experiencing this type of imbalance to ask for orange juice. He may complain about:

—heavy, difficult breathing,
—weakness with stomach pains,
—loss of appetite,
—aches in various places in his body,
—nausea and vomiting,
—increased thirst,
—increased urinary frequency and output,
—increased amounts (usually large) of sugar and ketones in his urine, and he may tell you he needs more insulin.

Care for the Client who has Diabetes

The daily care for your client centers on the need for "balance." Whenever your client's diet, insulin, and activity become out of balance, he will develop problems with his diabetes. It is your responsibility to:

- *Very Important:* Adhere closely to his meal plan; become familiar with the diabetic exchange diet in the Appendix and follow instructions from your nurse supervisor and dietician.
- Assist him to get enough exercise, without overexertion. The exercise must be in balance with his food intake.
- Assist him to test his urine as directed by your nurse supervisor.
- *Very Important:* Check his feet and legs for signs of infection, poor circulation, ingrown toenails, or sore areas. Be sure he always wears shoes that protect his feet. Gently wash his feet. You may soak them for a few minutes in warm water with mild soap. Thoroughly dry his feet, including between the toes. **NEVER** *cut his toenails!*

- Report any lumps or infections at insulin injection sites to the nurse supervisor.
- Protect him from skin damage that may lead to infections, such as sunburns, cuts, bruises, or pressure areas.
- Encourage him not to drink alcohol or smoke. Both can lead to heart disease. If your client does drink or smoke, do not lecture him. Report the situation to your nurse supervisor.
- Assist him as needed with grooming and hygiene, including teeth and gums.
- Avoid insulin imbalance (see section that follows). You may not be able to prevent your client from having an insulin imbalance. If he does have one, you must call your nurse supervisor and follow directions.

---

2) *Hypoglycemia:*

This condition may occur when there is too much insulin in the body, resulting in *low blood sugar.* Generally the client experiencing this imbalance will ask for hard candy or other sugar. It may occur when a client has exercised too long or actively, has not eaten enough food, or has taken too much insulin or oral medication for diabetes. If unattended, it can lead to an insulin reaction or shock. Signs of hypoglycemia are:

—increased profuse sweating,
—faint or dizzy feelings,
—pounding heart,

—trembling or shaking,
—headache,
—visual disturbances,
—inability to be awakened,
—irritable behavior or change in behavior and personality,
—hunger, and
—client telling you he is having a reaction.

Call your nurse supervisor, the physician, rescue squad or emergency unit

—if your client does not feel better within 15–20 minutes,
—if his symptoms worsen, or
—if he asks you to call.

F̶RACTURED HIP OR HIP REPLACEMENT SURGERY

Elderly clients tend to have more fractured hips and hip replacement surgeries than the rest of the population. Hip replacement surgery is the surgical removal of a fractured or diseased hip joint, which is then replaced with an artificial hip joint. Clients may have hip replacement surgery when the hip joint is damaged. See Figure 11-24 (a-d). Common causes include:

- arthritis;
- a tumor;
- necrosis or wearing away of the head of the femur;
- severe dislocation of the hip joint, with tears in the joint capsule;
- severe damage to the bony head of the femur; and

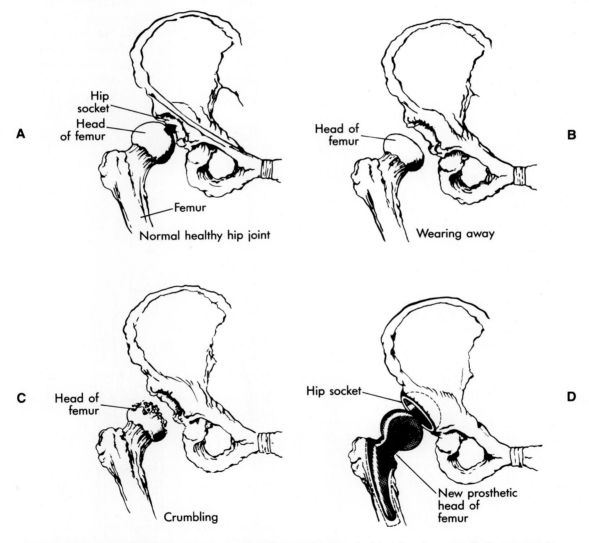

Figure 11-24. **A,** *The head of the femur bone fits smoothly into the hip joint of a normally functioning hip and leg.*

   B, *The early signs of hip damage include wearing away of the coverings and bone on the head of the femur.*

   C, *The head of the femur eventually crumbles and breaks off if left untreated.*

   D, *When the hip is "replaced" a new femur head prosthesis is constructed.*

● fractures, especially in older women who have fragile bones from osteoporosis. Even a minor fall can cause severe damage to the hip for these women.

Care is the same (Figure 11-25 a-b) whether a client has a fractured hip or a surgical hip replacement. If your client does not go to a rehabilitation center following his hospitalization, he will come home in 7–14 days after surgery. His surgeon will usually be a specialist in orthopedics. Each orthopedic surgeon has specific instructions about care for his clients. It is extremely important for you to consider the specific instructions for each client who has either of these conditions. Your nurse supervisor will review the instructions with you and supervise your practice of any new techniques before you care for the client.

You should discuss the care discussed in the following list with your nurse supervisor. This list is a guide that must be altered for each client's specific instructions. However, you should have instructions that cover each item on the list.

*1. Ability of the client to bear weight

Many clients who have had a hip replacement will be instructed to begin *(PWB) partial weight-bearing* activities a few days after surgery. A client who has had repair of a fractured hip generally will be *(NWB) non-weight-bearing* until the physician specifically orders activities. The nurse supervisor will give you precise instructions about weight-bearing.

The repaired hip fracture must heal sufficiently for the joint and bones to support even partial weight-bearing. You may have to remind and monitor your client not to bear

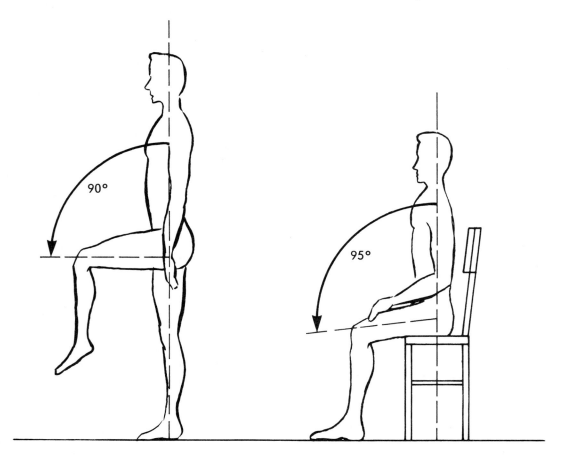

Figure 11-25. *A client who had hip replacement surgery should NEVER flex his leg so that the thigh comes close to the point where it joins his hip (thigh-hip joint). This means he must maintain an angle greater than 90 degrees betweent his hip and leg while standing, lying, or sitting. When his leg is fully extended straight, an angle of 180 degrees is created at the thigh-hip joint. At 90 degrees, his thigh-hip is in an L-shaped position. He may sit in a chair when the seat is elevated to create a tolerable angle greater than 90 degrees. Placing a pillow in the seat of the chair may elevate him sufficiently. Check the angle between his thigh and hip to be surre it is greater than 90 degrees.*

weight, or no more weight than allowable, especially as he feels better and ready to ambulate. If he begins to bear weight on his leg and hip too soon, it may cause infection, wearing of the femur head, or poor alignment of the fracture.

*2. Positioning of the client

A client who has had hip surgery should:

—Keep the hip in **abduction** to assure that the hip heals in the proper alignment by:

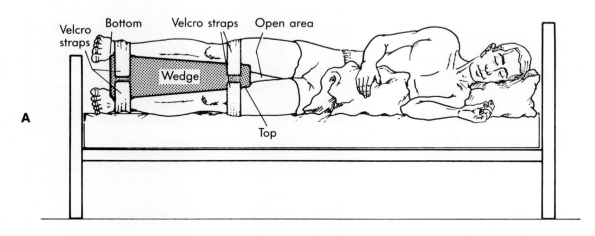

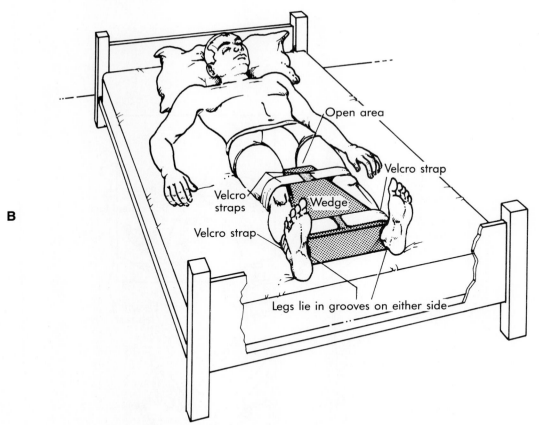

Figure 11-26. A, *A client who has a hip fracture or hip replacement surgery is positioned on his uninvolved side. His affected hip is slightly flexed. A foam wedge (or pillows) are used to keep his legs apart and abduct the hip joints. Note the 90-degree angle limit of flexion at the hip.*

    B, *The same client viewed from the front illustrates the use of the foam wedge (or pillows) between his knees and legs. These supports keep the hip joints abducted. The top or affected knee must be supported firmly and steadily. It must not fall off the wedge. His knees must not be allowed to touch one another.*

—keeping a specially designed foam wedge pillow between his thighs while he lies in bed, until the nurse supervisor tells you to discontinue using it (Figure 11-26).

—***Not*** crossing his legs at the knees or at the ankles.

—***Not*** allowing his hip joint to be flexed at an angle less than 90-degree (Figure 11-25 a-b).

—keeping his foot and ankle in 90–degree **dorsiflexion** while he is in bed.

—keeping his hip in a neutral, straight position, **not** rotating or turning inward or outward. Remind him to monitor the position of his leg and hip if he is able to do so.

—helping him to turn when he lies on his unaffected side. *Place a pillow between his legs so his knee cannot fall forward and cause his repaired hip to rotate out of position* (See Figure 11-26 a-b).

*3. Moving or Transferring the Client

—Use chairs that have firm seats, solid arm supports, and steady legs and be sure they do not move easily on the floor. Do not use deep, soft chairs that are difficult to get in and out of, or chairs that may slide.

—Use a raised toilet seat.

—Assist him to get out of his chair as shown in Figure 11-27 (a-c).

1) Assist him to move so he is sitting on the edge of the chair.

2) Place his *affected* leg slightly in front of the *unaffected* leg. The foot of his *unaffected* leg will be under the seat of the chair.

3) Assist him to rise while he pushes up, bearing weight on the *unaffected* leg. Make sure the weight is centered on the *unaffected* leg.

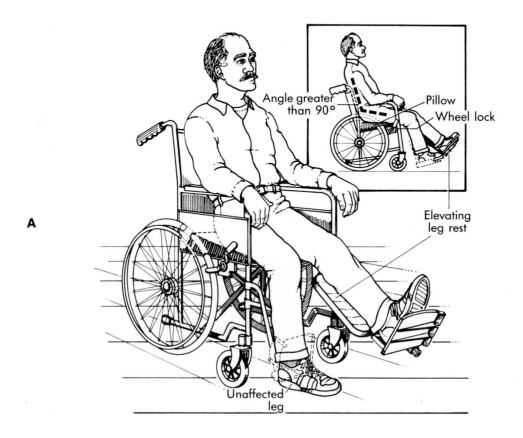

A

Angle greater than 90°

Pillow
Wheel lock

Elevating leg rest

Unaffected leg

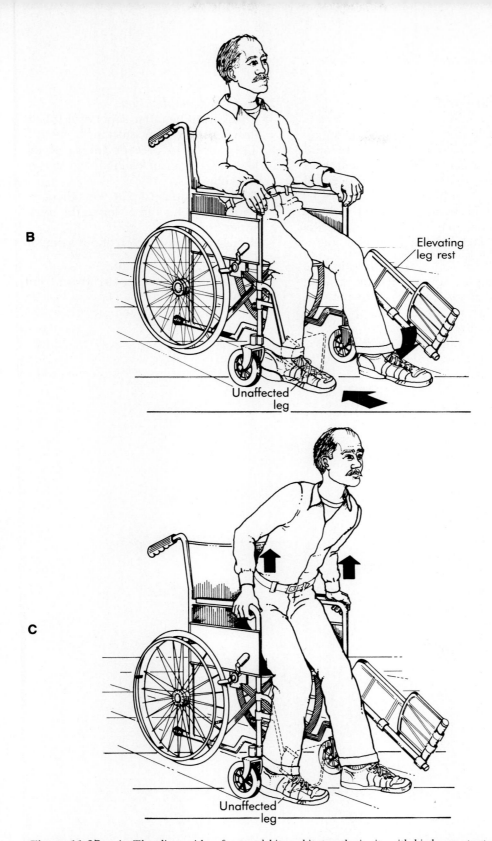

Figure 11-27. **A,** *The client with a fractured hip or hip prosthesis sits with his knees apart and feet supported flat on the floor. His hips are flexed greater than 90 degrees at the thigh-hip joint. Lock the wheels or casters on his chair and use a safety belt.*

B, *Bend his uninvolved knee. Place the uninvolved foot on the floor, but situated partially under the seat of the chair. Extend his affected leg slightly forward and check his balance.*

C, *When he is ready to move, he pushes himself up on his hands. At the same time, he places his weight on the uninvolved leg situated under the seat of the chair. Bending forward slightly at the waist, he can bring himself to a standing position.*

*4. Endurance and Exercise

—Remind him to perform ankle exercises to maintain and increase circulation.

—**DO NOT** allow him to bend over until you have cleared this movement with your nurse supervisor. Bending over will place stress on his hip joint.

—Consider his reduced level of exercise and activity; do not allow him to overextend his abilities, but keep him stimulated and alert.

*5. Prevent Complications

—Check with the nurse supervisor if he is instructed to wear stockings, such as TED socks, to prevent edema of the lower legs that can lead to blood clots or **thromboses.**

—Report any unusual pain your client experiences in his hip or leg to the nurse supervisor.

—Review the information about safety in Chapter 1.

PART II
Arthritic Conditions

ARTHRITIS

Arthritis is not a single disease but a group of diseases. This can be confusing because the word "**arthritis**" means inflammation of the joints. Arthritic diseases cause joints and connecting tissues to become painful, swollen, and inflamed. Several kinds of arthritic diseases also have other symptoms, however. For example, some kinds of arthritic diseases are **degenerative,** with progressive deterioration. Some do not cause inflammation and others do not involve the joints. There is also the word "**rheumatism,**" which is often used to refer to the aches and pains of muscles and joints. Some arthritic conditions can affect the kidneys, lungs, skin, eyes, blood vessels, and other parts of the body.

Although arthritis is usually thought of as an "old age disease," it can begin at any age. More than 250,000 children in the United States have juvenile arthritis. Different arthritic diseases thus affect the body in different ways. Your clients may have arthritic conditions in addition to other disabling problems.

A **joint** is a place where two bones meet. In this chapter we are most interested in moveable joints such as at the knee, hip, hands, or elbow. The ends of bones are covered with a tough elastic tissue called **cartilage.** The cartilage covering protects the bones from rubbing against each other as a joint is moved, such as when the elbow is bent. The cartilage and joint are lubricated with a fluid called **synovial fluid** which maintains smooth, painfree joint movements. It is slippery, clear, and thick, like the white of an egg. Small amounts of synovial fluid lubricate the spaces around the joint and between the car-

tilage. The fluid is produced by the synovial membrane. The membrane covers and encloses the entire inner joint area. The outside of the joint is covered by muscles, tendons, and ligaments which mobilize and support the joint.

A normal joint is shown in Figure 11-28. The following sections have pictures of the changes that occur within the normal joint when it is affected by a particular arthritic disease. Compare each type of arthritic joint

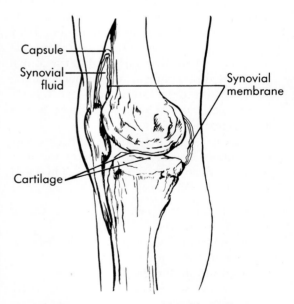

Capsule

Synovial fluid

Synovial membrane

Cartilage

Figure 11-28. *This is a functioning healthy joint. Notice the smooth rounded edges of the bone ends. They are cushioned in synovial fluid and covered with protective cartilage.*

303

with the normal joint and see if you can visualize the changes that cause disability and pain.

Arthritic conditions are classified to identify the person's expected level of independent function in daily activities. Your client's classification can be used to help you identify what he can and cannot do for himself. The American Rheumatism Association has developed the following classification system.

Class I. Complete ability to perform all activities of his daily living.

Class II. Normal activities can be performed with some discomfort.

Class III. Activities are limited to self-care and a few occupational duties.

Class IV. Person is bound to his bed or wheelchair.

RHEUMATOID ARTHRITIS

Rheumatoid arthritis is the most disabling and destructive type of arthritis. Rheumatoid arthritis is a hidden disease, beginning slowly with mild pain and inflammation. It may become progressive or non-progressive, or seem to appear and disappear. When severe, it may affect many joints at the same time, especially the hands and feet, elbow, shoulder, knee, hip, ankle, jaw, and shoulderblade areas. The affected joints become swollen, painful, stiff, and misshapen. They are warm and tender to the touch. This disease may not confine itself within the joints. It causes destruction in other parts of the body, including the lungs and heart. It leads to infections of many parts of the body and even death.

The early signs may follow a physically or emotionally stressful situation. Stress may trigger a flare-up of the disease. The early signs of rheumatoid arthritis are:

—early morning pain and stiffness for an hour or more;

—repeated pain, swelling, or stiffness in one or more joints;

—nodules under the skin;

—tingling sensations in the fingertips, hands, or feet;

—a general "run-down," tired feeling; and

—unexplained loss of weight and appetite.

Often it is difficult to make a diagnosis until more signs appear. A diagnosis may be con-

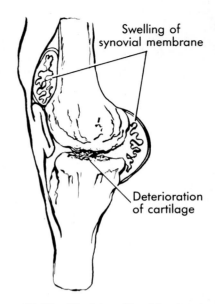

Figure 11-29 *The joint affected by rheumatoid arthritis develops a swollen inflamed synovial membrane. The protective cartilage is worn down, and the joint is poorly lubricated and painful.*

firmed with tests and after the signs persist for at least six weeks. There is no evidence that rheumatoid arthritis is hereditary.

Figure 11-29 shows the changes in the joint with rheumatoid arthritis.

The inner lining of the synovial membrane becomes thickened and inflamed. As this continues, the cartilage and bone protected by the cartilage are worn down and destroyed. The joint loses its protective lining and lubrication. The surrounding muscles and tissues eventually become diseased so they cannot support and move the joint. The joint becomes disabled, misshapen, and painful.

OSTEOARTHRITIS

Osteoarthritis is the most common type of arthritis. It is a non-inflammatory disease that affects only a few joints. It is called the "wear and tear arthritis" because it occurs in older persons and in persons who overuse or abuse a particular joint, such as the elbow of a baseball pitcher. Osteoarthritis affects the large weight-bearing joints of the body, the hips, knees, and spine. It also commonly occurs in the fingers and great toe.

The joint changes in osteoarthritis differ from those of rheumatoid arthritis. Com-

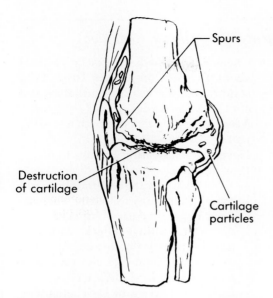

Figure 11-30. *Osteoarthritis affects the joint by destroying the cartilage covering the bone ends. Calcium spurs develop on the bones. They extend into the joint causing pain.*

pare Figure 11-30 below with the normal joint illustration.

In osteoarthritis, the cartilage that covers and protects the ends of the bones becomes so soft that it can be worn away. When the person moves the joint, the bones then rub together. The body reacts to protect the bones by building layers of calcium near the bones. The calcium does not do the same work as the cartilage and cannot be lubricated by the synovial fluid. Instead, the calcium accumulates, increasing the size until it forms hardened spurs. The spurs extend into the joint, making the joint painful and immobile.

The signs of osteoarthritis are:

—stiffness or pain in the mornings that lasts only a short while,
—stiffness or pain when moving after being in one position for a period of time,
—some limitation of joint motion,
—joint pain lasting longer than six weeks,
—cracking or grinding sounds when moving a joint,
—swelling or warm skin around a joint, and
—small bumps or nodules at the end of the finger joints if fingers are involved.

The client with osteoarthritis does not complain of an overall tired feeling as does the client with rheumatoid arthritis.

Care for Clients who have Rheumatoid or Osteoarthritis

Many clients who have arthritic conditions seek pain relief from a variety of sources besides medical care prescribed by a physician. For example, for a time, many persons with arthritis purchased copper bracelets to wear. They believed the copper bracelets would cure or ease their arthritic pain. If your client has a particular "cure" or favorite "treatment" for his arthritis, tell your nurse supervisor about it. The nurse, your client, you, and the family may discuss the client's use of the object or procedure.

Although the care for both rheumatoid and osteoarthritis is similar, each client's care plan is based on:

—his general health,
—his specific level of function,
—the severity of his arthritis, and
—his specific needs.

GOUT

Gout is the easiest form of arthritis to identify and care for at home. Gout is most often an inflammation of the great toe, although other body parts can be affected. The toe becomes very painful, swollen, hot, and tender. The problem occurs when excess uric acid builds up in the body. The uric acid forms needle-like crystals that settle in the joint spaces and causes pain. Nearly 90 percent of clients with gout are men.

Clients who have gout will have prescribed medications and may have special diets. You may have to assist the client to carry out the nurse supervisor's instructions for foot care. For example, keep pressure off his feet, including the weight of bed sheets. He may be told to elevate his feet during the day. The nurse supervisor may prepare a schedule that allows him to gradually begin to bear weight on his feet after the pain has subsided. When he has less pain you may also be directed to assist him with range-of-motion exercises for his toes, feet, ankles, and legs.

LUPUS ERYTHEMATOSUS

Lupus is a chronic disease that affects many body parts and systems. Treatment has im-

---

Guidelines for Assisting the Client With Arthritic Conditions

- Allow and encourage him to remain as independent as possible. The nurse supervisor or therapist may assist you to:
  —adjust the schedule of care activities to take advantage of his better times of day, and to
  —recommend or supply special assistive equipment or devices that may assist your client to maintain his independence (discussed in Chapter 6).
- Remind your client to take prescribed medications on time, as ordered by the physician.
- Use splints to help support the joints and keep them in proper position and alignment. Never use splints unless you have been instructed and supervised by the nurse or therapist. They will provide you with the schedule for splints and the correct techniques for your client's splints. Splints should benefit the client, not cause pain or discomfort.
- Assist and encourage correct body positions for your client while standing, sitting, and lying in bed.
- Balance rest, work, and exercise programs and activities. Rest helps reduce the inflammation of the joints. Resting too long in one position allows the joints to become stiff and the muscles to weaken.
- Assist your client, if directed by the nurse, to take a warm (never hot) shower or bath when first arising in the morning. This will help relax the joints and muscles that are stiff and painful in the morning.
- Place warm or cool moist compresses on the painful joints to reduce the pain, **if directed.** These procedures **must** be ordered by the physician. Follow instructions from the nurse supervisor exactly.

- Check heating pads for exact directions about use with compresses. Inspect the condition of the heating pad fabric and coils and the cord.
Never leave a client alone with a heating pad.
Never turn a heating pad on high.
- Provide exercise as directed:
  —Assist with range-of-motion and other exercises, following instructions from the nurse supervisor or therapist. Always check with the nurse supervisor before starting new exercises. Sample exercise programs are included in the Appendix.
  —*Exercise* is important for clients with arthritis because exercise:
    —helps maintain your client's overall physical strength,
    —helps maintain the strength of his bones,
    —increases the blood circulation throughout the body, and
    —improves his sense of well-being.
  —Consider your client when assisting with his exercises.
  —The client may apply heat to painful joints before exercise periods if ordered by the physician. Heat relaxes the joints and reduces pain for the exercises. *Be sure you understand what kind of heat you are to use and for what length of time.*
  —Begin exercises slowly, using small stretches and movements.
  —Repeat range-of-motion exercises to each joint (usually 3 times each joint, gradually building to 10 times each), as the nurse or therapist directs.
  —Conduct exercises 2–4 times a day as directed, for short periods, rather than exercising once a day for a long time.

---

proved so that fewer people die from the disease, but it causes pain and disability. Many people who have lupus also develop an arthritic condition called synovitis. **Synovitis** is an inflammation of the inner lining of the synovial membrane in the joint, similar to rheumatoid arthritis.

Lupus causes pain in the knuckles of the hands, at the middle and at the base of the fingers, in the knees, and sometimes in the

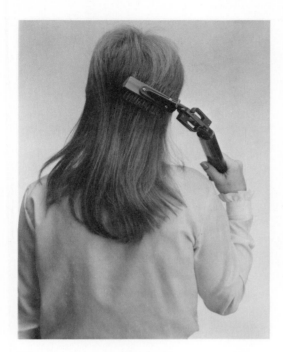

Figure 11-31. *Assistive devices, such as this extended, long-handled hairbrush, enable clients to maintain independent self-care.*
Reprinted by permission of © Bissell Healthcare Corporation/Fred Sammons, Inc.

hips. The joints appear normal, but are painful when moved or touched. Lupus is different for each person. Not all signs appear in every client, but several signs and symptoms usually appear together. In some cases, all symptoms of the disease may disappear after an initial flare-up of the disease. Lupus becomes a chronic problem in other cases. It periodically flares up or progressively worsens throughout the person's life.

The signs of lupus are:

—a reddened rash across the bridge of the nose extending onto one or both cheeks. It may extend onto the chest. The rash looks as if a butterfly were spread across the person's face,
—swelling and pain in the joints,
—low-grade fever,
—loss of appetite and weight loss,
—swollen glands,
—muscle aches,
—nausea and vomiting.

Later changes may include:

—inflammation of the linings of the heart, lungs, and abdominal cavity causing pain and discomfort.
—kidney disease in which the kidneys are unable to remove waste products from the blood. In severe cases the person may have kidney dialysis or a kidney transplant.
—inflammation of the central nervous system that can cause seizures or temporary memory loss.

Because lupus causes different signs and changes in each person, the care plan will be specifically designed for your client's needs. There are, however, some general rules for assisting a client with lupus.

Care for the Client who has Lupus

- Remind him to take his medications as prescribed.
- Balance his rest and exercise programs, avoiding overexertion.
- Limit exposure to the sun, which frequently causes skin irritations and worsening of symptoms.
- Follow the care for arthritic joints as discussed in the sections on rheumatoid arthritis and osteoarthritis.
- Keep him as independent as possible, including encouraging a good mental outlook.
- Report changes in his condition to the nurse supervisor.

PAIN CONTROL WITH ARTHRITIC CONDITIONS

Pain control is a major goal for persons who have arthritic conditions. A relatively new treatment for pain control, called the transcutaneous electrical nerve stimulator unit, or TENS unit, is discussed in the section on Chronic Pain in this chapter.

III
Progressive
Neuromuscular Diseases

Progressive neuromuscular diseases are diseases of the central nervous system that affect the functions and actions of the muscles. These diseases are typically chronic, develop slowly, have progressively worsening symptoms, and although treatable, are not curable. Their causes are not known. As the diseases progress, clients require assistance with their care and activities of daily living.

*P*ARKINSON'S DISEASE

Parkinson's disease is a slowly progressive, chronic disease. It is caused by damage to the part of the brain that produces the chemical dopamine. Dopamine helps nerves communicate to the body how and when it should move. When there is not enough dopamine, the messages between nerves are slowed and confused. Parkinson's disease symptoms are the result of this lost or slowed communication and damage to the brain. The person's symptoms become worse over time. The client may become dependent in many areas of self-care.

The person with Parkinson's disease has:

rigidity: The person has increased muscle tone. However, his muscles work against each other, causing stiffness and resistance to movement. The client therefore has difficulty changing positions and trying to start or stop moving. For example, a client will have difficulty starting his feet to take the steps to walk (Fig. 11-32, *A*). But once able to move, he has difficulty stopping again. He

typically walks with his trunk bent forward, taking short, rapid steps and shuffling his feet (Figure 11-32, *B*).

tremor: Tremors are shaking motions that the person cannot control. A tremor will begin in one part of the body while he is sitting or lying still. The tremor can gradually continue to involve the rest of the body and head. Tremors usually decrease when the client makes voluntary movements such as reaching for a cup or using a fork. They seldom occur during sleep. Tremors of the tongue and jaw can interfere with eating and talking. A motion called "pill rolling" may develop. The client appears to be rolling a small object between his fingers and thumb.

lack of expression: Clients who have Parkinson's disease cannot control the muscles that produce facial expressions. Therefore, they may develop blank looks on their faces. The client may appear not to blink or to react to conversations. *There is no mental deteriora-*

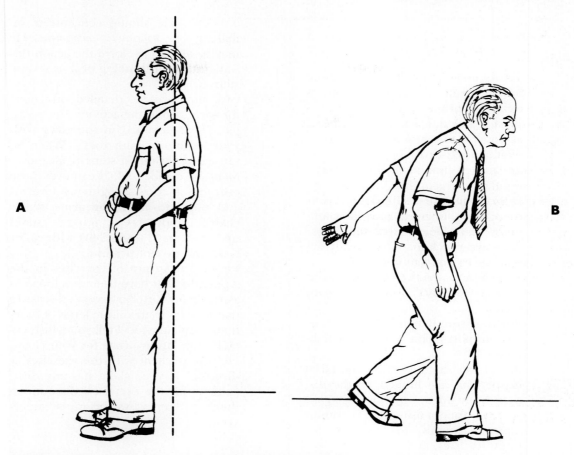

Figure 11-32. **A,** *The client who has Parkinson's disease may lean backwards, without knowing he is doing so, when he stands in one place.* **B,** *The client who has Parkinson's disease tends to lean forward with his body while walking and may shuffle his steps.*

tion with this disease. The lack of reaction is a result of damaged communication in the brain. *It is not a mental problem.*

other signs: Clients may have various signs common to the disease. For example, there may be drooling. The client does not have true dysphagia, but may have difficulty starting to swallow. While waiting to swallow, saliva collects in the mouth and causes drooling. Similarly, his speech may be slurred and the client may require time to respond verbally. This is because he needs time to start the muscles moving to talk. *But his mind is clear.* At times, clients may also experience **vertigo** or have difficulty catching themselves once they start to fall.

The client's care plan may include the following ways for you to assist your client.

Performing self-care activities boosts self-esteem. The person with Parkinson's disease should "do for himself" as long as possible, even when it takes more time. Assist him to use self-help devices when the nurse supervisor determines that he can no longer perform an activity without the assistive device. Encourage him, take the time, and be willing to work with your client's abilities. Praise, interest in his activities, and patience go a long way toward helping his outlook.

Care for the Client who has Parkinson's Disease

—Treat him as an adult. Remember he has no mental deficits. Be sure others treat him properly as well.

—Be sure he does as much for himself as possible to maintain his independence in self-care.

—Encourage him to do his exercises regularly.

—Inform your nurse supervisor if your client has changes in moods or attitudes, or becomes depressed.

—Allow time for him to react to instructions or respond to questions.

—Help him to practice techniques and routines to "start" and "stop" as directed.

—Provide stimulation, conversation, and support of his interests or hobbies.

—Remember that his verbal and facial expressions are limited by the disease. Your nurse supervisor may instruct you about using other communication modes to discover his interests, likes, and dislikes.

—Maintain his appearance, well-being, and personal hygiene.

—Provide a safe environment without unnecessary restrictions.

—Praise his efforts even when he is not successful.

Daily Exercises

The following techniques may be ordered for your client. Practice them with your nurse supervisor before trying them with your client. You may be directed to help your client practice them.

1. Encourage the client to use **one continuous motion** while completing an activity. For example, he may be able to pick up a fork, but cannot follow through to his mouth. Encourage the client to pick up the fork and move it to his mouth as

one step. He should concentrate on making *one continuous movement.* He may be able to perform the action this way instead of thinking of it as several steps.

2. Give him precise, detailed directions for each step in the activity. For example, "Lean forward in the chair with your 'nose over your toes'." When he can accomplish these steps in one movement, he can be told, "Lean over, nose over toes . . . now straighten your arms and push down on the arms of the chair . . . and, keep going . . . stand up." (See Fig. 11-33.) Start with easier tasks and do not tire him.

3. Review the group of exercises in the Appendix that have been developed to assist clients with Parkinson's disease to maintain their maximum levels of function. Your nurse will tell you which exercises are appropriate for your client. Help your client with the exercises as directed. If your client has any difficulties with the exercises, discontinue them and report to the nurse supervisor.

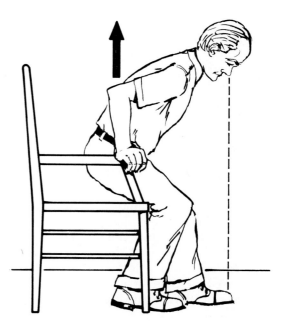

Figure 11-33. *The client who has Parkinson's disease can use specific techniques to help him move and ambulate.*

MULTIPLE SCLEROSIS

Multiple Sclerosis (M.S.) is a disease that causes disability among young adults during their productive working years and their childbearing/childrearing years. M.S. affects more women than men, and appears between the ages of 20 and 40. Clients are generally under age 60. There is a great deal of research on M.S. and new treatments are being developed. Neither the cause nor a cure have been found.

M.S. may begin with a single symptom that occurred years ago and went unnoticed. Double vision or tingling fingers are examples. Once the disease appears more fully, the earlier symptom may be remembered and recognized as having been an indication of the onset of the disease. Some clients have a mild form of the disease that does not cause disability. Others have recurring problems, but sometimes the disease apparently stays in **remission.** Most of the clients who need your care will have the progressive, disabling forms of M.S. Your client may not know which form of the disease he has because only time will tell the full extent of his disability.

M.S. is different for each client because of the way the disease affects the body. The disease affects the central nervous system by destroying the protective coverings (myelin sheaths) surrounding the nerve fibers in the brain and spinal cord. The destruction of the protective myelin leaves a hardened scar tissue (plaque). The plaque halts or disrupts the normal communication between the brain and nerves. This process may take years or occur quickly. Damage to nerves and myelin can occur in any place in the nervous system so that different activities are interrupted for each individual.

Common Disabling Conditions Associated with M.S.

1. *Bowel and Bladder Dysfunctions:* One of the earliest signs of M.S. is a **frequent and urgent need to urinate.** Incontinence and a tendency to develop urinary stones may develop later in the disease. A schedule that allows the client time to use the toilet frequently may prevent or minimize urinary incontinence.

Bowel problems may be successfully managed by following a consistent and careful dietary plan. Some will use stool softeners, suppositories, or perhaps an occasional enema. Your nurse supervisor will establish bowel and bladder programs with your client. Read about bladder and bowel training programs in Chapter 2.

2. *Fatigue:* All clients with M.S. experience **fatigue.** At times fatigue may become so overwhelming that a client will begin to do something and then become too tired to finish. You can assist by planning activities with several breaks scheduled early in the morning and after naps.

3. *Difficulty swallowing:* Clients may have **difficulty swallowing.** Your client needs fluids, even though they are difficult for him to swallow. He may have a special diet to assist him to swallow. Chapter 7, which discusses stroke, gives specific care methods for difficulty in swallowing.

4. *Sensory losses:* Clients may have **sensory losses,** such as visual difficulties and decreased sense of touch. If your client cannot read, you may offer books on cassette tapes or other reading aids. Be sure the visual problems do not alter his balance before walking with him.

5. *Sensitivity to heat:* Clients who have M.S. are **sensitive to heat.** When bathing your client, the temperature of the water must be lukewarm, even cool (**not over 84 degrees F.**). Fatigue is increased in hot and humid weather.

6. *Limitations:* The common limitations associated with M.S. will vary among clients. Generally, you may be directed to assist your client with:

—his self-care activities,
—moving and positioning,
—other needs according to his level of functioning,
—safe mobility,
—preventing skin breakdown,
—maintaining good circulation, and
—providing comfort measures for symptoms.

He may have:

—muscle weakness, tremors, or spasticity, and

—difficulty walking, carrying objects, or moving.

Your nurse supervisor or the physical therapist will instruct you about the client's specific exercises, walking activities, or range-of-motion exercises. Practice under their direction before you begin to work with your client.

7. *Emotional and psychological stresses:* The client and family can become emotionally and psychologically occupied with concerns about the outcome of the disease. They must cope with the grieving process common to disabling conditions, complications of the disease, and a stressful on-going anxiety about the future. M.S. can also alter the client's moods. For example, the disease can produce a euphoria that is not appropriate to the situation. You can assist in a number of ways.

Care for the Client who has M.S.

- Listen as an active and supportive listener.
- Keep him as independent as possible.
- Attend to his bladder problems as directed.
- Check water temperature and exposure to heat.
- Allow intervals of rest and plan to avoid fatigue.
- Provide the prescribed diet and remind him of medications.
- Encourage him, even in little things.
- Maintain good personal hygiene.
- Prevent skin breakdown and other problems of immobility.
- Assist with exercises as directed.
- Keep a safe environment.
- Report changes in his condition or behavior to the nurse.

PART IV

The Client with a Terminal Condition

THE CONCEPT OF HOSPICE FOR CARE

THE HOSPICE CONCEPT

Hospice is a concept for providing care so that clients who have terminal conditions can die at home or in a home-like setting. Many families want to care for their dying family members, but either cannot do so alone or fear caring for them at home. The hospice concept provides regular care assistance to families and dying clients. The amount of direct assistance varies with each situation. Usually the level of care increases as the client approaches death.

Hospice is not only for clients who have terminal cancer, although a large number of hospice clients do have cancer. Many people do not know that hospice programs provide service to clients with many terminal conditions. Hospice is included in many home care programs. It is often a free-standing agency, or it may include both hospital and home care services. The overall goals are to:

—provide 24 hour/day 7 days per week on-call service;
—care for the client who has a terminal condition;
—provide physical, emotional, and spiritual comfort to the dying client and his family;
—provide control of symptoms related to the terminal condition;
—assist the client to die peacefully in his home;
—provide relief from pain and suffering as possible; and
—maintain the client's dignity as a person.

Some hospice programs have a bereavement or aftercare program to assist a family to cope and adjust after a client's death.

The nurse supervisor will develop the care plan for the client and family in the hospice program. Each client will have individual physical and emotional needs. Each family will have special needs related to having the client die at home. The nurse supervisor will instruct you about working comfortably with the dying client and his family. In general you will consider:

—your own attitudes and beliefs about death and working with a dying client.
—the stages of grieving as part of the dying process.
—various means of providing comfort and physical care specific for each individual dying client.
—environmental influences on the client's level of comfort.
—the importance of quietly listening to the client and family if they express their fears, wishes, and ideas.
—advantages and stresses of a client dying in the home.
—how the age of the person influences the family reactions.
—differences in attitudes, beliefs, and customs about death in various cultural, religious, and ethnic groups.
—spiritual and emotional needs of the dying client.
—death as a stage in the life cycle.

The two most common activities in hospice care are keeping the client comfortable and assisting him with controlling unpleasant symptoms. Although you will be instructed about the emotional needs of the client and his family, your assistance is most important with comfort and symptom control. This is the essence of care.

COMMON CARE NEEDS ASSOCIATED WITH HOSPICE CLIENTS

- *Pain*—Pain control is the greatest and most common hospice need. The pain for many of these clients cannot be eliminated or relieved, but it may be controlled. Each person is the authority on his own pain. The idea is to give the pain reliever just before it is needed so that the client does not have to continually go in and out of pain. This means that the pain reliever may not be given on a set schedule or at certain hours.

  You may be directed to look for certain changes in your client so that you can notify the nurse supervisor before the client has pain. Pain control may be medications, special narcotic "cocktails," or other pain blocks used in conjunction with relaxation or other mental techniques. There need be no concern about the dying client becoming addicted to narcotic drugs.

- *Anxiety, fear, or emotional upsets*—The nurse supervisor will provide your client with assistance in these areas. If you are alone with the client or his family during an emotional upset, follow the instructions you have been given for that client and family. If in doubt, be a quiet listener. Contact your nurse supervisor as soon as possible and report what happened.

- *Comfort*—Most of your attention will be directed to assisting the client to be as comfortable as possible. As the dying process continues, many hospice clients have physical problems that produce discomfort or distress. Call the nurse supervisor and report any of these changes in the client's physical or emotional condition:
  —pain
  —nausea and vomiting
  —diarrhea
  —constipation
  —dry mouth sensations
  —coughing
  —difficulty breathing
  —difficulty swallowing
  —decreased appetite
  —skin breakdown leading to pressure sores
  —itching skin
  —body odor and "bad breath"
  —hiccoughs
  —swelling and congestion
  —weakness and dizziness
  —loss of contact with reality or hallucinations
  —difficulty getting to sleep and having restful sleep
  —anxiety and fears
  —restlessness and confusion

There are signs that may occur when a client is actively dying. The nurse supervisor will have informed the family about these signs. They may choose to call the clergy or minister and significant persons. Notify your nurse supervisor if you notice any of these changes occurring with your client:

—loss of body functions
—loss of muscle control
—"twitching" of the body or body parts
—changes in skin color
—hallucinations
—reduced respirations with periods of no respirations
—increased restlessness
—loss of consciousness
—"picking at the air" with his hands
—a "death rattle"
—gradual drop in blood pressure
—drop in pulse rate (pulse rate may increase on occasion)
—withdrawal from others, desire to be alone
—statements about fear, anger, or resentment that are changes in his behavior
—stops communication and may appear depressed
—statements that he "knows death is soon"

Courtesy Ann Liebers, RN, MSN, Exec. Dir. (Hospice of Morris County, New Jersey).

The hospice nurse is authorized in many states to pronounce death when the client dies. If you are alone with the client and you believe he has died, call the nurse supervisor.

You may have been instructed to call the rescue squad, emergency medical unit, the physician, and the clergy or minister. Stay calm and assist others to remain calm. Listen to the wishes of the family members. Remember that people express their grief in different ways. After the client dies, you may be instructed to assist with bathing and preparing the body.

Take time to discuss your feelings and reactions to the client's death. You may talk with your nurse supervisor or your own clergy or minister. This is important for you when you work with hospice clients. It will help you to assist your clients and their families in other hospice situations. It will also assist you to keep a positive attitude about living and dying.

AMYOTROPHIC LATERAL SCLEROSIS (ALS)

Amyotrophic Lateral Sclerosis (ALS) is a progressive terminal disease that affects the nerves in the brain and spinal cord. The disease occurs most often in white men between 40 and 80 years of age. The cause is still unknown. As with M.S. and Alzheimer's disease, the parts of the nervous system that are diseased will determine the first areas affected by the disease. The symptoms are:

—muscle weakness,
—difficulty chewing and swallowing,
—difficulty with speech,
—difficulty breathing, and
—emotional concerns, such as depression and anxiety.

Clients may live at home with little or no assistance until they cannot perform self-care. They often require a **tracheostomy** (Fig. 11-34) and a mechanical ventilator.

Clients become increasingly weaker and lose muscle functions, such as respiratory function or swallowing, causing aspirations. They eventually die within 2–10 years from complications. As this disease reaches its final stage, some clients and families may chose a *hospice* program, enabling the client to die at home. The family of a client who has ALS will experience stresses and grieving in response to this devastating disease.

Clients who have ALS do not lose their

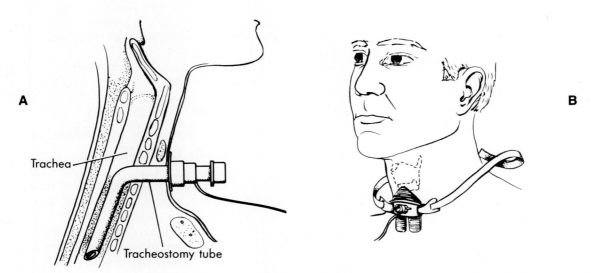

Figure 11-34. *A side view shows how a tracheostomy tube provides an airway from the trachea to the external neck.*

B, *A tracheostomy tube is secured around the client's neck with a gauze tie. The dressing and tracheostomy tube are cleaned by the nurse.*

cognitive abilities. They are very aware of what is happening with their conditions. Each client will respond and cope in his own way. The process of grieving is discussed in Chapter 1.

A nurse supervisor will be closely involved with this type of client. You may be responsible for specific care activities for a client with ALS, especially in the earlier stages of the disease. Many of the rehabilitation techniques in this book will be suitable for the home care of these clients. The nurse supervisor may include them in the client's care plan. For example, proper positioning, personal care, and prevention of pressure areas apply to all clients in your care.

*A*IDS

AIDS/ARC or Acquired Immune Deficiency Syndrome/AIDS Related Conditions: (Read about Universal Infection Control Precautions in Chapter 1).

Acquired Immune Deficiency Syndrome or **AIDS** is a disease caused by the HTLV-3 virus. AIDS is a syndrome because it is a group of signs and symptoms that include a number of other diseases and conditions. The virus attacks the **immune system.** This is the body system that fights off and resists infections and diseases. The virus weakens the body's resistance over several years and eventually destroys the immune system. Without the protection of the immune system, a client is susceptible to diseases and viruses that usually would not cause him to become ill or infected. It is these diseases and viruses that eventually cause him to die.

AIDS is transmitted from one infected person to an uninfected person by:

—sexual contact with an infected person. This includes oral/rectal, vaginal, and oral sexual encounters.
—sharing needles with an infected person.
—pregnancy and birth; infected mothers may transmit AIDS to their babies while pregnant or during the birth process.
—receiving a blood transfusion infected by AIDS.

Testing

A number of new blood tests are being developed to detect the presence of antibodies for the virus, but only one test is in general use at this writing. If this test is positive, it means that the person has been exposed to the virus at some time (HIV positive). Although it does not mean the person will contract AIDS, it does mean that he is able to spread the virus to others. But a negative test result does not mean that the person is free of the virus. It takes the body time to produce antibodies following exposure to the virus. If a person is tested before he has developed antibodies he may spread the virus without knowing he is doing so.

An AIDS carrier is a person who has the virus but may not become ill for a long time. He may never become ill. Other persons may develop ARC (AIDS Related Complex) years or months after the initial infection with the virus. The symptoms are persistent; although relatively mild, they can be fatal.

The person may develop AIDS years after the initial infection. The symptoms worsen as the body becomes overwhelmed with infections or disease. This is a terminal condition and you may care for your client in a hospice.

Concerns for Clients who have AIDS or ARC

AIDS is an emotionally upsetting and physically debilitating disease that results in death. At this time there is no cure for AIDS. AIDS clients need respect, care, attention, a sense of hope, and communication with others. The client, his family, and friends can all be expected to experience the grieving process. Additionally, the client or family may have feelings of guilt, embarassment, or anger about the client having the disease. Spiritual strength and assistance may be important resources for the client and his family. The diagnosis of AIDS may place a stigma on the entire family or group, isolating them from the rest of the community. Friends and family may fear contracting the disease. They may have a very real sense of loss of control of the situation. Confidentiality is very important.

Signs and Symptoms of AIDS

The signs and symptoms of AIDS are related to the damaged immune system. They will vary according to the type of bacterial or viral agent that invades the body. Clients who have AIDS can be expected to develop more than one infection at a time. They may have the symptoms and complications of several diseases. The common symptoms clearly indicate the need for a great deal of care. Your nurse supervisor will develop a care plan for your client and evaluate it as his condition changes. The common symptoms last two weeks or longer. They are:

—fatigue;
—fever;
—sweating at night;
—diarrhea (may become incontinent);
—nausea;
—weight loss, usually gradual at first;
—forgetfulness or other mental changes;
—shaking or seizures;
—speech or vision impairments;
—skin lesions and tendency for skin breakdown;
—pulmonary infections, may develop cough or Tuberculosis (TB);
—pain (varies); and
—loss of functional abilities over time until dependent and in bed for activities of daily living.

You will need to use the Universal Infection Control Precautions detailed in Chapter 1 to protect yourself from possible contamination. You will also use these precautions to protect your client from exposure to bacteria and viruses that will cause him to acquire additional infections. The Universal Precautions should be used for *all* clients. There is no way to know who has or who has not been infected.

Care for the Client who has AIDS

Most care for the client who has AIDS is directed at preventing transmission and spread of infection, and toward maintaining his maximum level of comfort and a postive attitude. Your nurse supervisor will inform you about the specific care plans for each client. As a general rule, follow the list below:

- Prevent skin breakdown. This may become more challenging as he loses his appetite, has increased nausea, reduces fluid intake, and has more diarrhea. Keep a schedule for turning your client.
- Provide excellent mouth care several times each day. The client's toothbrush, toothpaste, dental floss, waterpik, and other oral care products are kept for his own personal use. These items are never shared with others.
- Use an oral thermometer. Never share the thermometer with others. Wash with soapy water, rinse and wipe clean after each use. Use an axillary thermometer for a small child or infant. Soak for at least 10 minutes in a 70 percent alcohol solution.
- Maintain good grooming. Use an electric shaver rather than a blade to reduce transmission of the virus. The client should not share cosmetics.
- Assist with persistent diarrhea. Keep his skin clean and dry, follow dietary guidelines, add an incontinent pad as needed. Keep area odor-free and clean toilet or commode after each use.
- Exercise your client according to the instructions from the nurse supervisor. Prevent contractures, immobility, and poor circulation, and encourage relaxation.
- Provide nutritious meals according to prescribed diet. If he has a poor appetite or is nauseous, he may not be feeling well enough to eat foods that are difficult to chew.
  —Offer custards, eggnogs, and soups as healthful incentives.
  —Add lemon to season many foods. Present the food in an attractive manner. Add music and flowers if he enjoys them.

—Offer smaller meals, up to six each day, instead of large meals.

—Avoid fried foods.

—Offer dry toast, clear liquids, soft foods, or pureed foods if he is nauseated or has a sore mouth.

—Avoid talking about your client. Remember that communication can be verbal and non-verbal. Your client will read your body language and attitudes.

● Prevent further transmission of the infection:

—Wear gloves and a gown or apron when needed.

—Practice good personal hygiene for yourself.

—Inform the nurse supervisor if you develop a yeast infection.

—Inform your nurse supervisor if your client has any white deposits on his tongue or mucous membranes.

—Dispose of linens, products, and body fluids properly.

—Practice excellent handwashing techniques.

—Use the 1–10 Clorox solution.

—Wear gloves and a face mask when appropriate.

● Report any changes in the client's condition to the nurse supervisor.

Appendix A

*T*RAVELING WITH A DISABILITY

During the past ten years, the mechanisms for local and world travel have become opened to persons with disabilities. This has occurred almost without exception for the person's age or physical limitations. There are still barriers for persons with disabilities. For example, not all parts of the world have wheelchair accessible buildings and toilets. However, many changes have been made to make places more accessible to clients. Likewise, assistive devices and equipment have been designed to help a client with a disability to travel even when the environment is not as accessible as would be desired. (Figure A-1)

Many persons use tours designed for travel with disabilities and have specialized services while others decide to travel alone or with personal attendants. You may have the opportunity to accompany a disabled traveler. As a caregiver, there are certain precautions that you should be aware of, as well as some pointers that will make the travel easier and safer.

Discuss a client's special travel needs with the nurse supervisor. The client should visit his physician before embarking on a trip. The client and his family are primarily responsible for travel arrangements. Whether the trip is a long one or only a short one, the

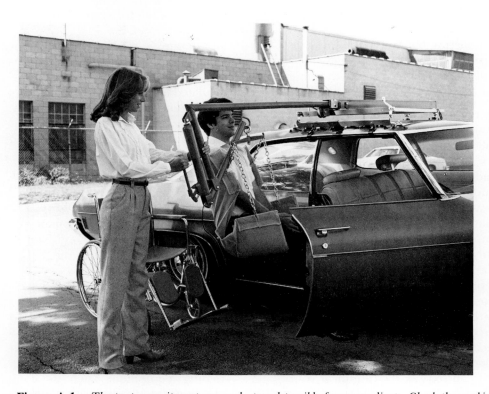

Figure A-1. *The proper equipment can make travel possible for many clients. Check the working order of equipment before traveling and be sure you or others know how to operate it safely.*

first step is to plan ahead and anticipate needs your client may have as you travel. You may wish to consult the following list of suggestions before traveling with a client:

1. Contact a reliable travel agent who:
   has worked with disabled persons before, and
   has full access to all forms of travel and accommodations.
2. Make reservations:
   as early as possible,
   state your client's specific special travel needs,
   specify special dietary needs
   arrange for points of departure and arrival,
3. Confirm reservations:
   indicate the clients needs when you confirm the reservations,
   confirm dietary orders for special meals,
   check arrival and departure times for changes and change other reservations accordingly.

   Examples:
   wheelchair to get on and off aircraft,
   crutches,
   precautions for blindness, deafness, or speech difficulties,
   or a disabled client who is traveling alone.

4. Carry necessary papers:
   physician's letter validating special needs,
   prescriptions for medications and aides, such as eyeglasses,
   health insurance papers, especially if traveling abroad and using international health insurance,
   complete personal identification and any Medic Alert tags for emergencies,
   telephone numbers of branch offices for equipment or care services.
5. Prepare for oxygen use if your client may require oxygen:
   specify oxygen when making reservations,
   notify an oxygen distributor at your destination,
   remind travel staff about your client's oxygen needs,

   remind travel staff of the special precautions necessary when oxygen is being used.
   liquid oxygen is the easiest for car travel. It can be refilled enroute.
   if you use a concentrator, a car battery and an oxygen concentrator can be adapted to operate together,
   carry oxygen tanks in the trunk of the car. The tanks should be securely tied and lie on their sides
6. Arrange to carry with you:
   medications and bottled water to take them,
   a small amount of supplies, about a week's extra supply if you are traveling internationally,
   small towels, soap, and pre-moistened wipes,
   urology or other specialty supplies, if used,
   a change of clothing for your client in case travel delays occur or your client has travel problems.
   motion sickness medications or skin patches, if prescribed.
   snacks suitable for your client's diet, in case of delays.
   an adaptor if electricity is used for equipment or heat cleaning of contact lens.
   insulated bags with reusable ice packs for items that require refrigeration.
   foam pillows if client is allergic to feather pillows or bedding.

   Carry these items with you onto the plane, train, bus, or car. **Do not allow them to be checked with other baggage.**

7. Consider special rental equipment for travel:
   —disposable supplies, including urology items,
   —gel cell batteries for motorized wheelchairs (These are the only ones airlines will allow. Check to see if your client's motorized wheelchair has a dual purpose charger for gel or water batteries.)
   —folding equipment such as commodes or tub benches with their own carry cases. (These will travel as baggage.)

—narrower wheelchairs for airline or other aisles; (wheelchairs are not counted as baggage although if too large, they are carried with the baggage. Clients use an airline wheelchair to enter and exit the aircraft).

8. Plan for changes:

be aware of the number of time zones you cross in travel and the effect this can have on your client.

prepare for climate changes with proper clothing changes, fluids, or medications,

anticipate your client's needs by securing necessary supplies when they are available.

where air pollution or ozone readings are high consider traveling early in the morning or later at night.

9. Some information to remember:

- Many bus lines allow a caregiver or companion to travel free of charge with a disabled person. A seeing eye dog may also travel along side the person.
- Trains are usually wheelchair access-ible, even allowing persons to use their own wheelchairs.
- Cruises are readily available for disabled travelers if requests for travel and accommodations are made early.
- At least two major rental car companies have rental cars equipped with driving hand controls for the disabled driver. Reservations must be made at least ten days in advance; in more remote locations, allow more time.
- Throughout the country, most facilities have or are creating wheelchair accessible accommodations. However, there is a wide range of variation as to what is considered accessible. When making reservations, check carefully about the accommodations. If your client has very specific needs, you may have to ask precisely about the accessibility. For example, a mechanical lift may make the hotel or cruise ship swimming pool accessible to your client (Figure A-2). Use the toll-free calling

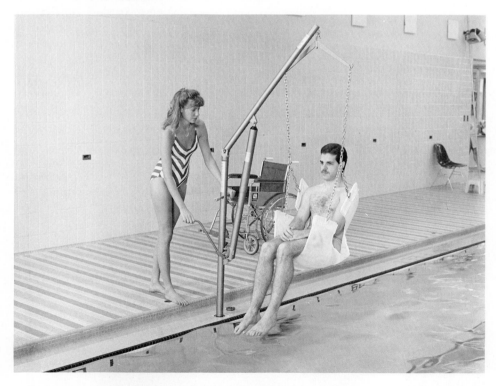

Figure A-2. *Planning ahead for a mechanical lift can make the pool available for a client who uses swimming as a form of recreation or relaxation.*

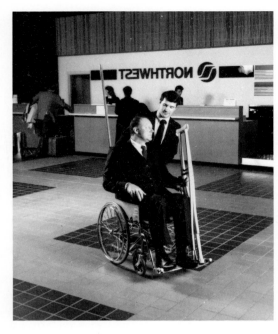

Figure A-3. *Airlines have many services available for clients who require assistance. It is advisable to call ahead to reserve for special needs. Improvements in air travel services and access for persons with disabilities are being developed.*

number when making reservations at hotel chains and requesting disabled facility information.

- A client will not be allowed to board an aircraft using his own wheelchair. He will be assisted to his seat in an airline "carry chair"; then he may slide or be lifted into the aircraft seat (Figure A-3).
- Most airlines reserve the bulkhead aisle seats for disabled travelers in order to give them as much room as possible and provide for safer exit in case of an emergency.

At this time the FAA is developing regulations about the types and locations of seating for persons with disabilities on aircraft. New access features and assistive equipment are being designed for commercial aircraft. These include accessible lavatory compartments, specialized crates for shipping wheelchair parts and batteries, and on-board wheelchairs with movable aisle armrests that permit seating in the standard space.

Wheelchairs and other equipment that are lightweight and compact are available for some persons. These are less burdensome and more maneuverable. Younger clients are often pleased with the style features of some new equipment. (Figure A-4).

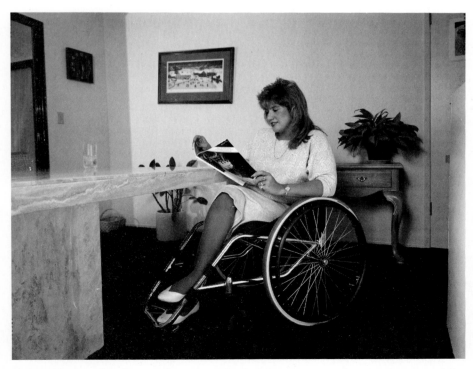

Figure A-4. *"Ultra-lite" weight and stylish wheelchairs are examples of the design and feature changes of wheelchairs. The new equipment can be maneuvered more easily.*

Appendix B

_T_HERAPEUTIC DIETS AND NUTRITION

General Guidelines

Fluids and foods are essential for all people. Clients who have chronic or debilitating conditions often require special therapeutic diets. Therapeutic diets may be designed to restore strength and energies, to maintain good health, to avoid a problematic food, to correct a deficiency, or to restrict or increase caloric intake. Therapeutic diets provide precise information about the fluids and foods to be served. Directions may include amounts and kinds of foods, times for serving foods or fluids, ways in which foods are to be prepared or combined, and foods to be avoided.

To assist your client with his therapeutic diet:

—Prepare only the foods that are ordered for his diet.
—Cook foods as ordered.
—Arrange foods so that they look attractive, and make sure they are hot or cold, as appropriate.
—Follow the meal plan completely; do not substitute.
—Serve meals at the designated times.
—Assist him with self-care or assistive devices as needed.
—Assist him to have food or fluids available with his medications when medications must be taken in combination with foods.
—See that he avoids prohibited foods; this will prevent food and medication interactions.
—Inform your nurse supervisor about changes in your client's:
  —eating habits
  —ability to chew or swallow foods
  —digestive upsets
  —potential food allergies

—amount of foods or fluids consumed
—bowel and bladder elimination patterns
—Read about nutrition in Chapter 2 and about special techniques for assisting clients who have difficulty with swallowing.

Dehydration

Dehydration can become a serious condition. It occurs when the amount of fluids in the body tissues is reduced, which also results in lost electrolytes. Stress or injury; debilitating conditions; illnesses causing vomiting, diarrhea, fever, cold-like symptoms with mucus production, or excessive perspiration; and reduced fluid intake may alter the volume of fluids and the electrolyte balance. Dehydration may not be suspected at first, especially if the client is drinking fluids.

Be alert and report the following signs of dehydration to the nurse supervisor:

—dry, itching skin
—reduced amount of urine output
—increased or excessive thirst
—abdominal cramping
—headache
—shortness or heaviness of breath
—constipation
—listlessness or mild discomfort

Types of Diets

Table B-1 offers general information about commonly ordered types of diets. With this information, you can identify foods on your client's diet and know why they are selected. This information _does not replace_ the instructions from your nurse supervisor or dieti-

Table B-1   Commonly Ordered Diets

Regular diet—A client on a regular diet does not require a special diet. He should eat a balanced selection of foods from all food groups. As a preventive measure, he should avoid a high fat intake and include high-fiber foods, complex carbohydrates, and plenty of fluids.

Bland diet—These foods are mild and easy to digest and contain little roughage. They are baked, poached, and boiled but are never fried. Nonirritating, bland foods tend to be served without spices or seasonings, at medium temperatures, and are often soft or creamed.

Liquid diets—Liquid diets are usually offered for short periods following illness or surgery. A client may eat a *clear liquid* diet followed by a *full liquid* diet until he has recuperated and can tolerate a soft diet.

Soft and mechanical diets—Soft diet foods are easily digestible semisolid foods such as eggs, pureed or creamed foods, or soft custards. Soft meals are given to clients progressing from liquid diets. Mechanical soft diets include many of the same foods as a regular diet except the foods have been chopped, pureed, or strained for clients who have difficulty swallowing, chewing, or digesting. Special *dysphagia diets* are offered in stages but are generally based on combinations of soft and mechanical diets.

Residue diets—Residue diets refer to the amount of bulk or residue they create in the colon. Low-residue diets are used for clients who have rectal or colon diseases or diarhhea. *Low-residue* foods are similar to soft and bland foods that do not irritate the colon. *High-residue* foods stimulate peristalsis and help prevent constipation. High-residue foods are high-fiber foods.

Diabetic and calorie diets—Clients may have diets that are designed to simply increase or decrease their caloric intake; these are high-calorie or low-calorie diets. A diabetic diet also requires you to measure caloric values of the foods. The amounts of carbohydrates, fat, and protein are also calculated in the diet. The insulin-dependent client with diabetes must coordinate his nutritional intake with his insulin. Other clients may be able to control their diabetes by careful food intake and recording.

Low-fat and low-cholesterol diets—Low-fat and low-cholesterol diets help reduce or control the amount of cholesterol in the bloodstream and assist clients who have difficulties with fat digestion. The relationship of fat and cholesterol is not clear, but fat intake may be related to increased cholesterol production in the body, even when cholesterol is not present in the food. This diet often corresponds with a low-calorie diet.

High-protein diet— The increase of protein in the diet promotes body tissue building and repair for debilitated clients and assists in healing wounds or pressure sores. High-protein diets may place a heavy load on the kidneys, so clients must drink plenty of fluids. Increased protein is usually added by supplementing regular meals or by using commercially prepared supplements.

Low-sodium or sodium-restricted diet—Many clients will be limiting the amount of sodium in their diets. Removing the salt shaker from the table and not adding salt during cooking are only beginning steps in reducing dietary sodium. You will be given explicit guidelines for the amount of sodium your client is allowed in his diet. Be alert for foods that contain hidden sodium. Assist your client and the family to learn to use herbs and spices as alternatives to salt for seasoning foods.

cian, who will direct you in detail about the specific diet for your client. Some clients may have more than one type of diet to follow. Special attention must be given to help these clients avoid restricted foods. Learn to read the labels of food products. You may be surprised at many of the ingredients in foods. For example, salt and sugar are both added to many brands of canned kidney beans. Canned soups and vegetables are high in sodium; however, new low-sodium soups and vegetables are now being offered by some companies. Fresh or frozen vegetables are still preferable nutritional choices.

If you, your client, or the family has questions about the diet or how to modify the diet to better suit your client's preferences, the nurse supervisor may request a dietitian to visit the home and plan specific meals. You may be instructed to assist your client and the family with a dietary diary, food log, or record of intake and output. As a general rule, you will be given a prepared dietary form or flow sheet and instructed to write down the foods and fluids your client consumes during the time you are with him. You will record the times and amounts he ate or drank and which foods or fluids. You may be directed to record other information, including measured urinary output. Review household measuring items with the dietitian, such as one cup or a glassful, to be sure the same measurements are used by everyone. If a client weighs his food on a food scale, learn to use

the scale accurately; some scales weigh in grams, and there are many versions.

Nutrients in Foods

When a client's body is under emotional or physical stress, he may require a diet high in a specific nutrient. Vitamins, minerals, fats, proteins, and carbohydrates are the types of nutrients in foods that are used by the body. Table B-2 lists foods that are high in specific vitamins or minerals. Foods that may affect the body in specific ways, such as laxative effects, are included also. Be sure a food is allowed in your client's therapeutic diet before buying or serving it. Remember to encourage your client to drink plenty of fluids unless they are specifically restricted.

Table B-2.   Nutrients in Foods

Foods high in sodium

—canned soups
—ham, bacon, smoked meats
—cheeses
—hot dogs, lunch meats
—commercial bakery items
—olives, pickles
—peanut butter
—crackers, pretzels, chips
—broths, bouillon
—canned vegetables
—salt added to foods
—soy sauce, Worcestershire sauce
—condiments, seasoning mixes
—croutons, other toppings

Foods high in potassium

—bananas
—oranges, orange juice
—coffee
—tomato juice
—certain cola beverages
—cereal grains

Foods high in fiber

—oats, oat bran
—raw fruits
—potatoes, brown rice
—nuts
—wheat bran, whole grains
—raw vegetables
—dried lentils, beans, peas
—popcorn

Foods high in calcium

—milk, cheese, yogurt
—dried fruits
—cheeses
—potatoes
—green and leafy vegetables
—calcium-fortified foods
—macaroni products
—molasses, brown sugar

Foods high in iron

—egg yolks
—liver, organ meats
—green leafy vegetables
—whole-grain breads, cereals

Continued.

Table B-2. Nutrients in Foods—cont'd

Foods high in fat or cholesterol

Read labels carefully. "No cholesterol" does not mean "low fat." A high-fat diet is undesirable: The fat may be converted to cholesterol in the body.

—saturated fats and lard
—marbled fatty red meats
—egg yolks
—coconut, macadamia nuts
—snack crackers
—chocolate, rich desserts

—sausages, fatty ground beef
—butter, whole dairy products
—pastries, Danish
—coconut or palm oil products
—liver, organ meats
—cream, whipped toppings

Foods low in fat or cholesterol

—fresh fruits
—soft "lite" margarine
—turkey, chicken: no skin
—skim milk products
—dried beans, lentils

—fresh vegetables
—fish (poached, broiled, or steamed)
—whole grains, especially oatmeal and oat bran
—rice, pasta

Notes on low fat and cholesterol:
- —check low-fat dairy products; some substitute undesirable ingredients such as palm or coconut oils
- —olive oil, nuts, unhydrogenated peanut butter, and avocados contain unsaturated vegetable fats
- —do not fry any foods; remove visible fat and skin from meat

Foods that may promote acidity of the urine

—cranberries, prunes, plums
—peanuts, walnuts, filberts
—corn, lentils, navy beans
—tapioca or rice puddings

—oil and vinegar dressing
—chicken, duck, lean beef
—whole-grain, enriched cereals
—macaroni products

Foods that may reduce the acidity of the urine

—orange or tomato juice
—almonds, chestnuts
—olives
—potatoes
—raisins, other dried fruits
—milk products, malts

—lemonade
—coconut, molasses
—cantaloupes, citrus fruits
—lima or soy beans
—spinach or beet greens
—flavored sodas

Foods that may produce flatus

—cabbage, sauerkrauts
—fried or fatty foods
—beer, carbonated drinks
—eggs
—cheeses

—broccoli, cauliflower
—onions
—some fish
—melons
—bean soups

Foods that may have a laxative effect

—prunes, prune juice
—fresh fruits
—fatty foods

—fresh fruits, watermelon
—chocolate
—coffee, teas

Foods that may have a constipating effect

—rice
—peanut butter
—some cheeses

—applesauce, apple peel
—bananas
—inadequate fluid intake

Table B-2. Nutrients in Foods—cont'd

Foods that may irritate the colon

—raw salad vegetables
—potato skins
—coarse grain products
—dried fruits
—mushrooms, corn, peas
—fried foods

—certain raw fruits
—nuts, seeds, coconut
—spicy seasonings, pepper, herbs
—pickles, olives
—tomatoes, dried beans
—smoked, processed meat items

Foods that are bland to the colon

—milk, yogurt
—puddings, custards
—gelatins
—soft noodles, macaronis
—clear liquids
—no fried foods

—creamed or egg-based dishes
—plain cooked potatoes
—ripe bananas
—cooked cream of rice
—pureed or strained vegetables
—soft white bread

Foods for a clear liquid diet

—plain tea, coffee
—apple, cranberry, or grape juices (unsweetened)
—clear soup broths (fat-free or fat removed)
—popsicles, frozen ices
—clear gelatins

—carbonated soda, water

Foods for a dysphagia diet

This diet is offered in stages beginning with very soft, textured foods and progressing to a regular diet.
—Beginning foods:
  —strained oatmeal, farina, cream of rice
  —yogurt, custard
  —pureed cottage cheese
  —mashed potato (gravy separate)
  —pureed fruit (no juices)
  —pureed vegetables as tolerated
—Intermediate foods include the above plus:
  —fruit nectars
  —poached, soft-cooked eggs
  —mechanical soft ground meats or fish
  —cream-style, pureed, thickened soups (not liquid broth)
  —thick milkshakes (preferably served cold)
  —ice cream or sherbert
  —soft cooked pasta dishes
—Progression foods include the above plus:
  —soft fruits, especially bananas
  —tuna, ham, or egg salad with mayonnaise only
  —cheeses, cheese casseroles
  —skinless baked potato or sweet potato
  —chopped carrots, peas, green beans
  —soups
—Regular foods as tolerated. Cut meats, vegetables, and sandwiches into small pieces. Note foods that cause difficulty and report to the nurse supervisor.

Appendix C

EXERCISE

Exercise is an important part of maintaining health and preventing further disabilities for your clients. However, exercises are not for all clients. Your nurse supervisor or the therapists will direct you about the specific exercises in the care plan for each client. The exercises in this section are generally used as indicated. No exercise or exercise program should be performed without supervision and practice with the nurse supervisor or therapists. Some exercises require a physician's order.

Generally, you should have your clients avoid these movements during exercises:

1. Straight knee situps . . . use bent-knee situps, raising their upper body only.
2. Locked knee toe touches are hard on the lower back.
   Instead, flex knees slightly when touching to the toes.
   Move slowly and smoothly.
3. Avoid fast and hard stretching and bouncing that can tear tendons or ligaments. Move slowly and rhythmically through stretches. Hold for a few seconds at the point of maximum extension and stretch.
4. Do not exercise without warming up.
5. Do not exercise soon after a meal.
6. Do not hold their breath during exercises.
7. Do not exercise in hot, humid weather.
8. If they cannot carry on a conversation, they are exercising beyond the point they should be.

RANGE OF MOTION EXERCISES (ROM)

Range of motion is the term for **a group of exercises** specifically designed to move a person's joints, muscles, and soft tissues through their full usual amount of movement. Although you will learn a complete set of range of motion exercises (ROM), the exercises must be individually tailored for each client's capabilities. Each client has a different residual range of motion following his disability or due to his chronic condition. For example, the client who has chronic pain or a muscle-joint contracture can expect to have some restrictions in range of motion. The client who has paresis following a stroke may perform ROM exercises to build and maintain functional abilities and to prevent contractures.

The nurse supervisor will instruct you about your activities for range of motion with each client. Nurses perform ROM exercises to maintain function, to prevent further disabilities or complications, and to promote mobility. A physical therapist may work with the client to increase the range of motion, or to build strength and endurance. Members of the client's family may also perform ROM.

ROM exercises are performed *actively, passively or with assistance*. **Active** means that the client is able to move through the steps of the exercises without assistance while using his own muscle power. **Active assistance** exercises occur when a client needs a piece of equipment or minimal assistance to perform ROM exercises as if they were active. **Passive** means that the client requires another person to move the muscles and joints through the exercises. A client may require both **active and passive** exercises. For example, both active and passive exercises are appropriate for the client with paresis on one side of his body. He may require passive exercises on the weakened side, while being able to perform active exercises on the other side of his body.

ROM exercises are joint movements. Joints in the body move or can be moved in the ways listed in the box on p. 327. All joints move differently; some joints move in more ways than others. Each client will have different amounts of movement in his joints depending on his condition and abilities (Figure C-1).

When reading instructions for ROM exercises pay close attention to the use of the following words which explain how to approach and assist the client:

- grasp
- support
- hold
- begin with, bring to, and end with
- turn
- roll
- return
- rest

For example, if the client has joint pain, grasp above or below the joint rather than at the joint. If he has muscular pain, position your hands at the joint to ease strain on the muscles.

Each word is specific in its meaning about the way you move your client.

Joint Movements and Terms

1. extension = straightening, extending

2. flexion = bending

3. *ad*duction = moving *toward* the middle of the body

4. *ab*duction = moving *away* from the middle of the body

5. pronation = "on the stomach," facing down

6. supination = "on the back," facing up

7. circumduction = moving in a circular motion

8. dorsiflexion = upward movement of the foot involving the ankle joint

9. plantar flexion = bending the foot downward involving the ankle joint

10. internal rotation = roll in toward the body

11. external rotation = roll out from the body

12. hyperextension = extend beyond a straight line

13. opposition = move thumb across the palm, in the direction of the little finger

14. ulnar deviation = move hand toward the little finger

15. radial deviation = move hand toward the thumb

Other important terms:

16. distal = farthest away from the middle of the body

17. proximal = closest to the middle of the body

18. cephalo = referring to the head

19. caudal = referring to the feet

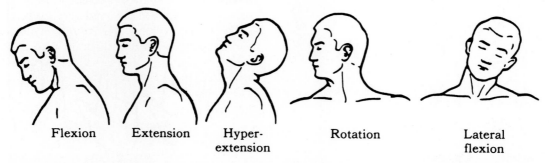

Flexion   Extension   Hyper-extension   Rotation   Lateral flexion

Figure C-1. *Active range of motion exercises that are performed by clients under the direction of the nurse supervisor or physical therapist.*

From Phipps, W.J., Long, B.C., and Woods, N.F.: Medical-surgical nursing, ed. 3, St. Louis, 1987, The C.V. Mosby Co.

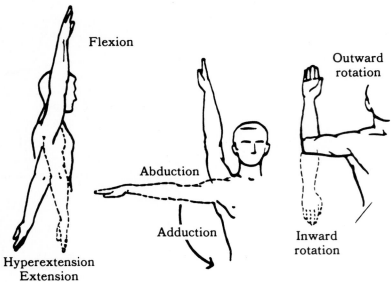

Range-of-motion exercises for the shoulder.

Range-of-motion exercises for the elbow.

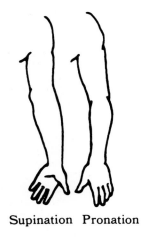

Range-of-motion exercises for the forearm.

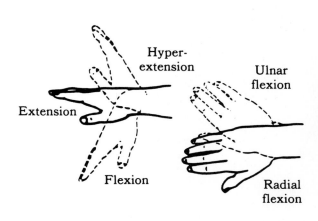

Range-of-motion exercises for the wrist.

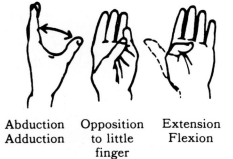

Range-of-motion exercises for the thumb.

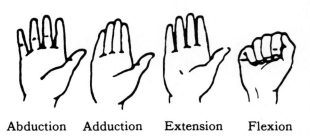

Range-of-motion exercises for the fingers.

Figure C-1, cont'd.

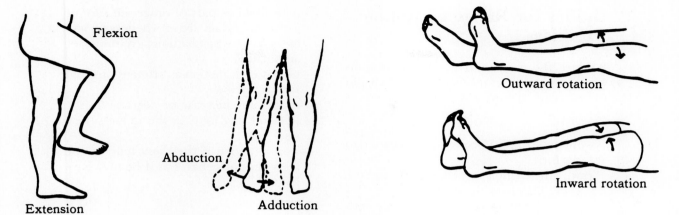

Range-of-motion exercises for the hip.

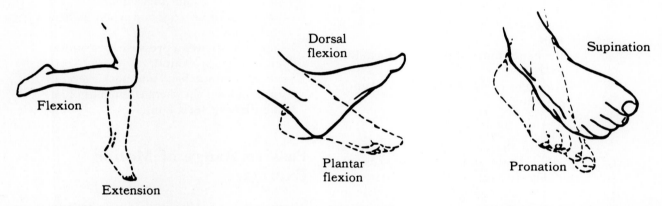

Range-of-motion exercises for the knee.   *Range-of-motion exercises for the ankle.*   *Range-of-motion exercises for the foot.*

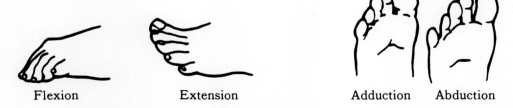

Range-of-motion exercises for the toes.

Figure C-1, cont'd.

Guides for Range of Motion Exercises

Be sure the client and family understand what you are doing and why before you begin the exercises (Figure C-2).

KNOW:

—the type of ROM exercises the client is to perform.
—why the client is receiving ROM and the overall goals of the exercises.
—the present range of motion in each joint.
—any precautions, such as pain, weakened bones, lost sensations, or contractures.
—the tolerance level for fatigue, endurance and stamina.
—what the client can do for himself or with assistance versus what must be done for him.
—the better times of day to perform ROM exercises.
—the client's level of awareness and understanding.

DO:

—inform the client about what you are going to do and explain what you are doing throughout the exercises.
—practice and perform ROM exercises under the direction and supervision of the nurse supervisor or physical therapist.
—use proper body mechanics.
—keep the client in proper alignment and position.
—perform exercises using slow, smooth motions and develop a sense of rhythm as each joint is moved.
—maintain a safe and comfortable work area for you and the client. For example, dress client in non-restrictive clothing, remove clutter from the area and lock wheels on the bed.

—plan ROM as part of other self-care or activities of daily living whenever possible, such as when bathing, grooming, or ambulating.
—repeat each motion as often as directed for each joint.
—report any increase or decrease in the ROM of any joint to the nurse supervisor.
—stop a motion if the client tells you he feels pain or behaves as if he may have pain.

NEVER:

—never perform ROM unless directed and supervised by the nurse supervisor.
—never go beyond the client's present range of motion for any joint.
—never force a joint movement.
—never continue a motion when a client feels pain.
—never grasp over a pressure sore or over an incision or wound.
—never continue head and neck exercises or motions if the client complains of being dizzy or feels faint.

Passive Range of Motion Exercises

All exercises must be individually tailored according to your client's capabilities. Never force a client to do an exercise that he or she is incapable of achieving. ROM exercises are performed under the direction and supervision of the nurse supervisor or the physical therapist.

Figure C-2 illustrates the steps that may be used as a reference when performing a complete set of ROM exercises for a client. You must learn and practice ROM exercises for each client under supervision from the nurse.

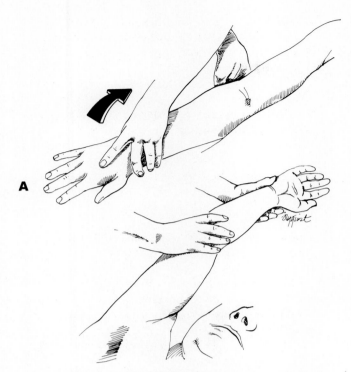

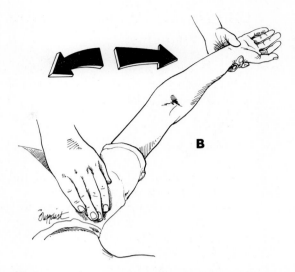

B, *Sliding arm toward body produces shoulder adduction. Sliding arm away from body produces abduction.*

A, *shoulder in extended position. Flexion occurs as arm is lifted up and back.*

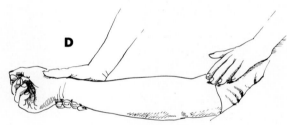

D, *Elbow extension.*

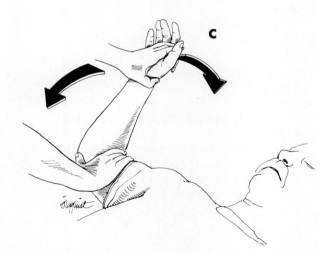

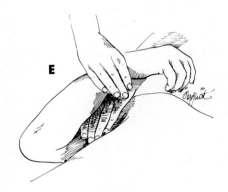

C, *As forearm is brought down, internal rotation occurs at shoulder joint. As forearm is brought up and back, external rotation occurs.*

E, *Elbow flexion.*

Figure C-2.
From Dittmar, S.: Rehabilitation nursing: process and application, St. Louis, 1989, The C.V. Mosby Co.

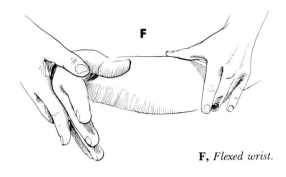

F, *Flexed wrist.*

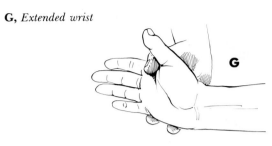

G, *Extended wrist*

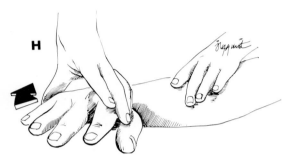

H, *Lateral movement of wrist produces radial and ulnar deviation.*

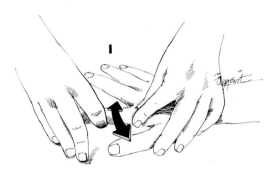

I, *Fingers abducted away from midline and adducted toward midline (of hand).*

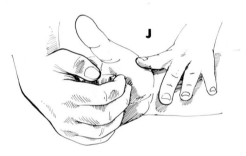

J, *Fingers flexed as group into closed fist.*

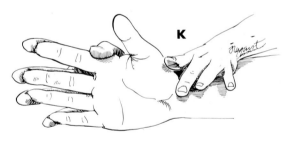

K, *Finger extension is described as open fist.*

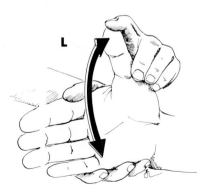

L, *Thumb flexed toward and extended away from fourth digit.*

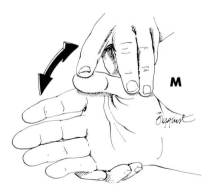

M, *Thumb abducted and adducted in relation to other fingers.*

Figure C-2. cont'd.

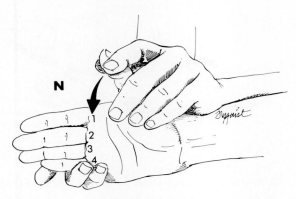

N, *Thumb moved in opposition to base of each of other four digits.*

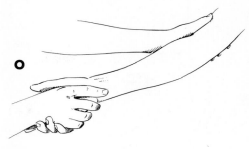

O, *Forearm in supination.*

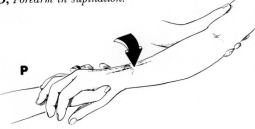

P, *Rolling forearm downward places it in pronation.*

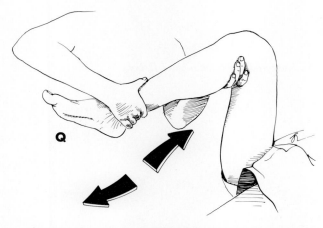

Q, *Caregiver can move hip in flexion by sliding leg back. Extension can be produced by sliding leg forward.*

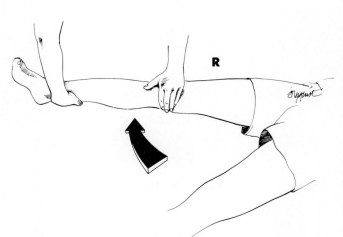

R, *Moving leg away from midline of body abducts hip.*

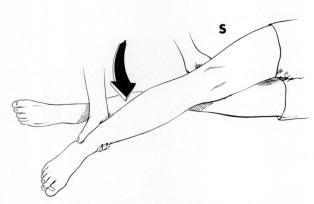

S, *Moving leg toward midline of body and crossing over it adducts hip.*

Figure C-2, cont'd.

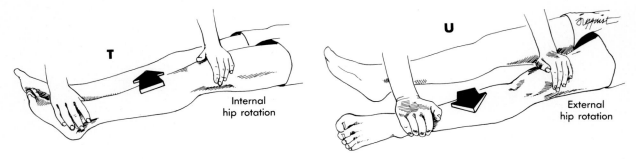

T, *Rolling leg inward causes hip joint to rotate internally.*   **U,** *Rolling leg outward causes hip joint to rotate externally.*

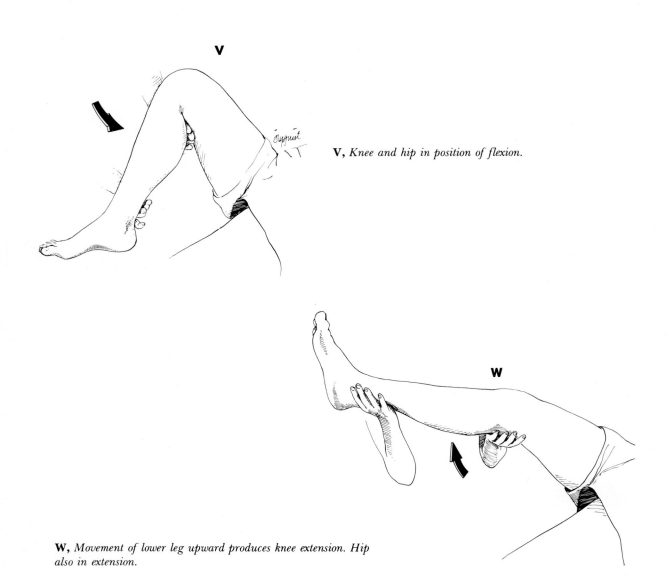

V, *Knee and hip in position of flexion.*

W, *Movement of lower leg upward produces knee extension. Hip also in extension.*

Figure C-2, cont'd.

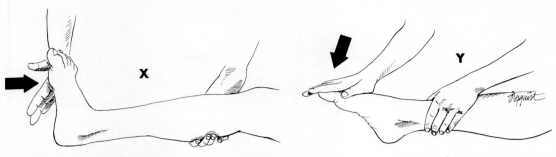

X, *Pressure with palm of hand against ball of foot causes ankle dorsiflexion.*

Y, *Pressure against top of foot causes ankle plantar flexion.*

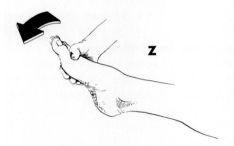

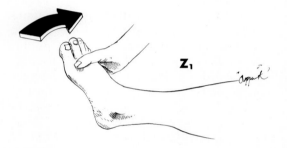

Z, *Turning foot inward produces ankle inversion.*

Z₁, *Turning foot outward produces ankle eversion.*

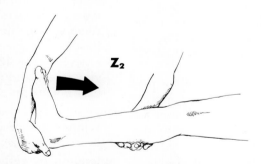

Z₂, *Heel cord stretching involves downward pull on heel cord and dorsiflexion of ankle.*

Figure C-2, cont'd.

Appendix D

GLOSSARY

abuse (verbal and physical) Physical abuse is physical harm or aggression, causing injury to another person. Verbal abuse is shouting, name-calling, and threatening or negative comments that may be obviously or subtly directed at another person.

activities of daily living (ADL) Activities that individuals perform in their daily personal care, such as dressing, grooming, eating, and personal hygiene.

affected versus unaffected Terms used to describe areas of the body that have deficits or losses. These terms are preferred over negative terms such as *weak* versus *strong* or *crippled,* which should never be used to describe an individual.

amyotrophic lateral sclerosis (ALS) A progressive neuromuscular disease affecting nerves in the brain and spinal cord, leading to paralysis and death.

alveoli Tiny air sacs that reach and extend into all areas of the lungs. Alveoli are necessary for the exchange of oxygen and carbon dioxide with the blood capillaries.

Alzheimer's disease A progressive, currently incurable disease producing mental changes due to chemical changes in the brain. It does not occur as part of the normal processes and changes often associated with aging.

amputation The removal of a limb or part of a limb such as a finger or toe. Amputations are classified as upper or lower extremity amputations. Lower extremity amputations of the leg are further designated as above or below the knee. Diabetes mellitus, trauma, and peripheral vascular conditions are the most frequent causes of amputations.

angina pectoris A cardiac condition characterized by heart pain in a radiated pattern. Angina pain is caused by a reduced supply of blood to the heart muscle.

arteriosclerosis A cardiac condition caused by "hardening of the arteries," which thickens the arterial walls so they lose elasticity and cannot contract and expand.

artery A blood vessel that carries oxygenated blood *away* from the heart to the body. (The pulmonary artery carries unoxygenated blood away from the heart to the lungs.)

arthritic conditions and diseases A group of diseases that cause various joint and connective tissue diseases and conditions. They usually produce inflammation, swelling, and pain in joints. Some are degenerative and progressive; others are related to lifestyle or age.

assistive device Innovative device or apparatus that assists or enables a person to perform activities by compensating for a deficit, disability, or impairment. They range from simple and homemade items to very sophisticated commercial products.

asthma A respiratory system disease causing spasms in the bronchial tubes. A serious asthma attack occurs when the air flow is restricted because the bronchial tubes have closed down or collapsed. Allergies, stress, and other individual stressors may initiate an asthma attack.

atrophy A wasting away of a normally developed muscle or tissue with a resulting decrease in size, function, and strength.

autonomic dysreflexia A high blood pressure crisis and emergency for the person who has a high-level spinal cord injury. It is the result of an irritating stimulus occurring below the level of injury.

bladder program or training A prescribed method for helping a client learn to control when and where he urinates.

bowel program or training A prescribed method for helping a client learn to control when and where he has a bowel movement.

bronchial tubes and bronchioles The branching portions of the air pathways in the lungs. The bronchial tubes are the transport systems connecting the nose and nasal passages through the trachea with the lungs. The bronchioles are finer divisions of the bronchial tubes and extend through the lungs until they become aveoli.

bronchiectasis A lung disease caused by scarring of the lung tissues following multiple and chronic bronchial infections; there may be blood or blood-tinged sputum and infection.

bronchitis An inflammation of the bronchial tree pathways of the lungs, usually accompanied by infection, coughing, and increased mucous production. The condition may become chronic leading to scarring and obstructed respirations.

cardiac pacemaker An electronic device that sends a controlled electrical stimulus to the heart node that initiates heartbeats. Cardiac pacemakers may be external or surgically implanted.

cardiac system The circulatory system of the body, including the heart, blood vessels, and capillaries.

cartilage A tough elastic tissue that covers the ends of bones providing protection during joint movements. The cartilage is within the synovial capsule and lubricated by synovial fluid.

cerebrum The largest portion of the brain, which is divided into the right and left hemispheres. The right hemisphere controls the left side of the body and the left hemisphere controls the right side of the body.

chronic condition A condition that lasts for three months or longer. The signs or symptoms may lie hidden or subtle for many years before the disease is recognized. The causes and cures may be unknown and they often require long-term care.

chronic obstructive pulmonary disease (COPD) A category of chronic respiratory diseases characterized by a resistance to air flowing out of the lungs and difficulty exhaling.

chronic restrictive pulmonary disease A category of chronic respiratory diseases characterized by difficulties inhaling and getting air into the lungs and similar difficulties exhaling due to muscle and nerve impairments.

colostomy A surgical opening through the skin of the abdomen into the colon, bypassing the anus, rectum, and other parts of the colon. Fecal wastes are excreted through the stoma. Colostomies may have one or two (double-barreled) stomas; they may be temporary or permanent.

concussion A minor head injury with a variety of predictable symptoms. Clients usually have a complete and rapid recovery; however, sometimes problems persist for years.

confidentiality An important and conscious effort to respect a client's privacy by not discussing his condition or personal life or giving out information to others (including friends and relatives) about the client. A part of ethical behavior.

congestive heart disease A cardiac condition in which venous blood does not return sufficiently from the heart to the body. The blood collects in the heart chambers, causing a congestion.

contractures An abnormal shortening of muscle tissue that makes the muscle highly resistant to stretching. The result is reduced function and malformed positioning.

contusion Damage to the brain, usually from a traumatic injury, similar to bruising the brain. A contusion may cause varying losses of consciousness and/or functional abilities.

degeneration A change in the form and function of body tissue that results in loss, usually progressive. Similar to deterioration, a worsening and breakdown of tissues or cells and function.

deficit A lack or deficiency characterized by less than normal range of function or competence. A deficit usually follows a disease, trauma, or other condition that reduces function.

dementia A change in the mental status of an elderly person that may result from a type of brain disease or may mimic other conditions. Medications may cause a client to appear as if he has a dementia.

diabetes mellitus   A chronic metabolic disease due to insufficient insulin production. Type I is insulin-dependent juvenile-onset diabetes; type II is adult-onset diabetes.

diaphragm   The musculomembraneous wall located between the abdomen and the chest cavity. It assists in breathing by contracting and expanding producing changes in the interthoracic pressure.

digestive system   The tract from the mouth, through the esophagus, stomach, intestines, and anus and all the glands and organs associated with taking in, digesting, and excreting foods.

disability   A physical, mental or emotional condition that inhibits a person from performing a function or activity for daily living or self-care.

donning and doffing   The processes of putting on and taking off a prosthetic device.

dysphagia   Difficulty swallowing and eating food and fluids; often a deficit following a stroke that may also involve speech.

dysarthria   Difficulties with the mechanics of speaking due to muscle dysfunctions necessary for clear speech.

embolism   A blood clot or air bubble floating freely in the blood stream that may lead to stroke or death.

emphysema   A type of COPD in which the lung tissues have a reduced capacity to expand and contract causing trapped air in the lungs. This reduces the oxygen exchange, increases mucous production, and causes disability or death.

exercises   A prescribed group of activities and movements for a client to maintain, promote, or improve his health or function. Exercises are performed under the direction and supervision of the nurse supervisor or physical therapist.

flaccid   A term that describes muscles that are weak, soft, floppy, or lax; usually a response to neurological impairments or deficits.

friction   Heat caused by rubbing two surfaces together; it is a major source of damage to the skin.

gastrostomy   A surgical opening through the abdominal wall into the stomach used to supply nourishment (special preparations of food) directly into the stomach when the upper digestive tract cannot be used or the client is not able to eat normally.

gout   Inflammation of the great toe caused by a buildup of uric acid in the body. Although chronic, gout responds well to treatment.

grieving process   Suggested stages of predictable responses to the crisis of disability and losses of function that many clients and families experience. Not all persons experience or express their grieving in the same ways; not all stages occur for all persons or in the same sequence.

Heimlich maneuver   A lifesaving maneuver designed to eliminate an obstruction from the upper airway.

hospice   A concept of care and support for a client with a terminal illness and his family. Hospice allows him to die at home as comfortably as possible and with health care management.

hyperglycemia   An insulin imbalance with *too little* insulin or high blood sugar.

hypertension   High blood pressurre resulting from the increased pressure of the blood against the walls of the arteries as the blood passes through; a risk factor for stroke.

hypoglycemia   An insulin imbalance with *too much* insulin or low blood sugar.

ileostomy   A surgical opening through the skin of the abdomen into the ileum, bypassing the colon, rectum, and anus to excrete fecal wastes through the stoma on the abdomen wall.

imbalance (insulin)   A condition in which there is either too much or too little insulin for metabolism; varies individually.

impaction   Used here as a bowel impaction: an immovable, tight accumulation of feces in the bowel that must be manually removed. (There are other types of impaction that may occur in the body, such as impacted wisdom teeth.)

incontinence   The loss of voluntary purposeful control of elimination, either bowel or bladder or both.

infection control (universal) Specific steps and procedures to prevent the spread of diseases. The precautions are based on knowledge of how diseases are caused and spread from one person to another. Good proper handwashing is a primary step in prevention.

insulin A natural hormone secreted by specialized cells in the pancreas. Insulin is essential for metabolism. Synthetic insulin has enabled insulin-dependent persons to survive diabetes mellitus.

integumentary system The body system composed of the skin and its parts, hair, and nails.

involuntary muscles Muscles that receive their messages from the brain and spinal cord but function without conscious decisions, such as the bowel and bladder actions.

isolation precautions The steps and procedures for keeping clean and solid or contaminated materials apart. Isolation may be protective in two ways: (1) keeping ill persons from spreading their diseases or infections and (2) keeping persons with reduced resistance or impaired immunological responses isolated from potentially harmful environmental contaminants or ill persons.

joint The points in the body where two bones meet; movable or unmovable. Usually surrounded by cartilage, connective tissues, synovial membrane and fluid, and supportive muscles and ligaments.

juvenile arthritis A chronic inflammatory type of arthritis that affects young people under 15 to 16 years of age. Although it is a systemic disease, disabling and damaging joints and connective tissues throughout the body, complete remission is possible in many cases with proper treatment.

juvenile diabetes Type I diabetes with onset in youth.

labile A term applied to emotional states, often following a stroke, during which a person has unstable and fluctuating emotional states. The person tends to alternate between cheerfulness and somberness.

limbic system The system of brain structures and their interconnecting/connecting nerves that influence and interpret behavior and feelings for the body's responses.

level of injury (spinal cord injury) The location of an injury in terms of location on the spinal cord. Described by the section of the cord and number of vertebra.

lupus erythematosus A chronic condition affecting many body parts and systems. The disease is different for each person and may become debilitating or flare up on occasion.

mechanical respirator or ventilator A breathing machine that replicates and substitutes for a client's paralyzed breathing muscles when the client cannot breathe on his own.

metabolism The physical and chemical activities that change food to energy and heat in the body. The building up and tearing down processes converting foods to simpler substances and excreting wastes. Metabolism uses enzymes, hormones, vitamins, and minerals.

multiple sclerosis A progressive neuromuscular disease, currently incurable, that affects young adults with varying degrees of severity. It may cause one problem or multiple problems or lead to death.

myelin sheath A protein and fatty substance that coats nerve fibers and axons with a sheathlike covering; may be protective or destructive.

neglect A form of abusive behavior in which an individual is not cared for, is ignored, or has his needs not cared for or excessively delayed. He may not be properly fed, cleaned, or given medical care or may be isolated from others.

nervous system The complex body system composed of nerves, nerve cells and axons, spinal cord, and brain structures that coordinate and direct the body's actions and functions and responses. There are two divisions: the central nervous system and the peripheral nervous system.

osteoarthritis The most common arthritic condition of old age. A painful, but noninflammatory condition caused by "wear and tear." The cartilage is worn away from protecting the bones and the body responds by producing painful calcium spurs.

pain   A state of discomfort that may become severe. Pain is acute or chronic, malignant or nonmalignant. Chronic pain that is nonmalignant tends to persevere, while malignant pain intensifies and becomes progressively worse as the disease progresses.

paralysis   Loss of movement or ability to voluntarily move muscles and body parts; it may involve sensory, circulatory, and other related losses.

paresis   A state of weakness, usually associated with a post-neurological or stroke aftermath. The paresis may be a slight or incomplete paralysis.

  paraparesis   A partial weakness of the lower extremities that may affect the body from below the thoracic region.

  quadriparesis   Weakness of all four body limbs.

  hemiparesis   Weakness affecting either the right or left side of the body.

  triparesis   Weakness affecting three of the body limbs.

Parkinson's disease   A progressive neuromuscular disease that chemically disrupts the communications betweeen the brain and the nerves that affect movement. The client remains mentally alert and active.

peer group counseling   A technique of therapeutic intervention and health education that uses trained persons who have disabilities or conditions to interact and teach others with the same or similar disabilities or conditions.

peripheral vascular conditions   Diseases or conditions related to poor circulation; often associated with heart diseases and complications for clients with diabetes mellitus.

plaque   A stiff substance that coats body parts causing reduced function and destruction such as plaque on teeth or plaque on nerve fiber endings in Alzheimer's disease.

plegia   Loss of ability to control movement and loss of sensation.

  hemiplegia   Plegia of one half the body, that is, an arm and leg on the same side; may involve deficits related to stroke.

  paraplegia   Plegia of the mid to lower back and below, causing varying losses in the legs, torso, bowel and bladder, and sexual function.

  triplegia   Plegia involving three limbs and parts of the body.

quadriplegia   Plegia involving both arms, both legs, torso, bowel, bladder, sexual functions, and respiratory functions in varying degrees according to level and severity of spinal cord injury.

phantom pain   A particular pain experience felt as if it were situated in an absent, amputated limb.

phrenic nerve pacemaker   A highly specialized electrode and transmitter device surgically implanted and designed to initiate breathing by stimulating the phrenic nerve(s).

postural hypotension   A decrease in blood pressure that occurs when a client who is lying down changes position to sit or stand. The condition is due to nervous system damage.

pressure sores   Preventable skin wounds caused by pressure on the skin, usually from prolonged sitting, lying in one place and position, or irritation. Some body areas, such as over bony prominences, are prone to developing pressure areas. Persons with chronic or disabling conditions are especially vulnerable to developing pressure sores.

progressive neuromuscular diseases   A category of chronic conditions involving the neuromuscular systems. These conditions are often incurable, have unknown causes, become progressively debilitating and disabling, and may lead to death.

prosthetic device   An "artificial" manufactured body part replacement usually for an arm, hand, foot, or leg. Other common prosthetic parts include hip joint replacements, artificial eyes, and dentures.

pulmonary system   The respiratory system responsible for respiration, carbon dioxide and oxygen exchange, blood transportation of oxygen, and coordination of respiratory and central nervous system functions.

range of motion   The full and normal extent of joint movement for any moveable joint. A set of exercises for passive, active assisted, and active range of motion is used (under direction and supervision of a nurse supervisor of physical therapist) to prevent further disabilities and complications and to promote well being.

rehabilitation The health care specialty that uses an interdisciplinary team approach to "restore an individual to the fullest physical, mental, social, economical, and vocational capacity to which he is capable." The goal of rehabilitation is to enable the individual to live to the fullest capacity possible, with optimal wellness and quality of life; focusing on his achievements, not on the disability; focusing on the person, not on the disability.

rehabilitation team The interdisciplinary team of health professionals who work together, including the client and his family, to evaluate a client's potential for achieving functional goals, to provide the education and services to achieve that potential and to provide comprehensive lifelong follow-up.

remission A period of time when the symptoms or severity of a chronic, progressive disease are lessened or cease; it may be temporary or permanent.

residual limb The portion of the limb that remains intact following the amputation of a body part. The residual limb may be fitted with a prosthesis. The word *stump* should be avoided.

respite care A program designed to provide temporary relief to caregivers from the stresses of caring for clients at home, such as adult day care centers, respite weekend services, or in-home live-in caregivers.

rheumatoid arthritis A destructive and disabling arthritic condition that may or may not progress. When severe, the disease affects many joints in the body simultaneously, causes a great deal of pain and general debilitation, and may destroy and infect body organs leading to death.

rheumatism A term referring to the group of inflammatory, painful and chronic conditions that include the arthritic conditions and others; a descriptive word, not a diagnostic term.

rigidity Increased muscle tone where muscles negatively work against one another producing stiffness and resistance to movement.

scanning A simple technique clients can learn to compensate for visual deficits following a stroke so they can increase their self-care and awareness of their surroundings.

sclerosed (sclerosis) A word meaning "hardened with thickening"; it often refers to the characteristics of unhealthy blood vessels and is associated with high risk for stroke or heart attacks.

severity of injury (spinal cord injury) The extent of injury to the spinal cord based on the evaluation of the loss of function and sensations among other body abilities.

shearing Stretching and pressure on the skin and underlying tissues caused when the skin tissues slide over one another damaging the skin; it often occurs during moving a client.

spasticity Muscle movements, usually following nervous system damage or disease, that are a response to increased muscle tone. Spastic movements are involuntary and generally uncontrolled; medications reduce spasticity in some clients. They may affect all body parts, usually occurring in the arms, legs, or trunk.

spinal cord The main bundle of the body's nerves located inside the vertebral column. The spinal cord extends from the base of the brain and brain stem to the lower back (tailbone).

sterile (sterilizing) Any method to destroy all microorganisms from an object, material, or food or liquid.

stoma An artificially created opening, in this case of an ostomy, that opens onto the skin of the abdomen through which body wastes are eliminated. Some stomas are used for feeding, such as a gastrostomy.

stroke (cerebrovascular accident, or CVA) An injury or damage to a part of the brain occurring when that part of the brain does not receive the blood it needs to function. Brain cells are damaged when the blood stream cannot supply necessary oxygen and they may die. The amount and type of losses and deficits depends on the area of the brain involved, the extent of the damage, and severity of the stroke.

stroke posture An undesirable position assumed by a client who has had a stroke with deficits in the sense of where his body parts are placed, hemiplegia, or other deficits. Rehabilitation positioning can prevent complications and further disabilities by not allowing this poor posturing.

"stump" shrinkers A method for shaping a residual limb in preparation for fitting a prosthesis. Purchased special socklike wraps that decrease edema following an amputation are alternatives to Ace wrapping techniques.

support group Groups of individuals and families who are dealing with the challenges of a family member with a specific condition, often incurable, chronic, or disabling. The main purposes are mutual support, sharing, developing resources, and problem solving among those with similar difficulties. Groups may have a health professional as a resource and often develop into social and friendship relationships.

synovial fluid A slippery, thick, clear fluid produced by the synovial membrane to lubricate the spaces around and between the cartilage of a joint.

terminal condition A condition, injury, or disease where the expected outcome is death.

thrombophlebitis An inflammation of a vein associated with a thrombus (blood clot). Prevention and early identification and treatment improve outcomes.

tracheostomy A surgical opening into the trachea performed to create or maintain a patent airway; permanent or temporary. A client may be connected to a mechanical ventilator via a tracheostomy.

transcutaneous electrical nerve stimulator (TENS) A small generator with wire leads and electrodes designed to temporarily relieve pain. Many units are portable or handheld units. Exact instructions and supervision is provided by the nurse supervisor or physical therapist.

traumatic brain injury (TBI) A severe head injury that involves damage to the brain. The location of the injury, part of the brain injured, and severity of the injury affect the level and type of dysfunction a client will experience. Serious brain injuries may occur with or without visible head injury.

tremor Uncontrollable, vibrating, shaking movements varying from severe to fine quivering that can affect one or many parts of the body, commonly associated with Parkinson's disease.

ureterostomy A surgical opening into the ureters of the urinary tract that bypasses the urethra and bladder. Urine is excreted through a stoma (or two stomas) opening through the skin of the abdominal wall, where it is collected in a special bag.

urinary system The body system formed by the kidneys, ureters, bladder, and urethra, which use involuntary muscles and some voluntary sphincter muscle controls. The urinary system filters fluid wastes from the blood stream, transports it to the bladder, and stores it until it is excreted through the urethra.

urinary drainage bag A urine collection bag attached to the terminal end of tubing that drains a client's urinary catheter or sheath. The bag can be hung from a bedside or wheelchair frame or secured to the client's leg as he ambulates.

urinary sheath A condom-like external urinary device worn over the penis and attached to a drainage catheter. A urinary sheath is designed to protect clients from urinary leaking or dribbling incontinence without an indwelling catheter.

varicose veins Enlarged, extended, and painful veins, usually in the legs. These occur when blood is not returned to the heart and collects in the veins, engorging them and causing the venous walls to out-pouch.

vein A blood vessel that carries carbon dioxide–laden blood from the body to the heart, where it is sent to the lungs to complete oxygen exchange. The pulmonary vein carries oxygenated blood to the heart.

vertebrae The flexible, hollow centered column of backbones, separated by discs, that extend from the base of the skull to the tailbone, housing the spinal cord.

vertigo Strong dizzy, lightheaded feelings that may be incapacitating. Disturbances may occur in the sense of balance, during which objects may seem to move inappropriately in space or the person may seem to move and turn in space, without a sense of control.

voluntary muscles Muscles that move when directed by the brain to perform intended actions, such as picking up a fork.

weight shifts Regularly scheduled exercises designed to shift a person's weight off a part of his body to prevent pressure areas from developing; they may be done while lying in bed or sitting in a wheelchair or chair.

Bibliography

Block, Ralph F., and Basbaum, Mel, editors: Management of spinal cord injuries, Rehabilitation Medicine Library Series, Baltimore, Williams & Wilkins.

Buchanan, Lorraine E., and Nawoczenski, Deborah A.: Spinal cord injury, Baltimore, 1987, William & Wilkins.

Caplan, Bruce, editor: Rehabilitation psychology desk reference, Rockville, Md., 1987, Aspen Systems Corp.

Dittmar, Sharon: Rehabilitation nursing: process and application, St. Louis, 1989, The C.V. Mosby Company.

DuVoisini, Roger: Parkinson's disease: a guide for patient and family, New York, 1984, Raven Press.

Engleman, Ephraim P., and Silverman, Milton: The arthritis book, Sausalito, Calif., 1979, Painter Hopkins Publishers.

Freeman, Julian: Arthritis: the new treatments, Chicago, 1981, Contemporary Books.

Friedman, JoAnn: Home health care: a complete guide for patients and their families, New York, 1986, W.W. Norton & Co.

Long, Kate, and Fries, James F.: The arthritis helpbook, Reading, Mass., 1980, Addison-Wesley Publishing Company.

Mace, Nancy L., and Rabins, Peter V.: The 36 hour day: a family guide to caring for persons with Alzheimer's disease, related dementing illnesses, and memory loss in later life, Baltimore, 1981, Johns Hopkins University Press.

Martin, Nancy, Holt, Nance B., and Hicks, Dorothy: Comprehensive rehabilitation nursing, New York, 1981, McGraw-Hill Book Co.

O'Brien, Mary T., and Pallett, Phyllis J.: Total care of the stroke patient, Boston, 1978, Little, Brown & Company, Inc.

Power, Paul W., and Dell Orto, Arthur E.: Role of the family in the rehabilitation of the physically disabled, Baltimore, 1980, University Park Press.

Rehabilitation nursing: concepts and practice: a core curriculum, Evanston, Ill., 1981, 1989, Rehabilitation Nursing Foundation.

Reisberg, Barry: A guide to Alzheimer's disease for families, spouses, and friends, New York, 1981, The Free Press.

Scheinberg, Labe C., editor: Multiple sclerosis: a guide for patients and their families, New York, 1983, Raven Press.

Sine, Robert, et al.: Basic rehabilitation techniques, ed. 3, Rockville, Md., 1989, Aspen Systems Corp.

Stryker, Ruth: Rehabilitative aspects of acute and chronic nursing care, Philadelphia, 1977, W.B. Saunders Company.

Trieschmann, Roberta B.: Aging with a disability, New York, 1987, Demos Publications.

Wright, Beatrice A.: Physical disability—a psychosocial approach, ed. 2, New York, 1983, Harper & Row, Publishers.

Ylvisaker, Mark, editor: Head injury rehabilitation: children and adolescents, Boston, Little, Brown & Company, Inc.

Zejdlik, Cynthia M.: Management of spinal cord injury, Belmont, Calif., 1983, Wadsworth Health Sciences Division.

Index

A

Abdominal thrusts for choking, 56–57
Above-the-knee amputation, 247–248
Absorbing devices for urine, 37, 39
Abuse of client, 10
Ace bandage wrappings of residual limb, 244–245
Acquired immune deficiency syndrome, 316–318
Active range of motion exercises, 328, 329–331
Activities of daily living, assistive devices for, 178–205
Acute pain, 282
Adjustments to spinal cord injury, 238–239
Adult-onset diabetes, 290
Aggressive client, 221–223
Aging, sensory changes with, 62
AIDS, 316–318
AIDS-related complex, 316–318
Air cushions for clients with lower extremity weakness, 197
Air filters, 278
Air mattress for client with lower extremity weakness, 197
Air purifiers, 278
Alcohol
  for client, 34
  and drugs, interactions of, 34
ALS; *see* Amyotrophic lateral sclerosis
Alzheimer's disease, 284–289
  caring for client with, 286
  nutrition and, 288–289
  signs or symptoms of, 285
  stages of, 285
Ambulation
  assistive devices for, 198–205
  with cane or one crutch, 199, 200
  with client, considerations in, 199
  on curbs and stairs, 200, 203–205
  with two canes or walker, 199–200, 201, 202–203
Amputation, 240
  above-the-knee, 247–248
  below-the-knee, 247, 248
  care for client with, 240–260
  changing dominant sides after, 247
  circulation problems after, signs and symptoms of, 246
  coping following, 246–247
  falling by client after, 246–247
  and fractured hip, 260
  and hemiplegia/hemiparesis, 259
  lower limb
    care with, 247–257
    standing transfer for client with, 118–119
  phantom pain after, 247
  reaction toward, 242–243
  special considerations following, 259
  successful management of, 242–243
  variations with, 259–260

Amyotrophic lateral sclerosis, 315–316
Anger by home health aide, dealing with, 11
Angina
  nitroglycerin for, 268
  rest for client with, 267
Angina pectoris, 265–266
Ankle, ROM exercises for, 331, 337
Ankle and foot supports, 177
Ankle foot orthosis, molded, 150
Aphasia, 78–80
  common deficits with, 79
  guidelines for working with client with, 80
Appliance cords, safety and, 21
ARC, 316–318
Architectural barriers in home, 20–21
Arm, Utah, 258
Armboards for wheelchairs, 159–162
Arteries, 264
  diseases of, 265
Arteriosclerosis, 265
Arthritic conditions, 303–307
  pain control with, 307
Arthritis, 303
  pain with, 103
  rheumatoid, 304
    assisting client with, 306
    care for client with, 305
    pain control for, 307
Artificial larynx, 70
Assisted standing transfer, 114–115
Assistive cough for spinal cord injured person, 232–233
Assistive devices
  for activities of daily living, 178–205
  for ambulation, 198–205
  for arthritic client, 307
  for communication for aphasic clients, 81
  for dressing, 179–188
  for eating, 193–195
  for grooming, 189–192
  for spinal cord injured persons, 231
Asthma, 277–280
Atherosclerotic cardiovascular heart disease, 265
Atrophy, muscle, after stroke, 211
Attachments, wheelchair, 159–163
Auditory clues for visually impaired person, 65
Autonomic dysreflexia in spinal cord injured person, 236–237

B

Back braces for trunk support, 195–196
Bags
  ostomy, 51–52
    cleaning, 52
  urinary drainage, 45–47

Balance after stroke, 211
Bar(s)
  around toilet, 168
  trapeze, 165
Base of support and body mechanics, 86, 88
Basic needs and emergency situations, 26–60
Bath, aids for, 169–170
Bath mitt, 169–170, 191
Bathing client, considerations in, 196
Bathroom, safety in, 23–24
Bathroom equipment for home care, 167–170
Bathtub; *see* Tub
Batteries, wheelchair, 158–159
Battery charger, 159
Bed
  to bedside commode, transfer board from, 124
  client in, placing sling for mechanical lift under, 130
  for home care, 163–164
  returning client to, 106
  short-sitting in, in preparation for transfer for persons with
    spinal cord injuries, 105–106
  siderails for, 164–165
  sitting position on, moving to, 103–105
  standing transfer from, to chair, 116–117
  turning of client in, 97–99
  wheelchair to, transfer board to, 121–123
  to wheelchair, transfer board from, 121
Bed cradles, 92
Bed extenders, 164
Bed shampoo tray, 191
Bedboards, 163, 164
Beddings for clients with lower extremity weakness, 197–198
Bedrest, excessive, negative effects of, 232
Bedroom, safety in, 24
Bedroom equipment for home care, 163–167
Bedside commodes, 165–166
  bed to, transfer board from, 124
  with wheels, 166–167
Bedsores, 28–30
Below-the-knee amputation, 247, 248
  ace bandage wrappings of, 244
Belt, pelvic, with above-the-knee prosthesis, 257
Binders for trunk support, 195
Bladder
  difficulties with, after stroke, 216
  function and dysfunction of, 36–47
  problems with, with multiple sclerosis, 311
  retraining of, after spinal cord injury, 233
  training of, 36, 37
Bland diet, 324
Bleach and water disinfectant, 16
Bleeding, 60
  in brain and stroke, 207
Blindness, 63
Blood clots causing strokes, 207
Blood glucose meter, 294–295
Blood glucose monitoring, 294–295
Blood isolation precautions, 18
Blood pressure, high, 265
  and stroke, 207
Blood sugar
  high, 295
  low, 296
Blood tests for clients with diabetes mellitus, 292, 294
Blouses, dressing in, 180–182
Bobath principle for pulling up of client in chair or wheelchair,
  110–111

Body language, 74
Body mechanics for moving clients, 85–88
Body positions, 89–96
Body stocking, care of, 187
Boiling water for sterilization, 16
Bowel
  difficulties with, after stroke, 216
  function and dysfunction of, 47–53
  problems with, with multiple sclerosis, 311
  retraining of, after spinal cord injury, 233
  training of, 47–48, 49
Brace(s)
  back, for trunk support, 195–196
  leg, 149–151
    care and storage of, 150–151
    shoes for, 151
  molded, for trunk support, 196
Brain
  bleeding in, and stroke, 207
  communication deficits and, 76–78
  contusion of, 218
  diagram of, 77
  function of, 208, 209
Brain injuries; *see also* Head injuries
  communication deficits after, 78–80
  location of, and disability, 218–219
  traumatic
    care for client with, 217–223
    home care for client after, 219–220, 221
Brassieres, dressing in, 182
Breathing, exercises to assist, 274–277
Bridging
  for dressing, 184
  position, 96
Bronchitis, chronic, 274–277
Brushes, long-handled, 189
Built-up handles for utensils, 193–194
Burns, 54–55
Button hooks, 180

C
Calcium, foods high in, 325
Canes, 147, 148–149
  ambulation with, 199, 200
  with base, 147
  two, ambulation with, 199–200, 201, 202–203
Cap turner, 191
Car
  loading wheelchair into, 143
  standing transfer into, 140–143
  transfer board to get into and out of, 140
  transfers into and out of, 132–139
  trunk of, loading wheelchair into, 144
Car top lift, 172, 174
Cardiac condition, care of client with, 263–270
Cardiac pacemaker, 268–269
Cardiovascular accident; *see* Stroke
Cardiovascular heart disease, atherosclerotic, 265
Caregivers, injuries among, 19
Carpets, safety and, 21
Casters with brake locks for bed, 164
Catheters, 40, 42–47
  external, 39
  indwelling urinary (Foley), 42–45
    obtaining urine specimen from, 292, 293–294
  suprapubic, 46
  Texas, 39

Catheterization, intermittent, 46
C-clip glass, 195
Center of gravity and body mechanics, 85–86
Central hearing loss, 68
Central nervous system, injury to, 225
Certified rehabilitation nurse (C.R.R.N.), 5
Chair
  pulling up client in, 108–111
  sitting in, moving person with one-sided weakness from, 106–107
  standing transfer from bed to, 116–117
Chair commodes, 165–166
  with wheels, 166–167
Chest-strengthening exercise to assist breathing, 276–277
Chewing, difficulty with, 34–35
Children as clients, 8–9
Choking, 34–35, 56–57
Cholesterol, foods containing, 326
Chronic bronchitis, 274–277
Chronic conditions, 261
  care of clients with, 261–318
  causes of, factors influencing, 2–3
Chronic obstructive pulmonary diseases, 272–280
Chronic pain, 281–283
Chronic restrictive pulmonary diseases, 280–281
Circulation, 263–265
  problems with, after amputation, signs and symptoms of, 246
Circulatory system, functions of, 263–265
Cleaning to remove pathogens, 14–16
Clear liquid diet, 324
  foods for, 327
Clergy as member of rehabilitation team, 7
Clothing after amputation, 257
Clots, blood, causing strokes, 207
Coats, dressing in, 182
Colon, foods affecting, 326–327
Colostomy, 49, 50
  bowel training program after, 52
  irrigating, 53
Coma, 218
Combs, long-handled, 189
Commode(s)
  bedside, 165–166
    bed to, transfer board from, 124
    with wheels, 166–167
  standing transfer from bed to, 116–117
Communication
  assigning meaning to, 74–75
  clearer, tips for, 75–76
  deficits in, 76–82
    brain and, 76–78
  of emotions, deficits in, following stroke, 82–83
  with nurse supervisor, 10
  and sensory disorders, 61–83
  verbal and non-verbal, 73–74
Communication safety, 25
Communication process, pattern of, 74
Concussion, 218
Conductive hearing loss, 68
Confidentiality, 8
Confusion with memory loss after stroke, 83
Congestive heart disease, 265
Constipating effect, foods having, 326
Constipation, 48–49
Contact lenses, 66–67
Contoured cushions for clients with lower extremity weakness, 197

Contractures after stroke, 211
Control, loss of, fear of, by client, 9
Controlled diet for cardiac client, 267
Contusion, brain, 218
Cooling system, safety and, 22
Coordination after stroke, 211
COPD; *see* Chronic obstructive pulmonary disease
Coping following amputation, 246–247
Corsets for trunk support, 195
Cough, assistive, for spinal cord injured person, 232–233
Coughing exercises to clear mucus, 276, 277
Covering, bed, for clients with lower extremity weakness, 197–198
Cramps, heat, 59
Crutch(es), 149
  Loftstrand forearm, 149
  one, ambulation with, 199, 200
  platform walking, 149
  rubber tips for, 148
  two, ambulation with, 199–200, 201, 202–203
Crying, inappropriate, 82
Cup holder, 195
Curbs, ambulation on, 200, 203–205
Cursing, uncontrollable, 82–83
Cutting food, assistive devices for, 194–195
CVA; *see* Stroke

D

Daily living, activities of, assistive devices for, 178–205
Decubitus ulcers, 28–30
Deficits following stroke, 210
Dehydration, 323
Dementias, 284
Dental care, 32–33
Dentures, care of, 32–33
Depression
  signs of, 82
  after stroke, 82
Diabetes mellitus, 289–296
  blood testing for clients with, 292, 294
  care for client with, 296
  complications of, 290
  signs of, 290
  type I, 290
  type II, 290
  urine tests for client with, 292
Diabetic diet, 324
Diaphragm-strengthening exercise to assist breathing, 274–275
Diarrhea, 48–49
Diet(s)
  commonly ordered, 324
  controlled, for cardiac client, 267
  therapeutic, and nutrition, 323–327
Dietitian as member of rehabilitation team, 7
Dietary instructions, 33–34
Digoxin for cardiac client, 267–268
Directel, 70
Disability, 1–2
  clients with, equipment for, 145–177
  vs disease, 1–2
  grieving about, 9
Disabled persons
  traveling by, 319–322
  turning, 97
    with turning sheet, 100

Disease
  Alzheimer's, 284–289
  vs disability, 1–2
  heart, congestive, 265
  infectious, spreading of, 12–13
  neuromuscular, progressive, 308–312
  Parkinson's, 308–310
    communication deficits with, 78–80
  peripheral vascular, 266
  pulmonary
    obstructive, chronic, 272–280
    restrictive, chronic, 280–281
Dish stop, 193, 194
Disinfectant, home, 16
Diuretics for cardiac client, 268
Doffing of lower limb prosthesis, 251
Dogs, seeing-eye, 66
Dominant sides, changing, after amputation, 247
Donning of lower limb prosthesis, 251–253
Doors, lever handled, 147
Double vision, 62
Drainage bags, urinary, 45–47
Draw sheet, pulling client up in bed using, 101
Dressing
  assistive devices for, 179–188
  lower-body, 182–188
  after stroke, 215
  upper-body, 180–182
Drugs
  and alcohol, interactions of, 34
  and food, interactions of, 33–34
Dying patients, 313–317
Dysarthria, 80, 82
Dysphagia, 34
  with multiple sclerosis, 311
  after stroke, 215
Dysphagia diet, 324
  foods for, 327
Dysreflexia, autonomic, in spinal cord injured person, 236–237

E

Ear, anatomy of, 69
Earwax, buildup of, 71
Eating, 33–36
  assistive devices for, 193–195
  difficulties with, after stroke, 215
  and person with impaired vision, 63–64
Education for cardiac client, 269–270
Elbow, ROM exercises for, 330, 333
Electrical cords, safety and, 21
Embolus, 266
Emergency care, 53–60
Emergency response unit for cardiac client, 268–269
Emergency situations, basic needs and, 26–60
Emotional changes after stroke, 82
Emotional lability after stroke, 82–83
Emotions, deficits in communicating, after stroke, 82–83
Emphysema, 272–273
Enteric precautions, 18
Equipment
  for care in home, 163–177
  for clients with disabilities, 145–177
  to help clients move, 146–163
  for home care
    bathroom, 167–170
    bedroom, 163–167

  safety and, 20, 21
  for moving clients, specialized, 170–175
  causing skin pressure, 30
  sterilizing, 291
  for walking, 146–151
Equipment vendors as members of rehabilitation team, 7
Exercise, 328–337
  to assist breathing, 274–277
  for Parkinson's disease client, 310
  range of motion, 328–331
    guides for, 332
    passive, 332–337
  respiratory, for spinal cord injured person, 232–233
Exercise program for cardiac client, 267
Exhaustion, heat, 59
Expression, lack of, with Parkinson's disease, 308–309
Expressive aphasia, 78, 79
Expressive-receptive aphasia, 79
Extended-wear soft contact lenses, 66–67
External catheters, 39
Eye prosthesis, care of, 67–68
Eyeglasses, care for, 68

F

Fainting, 54
Fall, proper way to, after amputation, 246–247
Family of client
  as member of health team, 3, 5
  with traumatic brain injury, stresses on, 220
Fat, foods containing, 326
Fatigue with multiple sclerosis, 311
Fear, feelings of, by client, 9
Fecal impaction, 48, 49
Fecal isolation precautions, 18
Feeding of self, 35–36
Fever, rheumatic, 265–266
Fiber, foods high in, 325
Filters, air, 278
Fingernails, care of, 31
Fingers, ROM exercises for, 330, 334
Fire extinguisher, 21
First degree burns, 54
Flaccid muscles after stroke, 211
Flatus, foods producing, 326
Flotation mattresses for clients with lower extremity weakness, 197–198
Fluids, 34
Foam cushions for clients with lower extremity weakness, 197
Foley catheter, indwelling, 42–45
Food
  cultural considerations with, 35
  cutting of, 194–195
  difficulty chewing or swallowing, 34–35
  and drugs, interactions of, 33–34
  nutrients in, 325–327
Foot
  care of, 31
  ROM exercises for, 331, 337
Foot and ankle supports, 177
Forearm, ROM exercises for, 330, 333, 335
Forgetting and losing by Alzheimer's client, 288
Fowler's position, 92, 93–94
Fractured hip, 297–302
  amputation and, 260
Friction, skin, 30–31
  of spinal cord injured person, 234

Frustration
  dealing with, by home health aide, 11
  feelings of, by client, 9
Full liquid diet, 324

G

Gel cushions for clients with lower extremity weakness, 197
Gel mattresses for clients with lower extremity weakness, 198
Global aphasia, 79
Glucose, blood, monitoring of, 294–295
Gout, 305
Grab bars for tub, 129
Gravity
  center of, and body mechanics, 85–86
  line of, and body mechanics, 85–86
Grieving after spinal cord injury, 238–239
Grieving process, 9
Grooming, assistive devices for, 189–192

H

Hair, releasing, from grasp of client, 223
Half-standing transfer, 120
Hand cones, 95
Hand rolls, 95
Hand splints, 176–177
Handles for utensils, built-up, 193–194
Hands, care of, 31
Handwashing to prevent infection, 11, 12
  proper, 13–14
Hard contact lenses, 66
  removing, 67
Harnesses for upper limb prosthesis, 258
Head injuries, 218, 219; *see also* Brain injuries
Hearing, 68–73
  diminished, signs of, 69, 71–72
  loss of
    caring for client with, 72, 73
    signs of, 69, 71–72
    types of, 68
  normal aging changes in, 62
Hearing aid
  care of, 71
  for conductive hearing loss, 68
  diagram of, 70
  inserting, 72
  removing, 72
  working of, 69, 71
Heart, 263–264
Heart attack, risk factors for, 266
  reducing, 266–270
Heart disease
  atherosclerotic, 265
  congestive, 265
Heat, sensitivity to, and multiple sclerosis, 311
Heat cramps, 59
Heat exhaustion, 59
Heat reactions, 58–59
Heat sources, safety and, 22
Heatstroke, 59
Heimlich maneuver, 56–57
Hemianopia, homonymous, 62–63
Hemiparesis, 228
  amputation and, 259
  after stroke, 211
Hemiplegia
  amputation and, 259

and aphasia, 78
  client with, shoe tying by, 188
  after stroke, 211–213
Hemorrhage, 60
High blood pressure, 265
  and strokes, 207
High-calorie diet, 324
High-protein diet, 324
High-residue diet, 324
Hip
  fractured, 297–302
    amputation and, 260
  ROM exercises for, 331, 335, 336
Hip prosthesis, 297–302
Hip replacement surgery, 297–302
Home
  architectural barriers in, 20–21
  care of client in
    equipment for, 163–177
    special considerations in, 8–11
Home health aide
  anger or frustration of, 11
  as member of rehabilitation team, 5
Home oxygen safety, 279–280
Home setting, safety in, 18–25
Homonymous hemianopia, 62–63
Hospice clients, care needs of, 314–315
Hospice concept, 313–315
Household supplies and products, safe handling of, 19, 20, 21
Humidifiers, 278
Hydraulic lift, 171
Hyperglycemia, 295
Hypertension, 265
  and stroke, 207
Hypoglycemia, 296
Hypotension, postural
  signs and symptoms of, 236
  after spinal cord injury, 235–236

I

Identification picture board, 81
Ileostomy, 49, 50
Immobility, negative effects of, 232
Immune deficiency syndrome, acquired, 316–318
Impaction, fecal, 48, 49
Incontinence, 36–37
  after stroke, 216
Indwelling urinary (Foley) catheter, 42–45
  obtaining urine specimen from, 292, 293–294
Infarction, myocardial
  post, 265
  risk factors for, 266
    reducing, 266–270
Infection control, 11–18
  steps in, 13–18
  measures for, 14–18
Infection process, steps in, 12–13
Infectious disease, spreading of, 12–13
Injury
  brain; *see* Brain injuries
  head; *see* Head injuries
  spinal cord; *see* Spinal cord injuries
Insulin, 290–292
  imbalance of, 295–296
  injection of, rotating, 291
  metabolism of, 289

Insulin-dependent diabetes, 290
Insulin holders, 291
Intermittent catheterization, 46
Involuntary muscles and spinal cord injury, 226
Iron, foods, high in, 325
Isolation precautions, 16–18

J

Jackets, dressing in, 182
Jeans, dressing in, 183–184
Jogging suits, 183
Joint
  anatomy and physiology of, 303–304
  movements of, terms describing, 329
Juvenile diabetes, 290

K

Kitchen, safety in, 22–23
Knee, ROM exercises for, 331, 336
Knives, rounded, 194–195

L

Labels, 2
Language
  body, 74
  negative, 2
  problems with, 76, 78–80
  and speech communication, deficits in, 73–76
Lanoxin for cardiac client, 267–268
Lapboards for wheelchairs, 162–163
Larynx, artificial, 70
Lateral sclerosis, amyotrophic, 315–316
Laughing, inappropriate, 82
Laxative effect, foods having, 326
Leg braces, 149–151
  care and storage of, 150–151
  shoes for, 151
Lever handled doors, 147
Leverage, body used for, 88
Lifeline Unit, 268
Lift
  car top, 172, 174
  mechanical, 170–172
    transfers using, 130–131
  and slings, 170–172, 173, 174
  specialty, 172, 173
  tub, 172, 173
Lifting, 86–87
Lighting, safety and, 21–22
Limb, residual, 240
  ace bandage wrappings of, 244–245
  care of, 254
  "stump" shrinkers for, 245–246
Line of gravity and body mechanics, 85–86
Liquid diet, 324
Loading wheelchair
  into car, 143
  into car trunk, 144
Loftstrand forearm crutch, 149
Long leg braces, 149–150
Losing and forgetting by Alzheimer's client, 288
Loss and grieving process, 9
Lost teeth, 55
Low-calorie diet, 324
Low-cholesterol diet, 324
Low-fat diet, 324

Low-residue diet, 324
Low-sodium diet, 324
Lower-body dressing, 182–188
Lower extremity weakness, clients with
  paddings, coverings, and bedding for, 197–198
  seating for, 196–197
  supports for, 196–198
Lower limb amputation
  care with, 247–257
  standing transfer for client with, 118–119
Lower limb prosthesis
  care of, 254–256
  diagram of, 255
  donning and doffing of, 251–253
  pivot transfer for client wearing, 119
Lung(s)
  anatomy and physiology of, 270–272
  chronic diseases of
    obstructive, 272–280
    restrictive, 280–281
Lupus erythematosus, 305–307
Lying down from sitting position, 107

M

Malignant pain, chronic, 282–283
Mattress, 163–164
  for clients with lower extremity weakness, 197–198
  to prevent pressure areas, 103
Mattress covers for clients with lower extremity weakness, 197
Meaning, assigning, to communication, 74–75
Mechanical diet, 324
Mechanical lift, 170–172
  transfers using, 130–131
Mechanical ventilator, 280–281
Medications for cardiac client, 267–268
Memory loss
  care for client with, 83
  confusion with, after stroke, 83
Mental health activities for visually impaired person, 65–66
Microorganisms, 11
Mixed hearing loss, 68
Mobility
  after amputation, 246–247
  and client with impaired vision, 65
Molded ankle foot orthosis, 150
Molded braces for trunk support, 196
Molded cushions for clients with lower extremity weakness, 197
Monitoring, blood glucose, 294–295
Monkeys to assist handicapped persons, 66
Motorized wheelchairs, 157–159
Mouth, care of, 32–33
Mouthstick, 231
Movement, loss of, after spinal cord injury, 231–232
Moving
  of client
    on bed, 97
    body mechanics for, 85–88
    general rules for, 89
    after hip surgery, 300–301
    with one-sided weakness to sit in chair, 106–107
  to sitting position on bed, 103–105
    specialized equipment for, 170–175
    turning and positioning and, 84–144
  pain with, clients having, 103
M.S.; *see* Multiple sclerosis

Multiple sclerosis, 311–312
  communication deficits with, 78–80
Muscle
  atrophy of, after stroke, 211
  flaccid, after stroke, 211
  voluntary and involuntary, and spinal cord injury, 226
  weakness of, after stroke, 211–213
Myocardial infarction
  post, 265
  risk factors for, 266
    reducing, 266–270

N

Nail brush, 191
Nasal prongs for oxygen use, 281
Needs, basic, and emergency situations, 26–60
Neglect of client, 10
Nerve damage causing hearing loss, 68
Neuromuscular diseases, progressive, 308–312
Nitroglycerin for angina, 268
Non-malignant pain, chronic, 282
Non-verbal communication, 73–74
Nosebleeds, 55
Nourishment, 33–36
Nurse
  certified rehabilitation (C.R.R.N.), 5
  registered professional, as member of rehabilitation team, 5
  rehabilitation insurance, 5
Nurse supervisor, communication with, 10
Nutrients in foods, 325–327
Nutrition
  and Alzheimer's disease, 288–289
  therapeutic diets and, 323–327
Nutritional difficulties following stroke, 215
Nutritionist as member of rehabilitation team, 7

O

Obstructive pulmonary diseases, chronic, 272–280
Occupational therapist as member of rehabilitation team, 6
Oral communication, 73–74
Orientation, reality, 83
Ortho cane, 148
Orthosis, molded ankle foot, 150
Orthotist as member of rehabiliation team, 7
Osteoarthritis, 304–305
  assisting client with, 306
  care for client with, 305
  pain control for, 307
Ostomy, 49–53
  negative reactions to, 52
Ostomy bag, 51–52
  cleaning, 52
Otosclerosis, 68
Overbed tables, 167
Overhead trapeze bars to assist in turning of clients, 101–102
Oxygen safety at home, 279–280
Oxygen therapy, 278–279

P

Pacemaker
  cardiac, 268–269
  phrenic nerve, 281
Paddings
  for clients with lower extremity weakness, 197–198
  to prevent pressure sores, 30–33

Pain
  acute, 282
  chronic, 281–283
  control of, 282
    attitudes toward, 283
  and hospice client, 314
  malignant, chronic, 282
  non-malignant, chronic, 282
  phantom, after amputation, 247
  shoulder, after stroke, 213–215
  tolerance to, 283
  on turning or moving, clients having, 103
Pants, dressing in, 183–185
Paralysis after spinal cord injury, 231
Paraparesis, 228
Paraplegia, 226, 228
  turning client with, 97, 100
Paresis, 228
  after stroke, 211–213
Parkinson's disease, 308–310
  communication deficits with, 78–80
  pain with, 103
Passive range of motion exercises, 332–337
Patches, medication, for cardiac client, 268
Pathogens, 11
  removal of, 14–16
Pelvic belts with above-the-knee prosthesis, 257
Peripheral vascular diseases, 266
Personal adjustments to spinal cord injury, 238–239
Personal care attendant; *see* Home health aide
Personal safety, 19
Phantom pain after amputation, 247
Phrenic nerve pacemaker, 281
Physical abuse of client, 10
Physical difficulties following stroke, 211–216
  related to movement, 211-215
Physical therapist as member of rehabilitation team, 6
Physician as member of rehabilitation team, 6
Physiatrist as member of rehabilitation team, 6
Pick 'N Stick identification stickers, 81
Picture boards for aphasic clients, 81
Picture stickers, 81
"Pill rolling" with Parkinson's disease, 308
Pivot transfer for client with lower limb prosthesis, 119
Place, sense of, normal aging changes in, 62
Plastic sheet coverings for clients with lower extremity weakness, 197
Plateguards, 193, 194
Platform walking crutch, 149
Poison Control Center, contacting, 58
Poisoning, 58
Position(s)
  body, 89–96
  of client after hip surgery, 299–300
  changes in, to prevent pressure sores, 29–30
  sense of
    loss of, after spinal cord injury, 233
    normal aging changes in, 62
Positioning of client, 89–96
  general rules for, 89
  with lower limb amputation, 248, 249–250
  and turning and moving, 84–144
Positioning bridging, 96
Postural hypotension
  signs and symptoms of, 236
  after spinal cord injury, 235–236

Potassium, foods high in, 325
Power, feelings of lack of, by client, 9
Pressure on skin, preventing, 29–30
Pressure sores, 27–28
    prevention of, 28–30
    after spinal cord injury, 230, 234
Products, household, safe handling of, 19–20, 21
Profanity, uncontrollable, 82–83
Progressive neuromuscular diseases, 308–312
Prone position, 89, 90
Prosthesis
    care of, 254–256
    eye, care of, 67–68
    hip, 297–302
    lower limb
        care of, 254–256
        diagram of, 255
        donning and doffing of, 251–253
        pivot transfer for client wearing, 119
        standing transfer for client with, 118–119
    upper limb, harnesses for, 258
    walking, falling by client with, 246–247
Prosthetic device, 240–241
Prosthetic socks, 256–257
Prosthetist, 241
    as member of rehabilitation team, 7
Protein, need for, 33
Psychologist as member of rehabilitation team, 7
Ptosis, 62
Pulling up of client in chair or wheelchair, 108–111
Pulmonary diseases
    obstructive, chronic, 272–280
    restrictive, chronic, 280–281
Purifiers, air, 278
"Pursed-lip" breathing exercises, 274

Q

Quadraparesis, 228
Quadriplegia, 228
    turning client with, 97, 100

R

Rails for toilet, 167–168
Range of motion exercises, 328–331
    guides for, 332
    passive, 332–337
Reachers, 191
Reagent strips for blood glucose monitoring, 295
Reality, orientation of client to, 83
Receptive aphasia, 78–79
Registered professional nurse as member of rehabilitation team, 5
Regular diet, 324
Rehabilitation
    goal of, 2
    principles of, 1–25
Rehabilitation insurance nurse, 5
Rehabilitation team, 3–7
Reimplantation of teeth, 55
Residual limb, 240
    ace bandage wrappings of, 244–245
    care of, 254
    "stump" shrinkers for, 245–246
Residue diet, 324
Respiratory exercises for spinal cord injured person, 232–233
Respiratory isolation precautions, 17–18

Respiratory problems, chronic, 270–281
Respiratory system, 270–272
Respiratory therapist as member of rehabilitation team, 6
Respite care, 289
Rest for cardiac client, 267
Restrictive pulmonary diseases, chronic, 280–281
Retraining, bowel and bladder, after spinal cord injury, 233
Returning client to bed, 106
Rheumatic fever, 265
Rheumatism, 303
Rheumatoid arthritis, 304
    assisting client with, 306
    care for client with, 305
    pain control for, 307
Rigidity with Parkinson's disease, 308
Rolls, trochanter, 91
Rounded knives, 194–195
Rubber tips for walker and crutches, 148
Rugs, safety and, 21
Runners, carpet, safety and, 21

S

Safety, 18–25
    oxygen, at home, 279–280
    for visually impaired person, 66
Safety siderails for bed, 164–165
Safety strap for trunk support, 196
Scanning, 63
Sclerosis
    amyotrophic lateral, 315–316
    multiple; *see* Multiple sclerosis
Scooter, three-wheeled, 159, 160
Seating of client
    considerations in, 197
    with lower extremity weakness, 196–197
Second degree burns, 54
Seeing-eye dogs, 66
Seizures, 55
Semi-prone position, 89, 90, 91
Semi-standing transfer, 120
Sensation
    loss of, after spinal cord injury, 233
    phantom, after amputation, 247
Sensorineural hearing loss, 68
Sensory changes, normal in aging, 62
Sensory and communication deficits, 61–83
Sensory losses with multiple sclerosis, 311
Shampoo tray, bed, 191
Shearing and skin damage, 30–31
    in spinal cord injured person, 234
Sheath, urinary, 39–40, 41
Sheepskins
    for bedding for clients with lower extremity weakness, 197, 198
    to prevent pressure sores, 31
Sheet
    draw, pulling client up in bed using, 101
    turning, use of, 100
Shirts, dressing in, 180–182
Shock, 59–60
Shoe horn, long-handle, 187
Shoelaces, tying, 188
Shoes
    after amputation, 257
    applying, 187–188
    for leg braces, 151

Short leg braces, 149–150
Short-sitting in bed in preparation for transfer for persons with
   spinal cord injuries, 105–106
Shoulder
   pain in, after stroke, 213–215
   ROM exercises for, 330, 333
Shower, stall, 170
Shower hose, 169
Shower stall, standing transfer into, 128
Side-lying position, 94
Siderails for bed, 164–165
Sitting in chair, moving person with one-sided weakness for,
   106–107
Sitting position
   on bed, moving to, 103–105
   lying down from, 107
Skin
   care of, 27–31
      basic rules for, 30
      in spinal cord injured person, 233–234
   diagram of, 27
   pressure on, preventing, 29–30
Skin isolation precautions, 18
Slings
   and lifts, 170–172, 173, 174
      care of, 172
   for mechanical lift, placing, under client in bed, 130
   for shoulder pain after stroke, 213
Smell, sense of
   loss of, 73
   normal aging changes in, 62
Smoke detectors, 21
Social service worker as member of rehabilitation team, 7
Sock puller, 187
Socks
   prosthetic, 256–257
   putting on, 185–187
Sodium, foods high in, 325
Sodium-restricted diet, 324
Soft contact lenses, extended-wear, 66–67
Soft diet, 324
Sores, pressure; *see* Pressure sores
Spasticity
   after spinal cord injury, 234–235
   after stroke, 211
Specialized equipment for moving clients, 170–175
Specialty lifts, 172, 173
Specialty wheelchairs, 157–159
Speech, problems with, 76, 78–80
Speech and language communication, deficits in, 73–76
Speech-language, hearing therapist as member of rehabilitation
   team, 6
Speech pathologist as member of rehabilitation team, 6
Spinal cord, 225, 226
Spinal cord injuries
   assisting client with, 229
   assistive devices for person with, 231
   bowel and bladder retraining after, 233
   care for client with, 224–239
   communication deficits with, 78–80
   level of
      and abilities, 226–228
      and disabilities, 225–226
   loss of movement after, 231–232
   personal adjustments to, 238–239
   postural hypotension after, 235–236

principles of care for, 229
severity of, 226–228
skin care of person with, 233–234
spasticity after, 234–235
special care for person with, 230–238
transfer for persons with, short-sitting in bed in preparation
   for, 105–106
Splints, hand and wrist, 176–177
Stairs
   ambulation on, 200, 203–205
   considerations in using, 204
Stall showers, 170
Standing transfers, 112–115
   assisted, 114–115
   from bed to chair, 116–117
   into car, 140–143
   for client with lower limb amputation, 118–119
   into shower stall, 128
   to tub seat, 128, 129
Sterilizing, 14, 16
   in home, 291
Stocking
   body, care of, 187
   pulling on, 185–187
   support, care of, 185
Stoma, 51
Strap, safety, for trunk support, 196
Stress reduction for cardiac client, 269
Stresses of multiple sclerosis, 312
Stroke
   assisting recovery from, 210
   care of client after, 206–216
   causes of, 207–210
   communication deficits after, 78–80
   deficits following, 210
      in communicating emotions, 82–83
   physical difficulties following, 211–216
      related to movement, 211–215
   visual deficits after, 62–63
   warning signs of, 208
"Stroke posture," 212
"Stump" shrinkers, 245–246
Suicide, potential for, 54
Supine position, 90, 91, 93
Supplies, household, safe handling for, 19–20, 21
Supply vendors as members of rehabilitation team,
   7
Support
   base of, and body mechanics, 86, 88
   for clients
      with lower extremity weakness, 196–198
      with trunk weakness, 195–196
   foot and ankle, 177
Support groups
   for cardiac clients, 270
   for client after traumatic brain injury, 220
Support stockings, care of, 185
Suprapubic catheter, 46
Surgery, hip replacement, 297–302
Swallowing, difficulty with, 34–35
   with multiple sclerosis, 311
   after stroke, 215
Sweaters, dressing in, 180–182
Swivel spoon, 193
Syndrome, acquired immune deficiency, 316–318
Synovitis, 306

T

Tables, overbed, 167
Taste, sense of
  loss of, 73
  normal aging changes in, 62
TDD; *see* Telecommunications devices for disabled
Team, rehabilitation, 3–7
Teeth
  care of, 32–33
  lost, 55
  reimplantation of, 55
Telecommunications devices for disabled, 70, 71–72
Telephone cords, safety and, 21
Telephone holder for spinal cord injured persons, 231
Telephones
  for hearing impaired persons, 71–72
  for visually impaired person, 66
Television sets for hearing-impaired persons, 72
Temperature, sense of
  loss of, 73
    after spinal cord injury, 233
  normal aging changes in, 62
TENS unit, 283, 284
Terminal condition, client with, 313–318
Test(s)
  for AIDS, 316
  blood, for clients with diabetes mellitus, 292, 294
  urine, for clients with diabetes mellitus, 292
Texas catheter, 39
Therapeutic diets and nutrition, 323–327
Third degree burns, 54–55
Thrombophlebitis, 266
  spinal cord injured person, 237–238
Thrombosis after spinal cord injury, 230
Thrombus, 266
Thrusts, abdominal, for choking, 56–57
Thumb, ROM exercises for, 330, 334, 335
Toenails, care of, 31
Toes, ROM exercises for, 331
Toilet paper holder, 192
Toilet seat, elevated, 167
Toilets, home, 167–168
Toothbrushing, 32
Touch, sense of
  and client with impaired vision, 65
  and communication, 74–77
  loss of, 73
    after spinal cord injury, 233
  normal aging changes in, 62
Touch 'N Talk picture board, 81
Tracheostomy, 315
Training
  bladder, 36, 37
  bowel, 47–48, 49
Transcutaneous electrical nerve stimulator unit, 283, 284
Transfer(s), 111–144
  into and out of car, 132–139
  after hip surgery, 300–301
  using mechanical lift, 130–131
  for persons with spinal cord injuries, short-sitting in bed in preparation for, 105–106
  semi- or half-standing, 120
  standing; *see* Standing transfer
  using transfer board, 120–127
    from bed to bedside commode, 124
    from bed to wheelchair, 121

    into and out of cars, 140
    out of tub, 126
    from wheelchair to bed, 121–123
    from wheelchair to tub, 124–127
Transfer board, 120
  for home use, 172, 175
    making, 175, 176
  transfers using, 120–127
Trapeze bar, 165
  overhead, to assist in turning of clients, 101–102
Traumatic brain injury
  care for client with, 217–223
  home for client after, 219–220, 221
Traveling by disabled persons, 319–322
Tremor with Parkinson's disease, 308
Triparesis, 228
Trochanter rolls, 91
Trunk weakness, clients with, supports for, 195–196
Tub
  grab bars for, 129
  home, 168–169
  transfer board out of, 126
  wheelchair to, transfer board from, 124–127
Tub bench, 169
Tub lift, 172, 173
Tub seat, 169
  leaving, 128
  standing transfers to, 128, 129
Tumors, communication deficits in clients with, 78–80
Turning
  of client
    in bed, 97–99
    moving and positioning and, 84–144
    using overhead trapeze bar, 101–102
    to prevent pressure sores, 29–30
    with turning sheet, 100
  pain on, clients having, 103
Turning sheet, use of, 100
Turns and turning of client, 97–103

U

Ulcers, decubitus, 28
  prevention of, 28–30
Underwear, dressing in, 182
Universal cuff, 190, 192
Upper-body dressing, 180–182
Upper extremity weakness, assistive devices for grooming by client with, 189–192
Upper limb prosthesis, harnesses for, 258
Ureterostomy, 49, 50
Urinary catheter, indwelling, 42–45
Urinary devices, specialized, 37–47
Urinary drainage bags, care of, 45–47
Urinary sheath, 39–40, 41
Urine, 36
  absorbing devices for, 37, 39
  acidity of, foods affecting, 326
Urine specimen, obtaining, from indwelling catheter, 292, 293–294
Urine tests for clients with diabetes mellitus, 292
Utah arm, 258
Utensils, built-up handles for, 193–194

V

Vaporizers, 278
Varicose veins, 266

Vascular diseases, peripheral, 266
Veins, 264
    varicose, 266
Vendors as members of rehabilitation team, 7
Venous conditions, 266
Ventilator, mechanical, 280–281
Verbal abuse of client, 10
Verbal communication, 73–74
Violent client, caring for, 221–223
Viruses, 11–12
Vision, 62–68
    double, 62
    impaired, working with person with, 63–66
    normal aging changes in, 62
Vocational counselor as member of rehabilitation team, 7
Voluntary muscles and spinal cord injury, 226

W

Walk-cane, folding, 148
Walker(s), 147–148
    ambulation with, 199–200, 201
    folding, with wheels, 147
    rubber tips for, 148
Walking, equipment for, 146–151
Walking prosthesis, falling by client with, 246–247
Wandering by clients with Alzheimer's disease, 287
Water, boiling, for sterilization, 16
"Water pills" for cardiac client, 268
Water mattresses for clients with lower extremity weakness,
    197–198
Waterproof mattress covers for clients with lower extremity
    weakness, 197
Weakness
    lower extremity, clients with

paddings, coverings, and beddings for, 197–198
    seating for, 196–197
    supports for, 196–198
    muscle, after stroke, 211–213
    one-sided, client with, moving, to sit in chair, 106–107
    trunk, clients with, supports for, 195–196
    upper extremity, assistive devices for grooming by client with,
        189–192
Wheelchair(s), 151–159
    armboards for 159–162
    armrests of, 151, 153
    attachments for, 159–163
    batteries for, 158–159
    bed to, transfer board from, 121
    to bed, transfer board to, 121–123
    brakes of, 154, 155
    care of, 155, 157
    footrests of, 153, 155
    hand rims for, 156
    lapboards for, 162–163
    loading
        into car, 143
        into car trunk, 144
    pulling up client in, 108–111
    seat of, 151
    specialty and motorized, 157–159
    standing transfer from bed to, 116–117
    to tub, transfer board from, 124–127
    wheels of, 155
Wheelchair cushions to prevent pressure sores, 31
Wound precautions, 18
Wrappings, ace, bandage, of residual limb, 244–245
Wrist, ROM exercises for, 330, 334
Wrist splints, 176–177